NEWER TRACE ELEMENTS IN NUTRITION

NEWER TRACE ELEMENTS IN NUTRITION

edited by Walter Mertz and W.E. Cornatzer

HUMAN NUTRITION RESEARCH DIVISION
AGRICULTURAL RESEARCH SERVICE
U.S. DEPARTMENT OF AGRICULTURE
BELTSVILLE, MARYLAND 20705

IRELAND RESEARCH LABORATORY
DEPARTMENT OF BIOCHEMISTRY
SCHOOL OF MEDICINE
THE UNIVERSITY OF NORTH DAKOTA
GRAND FORKS, NORTH DAKOTA 58201

1971

MARCEL DEKKER, INC. New York

LIBRARY OF CONGRESS CATALOG CARD NUMBER: 70-157834
ISBN NO.: 0-8247-1110-6

The dedication of the Human Nutrition Laboratory in Grand
Forks, North Dakota, is an expression of the growing public
awareness of the problems of nutrition, particularly those of
trace element nutrition. It was fitting that the operation of
this Laboratory, devoted to research into the health effects and
requirements of trace elements in man, should be inaugurated by
an International Symposium on the Newer Trace Elements in
Nutrition. The joint sponsorship of this symposium by the U. S.
Department of Agriculture and the University of North Dakota
reflects the close collaboration that the new Laboratory hopes
to have not only with the University but also with other regional
institutions.

The topics of the symposium and consequently its proceedings
were organized in five sessions, each directly related to
microelements for which essentiality or new functional aspects
have been discovered only recently. The first session, representing the first three chapters of this book, present the
macro- and the microcosmos of which our endeavor is part. For
the trace element researcher whose main tool is a more and more
restricted, purified and therefore artificial environment it is
necessary to understand that any one micronutrient is but one of
a great number of factors essential for health and life and that
its effects are dependent on and influenced by many other
nutrients. On the other hand, the knowledge of the function
of a trace element is not complete until we understand the
mechanism by which it interacts at the molecular level with
components of metabolism such as proteins, nucleic acids, or
hormones, either as a catalyst or as a part of structure, or in
both ways.

272394

Against this background the following two sessions, represented in chapters four to nine, discuss the latest knowledge of
two elements, selenium and chromium, whose essentiality has
been known for more than a decade. Both of these elements may
have a considerable impact on public health: selenium not only
because of the great differences of concentration in the environment, ranging from deficient to toxic levels but also through
its potential to counteract the toxic effects of several heavy
metals such as cadmium, mercury, and lead to which an increasing
number of people are exposed through environmental pollution.
Chromium appears to present a nutritional problem in the U. S.,
particularly in pregnancy and old age.

The following session presented evidences for an essential
function of three new trace elements: nickel, vanadium, and tin.
Even though all three discoveries were made using a strictly
controlled environment, it is possible that any one may have
considerable implications in human nutrition, as past experience
with other trace elements has demonstrated. For example, the
study of zinc nutrition was academic until the 40's when
practical problems in animal nutrition arose. The recent
discovery of the implication of zinc in taste acuity is but
one example of how zinc nutrition has become a problem for man.

Progress in trace element research has always depended on
advances in trace analysis. The intensified research with the
"new" trace elements which are present and active in very small
concentrations emphasizes the need for a continuing development
of even greater precision and refinement of analytical method-
dology. The last session gave promising examples of such a
development.

W. Mertz

E. W. Cornatzer

CONTRIBUTORS TO THIS VOLUME

A. BABICKÝ, Institute of Physiology and Radioisotope Laboratories
   of the Institutes for Biological Research, Czechoslovak
   Academy of Sciences, Prague, Czechoslovakia

J. BENEŠ, Institute of Physiology and Radioisotope Laboratories
   of the Institutes for Biological Research, Czechoslovak
   Academy of Sciences, Prague, Czechoslovakia

G. G. CLEMENA, Department of Chemistry, University of Virginia,
   Charlottesville, Virginia

L. D. COOPER, Department of Chemistry, University of Virginia,
   Charlottesville, Virginia

T. G. DALAKOS, Departments of Biochemistry and Medicine,
   State University of New York, Upstate Medical Center,
   Syracuse, New York

R. J. DOISY, Departments of Biochemistry and Medicine, State
   University of New York, Upstate Medical Center,
   Syracuse, New York

W. A. GORDON, National Aeronautics and Space Administration,
   Lewis Research Center, Cleveland, Ohio

K. M. HAMBIDGE, B. F. Stolinsky Research Laboratories,
   Department of Pediatrics, University of Colorado Medical
   Center, Denver, Colorado

W. W. HARRISON, Department of Chemistry, University of Virginia,
   Charlottesville, Virginia

D. M. HEGSTED, Department of Nutrition, Harvard School of Public
   Health, Boston, Massachusetts

R. I. HENKIN, Section on Neuroendrocrinology, Experimental
   Therapeutics Branch, National Heart and Lung Institute,
   Bethesda, Maryland

L. L. HOPKINS, JR. , Human Nutrition Research Division, U. S.
   Department of Agriculture, Agricultural Research Service,
   Beltsville, Maryland

J. M. HSU, Biochemistry Research Laboratory, Veterans
Administration Hospital, The John Hopkins University and
the Department of Biochemistry, Baltimore, Maryland

M. E. KALAFER, Departments of Biochemistry and Medicine, State
University of New York, Upstate Medical Center,
Syracuse, New York

J. KALOUSKOVA, Institute of Physiology and Radioisotope
Laboratories of the Institutes for Biological Research,
Czechoslovak Academy of Sciences, Prague, Czechoslovakia

O. A. LEVANDER, Human Nutrition Research Division, U. S.
Department of Agriculture, Agricultural Research Service,
Beltsville, Maryland

W. MERTZ, Human Nutrition Research Division, U. S. Department
of Agriculture, Agricultural Research Service,
Beltsville, Maryland

H. E. MOHR, Human Nutrition Research Division, U. S. Department
of Agriculture, Agricultural Research Service,
Beltsville, Maryland

F. H. NIELSEN, Human Nutrition Laboratory, Agricultural Research
Service, U. S. Department of Agriculture, Grand Forks,
North Dakota

I. OSTADALOVA, Institute of Physiology and Radioisotope
Laboratories of the Institutes for Biological Research,
Czechoslovak Academy of Sciences, Prague, Czechoslovakia

J. PARIZEK, Institute of Physiology and Radioisotope Laboratories
of the Institutes for Biological Research, Czechoslovak
Academy of Sciences, Prague, Czechoslovakia

S. I. REKANT, Departments of Biochemistry and Medicine, State
University of New York, Upstate Medical Center,
Syracuse, New York

E. E. ROGINSKI, Human Nutrition Research Division, U. S.
Department of Agriculture, Agricultural Research Service,
Beltsville, Maryland

M. A. RYAN, Department of Chemistry, University of Virginia, Charlottesville, Virginia

K. SCHWARZ, Laboratory of Experimental Metabolic Diseases, Medical Research Programs, Veterans Administration Hospital, Long Beach, California, and Department of Biological Chemistry, School of Medicine, University of California, Los Angeles, California

M. L. SCOTT, Department of Poultry Science and Graduate School of Nutrition, Cornell University, Ithaca, New York

M. L. SOUMA, Departments of Biochemistry and Medicine, State University of New York, Upstate Medical Center, Syracuse, New York

D. H. P. STREETEN, Departments of Biochemistry and Medicine, State University of New York, Upstate Medical Center, Syracuse, New York

M. L. TAYLOR, USAF, BSC, 6570 Aerospace Medical Research Laboratory, Toxic Hazards Division (MRTC), Wright-Patterson Air Force Base, Dayton, Ohio

E. J. UNDERWOOD, Institute of Agriculture, University of Western Australia, Nedlands, Australia

B. L. VALLEE, Biophysics Research Laboratory, Department of Biological Chemistry. Harvard Medical School, and the Division of Medical Biology, Peter Bent Brigham Hospital, Boston, Massachusetts

CONTENTS

Chapter 8.   METABOLISM OF ^{51}CHROMIUM IN HUMAN SUBJECTS
             NORMAL, ELDERLY, AND DIABETIC SUBJECTS

             R. J. Doisy, D. H. P. Streeten,
             M. L. Souma, M. E. Kalafer,
             S. I. Rekant, and T. G. Dalakos

Chapter 9.   CHROMIUM NUTRITION IN THE MOTHER
             AND THE GROWING CHILD

             K. M. Hambidge

Chapter 10.   THE BIOLOGICAL ESSENTIALITY
              OF VANADIUM

              L. L. Hopkins, Jr. and H. E. Mohr

NEWER TRACE ELEMENTS IN NUTRITION

Chapter 1

THE HISTORY AND PHILOSOPHY OF TRACE ELEMENT RESEARCH

E. J. Underwood

Institute of Agriculture
University of Western Australia
Nedlands, Australia

I. EARLY HISTORY

The first indications that trace elements may be of
physiological importance to animals came over a century ago in
Europe when several investigators independently demonstrated
their presence in significant quantities in a variety of
special compounds present in living tissues. As early as 1847
copper was shown to exist in combination with the blood
proteins of snails[1] and 30 years later the copper-containing
pigment, hemocyanin, was found to behave as a respiratory
compound in various marine organisms[2]. In 1869 also

Church[3] identified the red pigment, turacin, which occurs in
the feathers of the South African bird, turaco, as a copper
compound containing no less than 7% copper. A few years later
a zinc-containing blood pigment named "sycotypin" was
demonstrated in the blood of mollusca[4] and a vanadium-
containing protein compound named "hemovanadin" was found in
the blood of ascidians[5].

At that time these substances were regarded as little
more than scientific curiosities and their discovery did little
to stimulate studies of the possible wider significance of the
component elements. Even today it is not known if hemovanadin
performs any vital respiratory or other function, or in what
manner or for what purpose in the evolution of certain ascidian
worms vanadium came to be concentrated in this way. Actually
these early workers could hardly have been expected to think of
these elements in terms of respiratory or oxidative processes
because it was not until MacMunn[6] published his pioneer
observations on iron and cell respiration in 1885 that the
concept emerged that trace element-containing metalloenzymes
are of profound importance to the functional integrity of the
cells. Fifty years later this was to prove an exceptionally
fruitful area of trace element research, as we shall see.

In this early period the French botanist Chatin[7]
published his remarkable observations on the iodine content of
soils, waters, and foods and concluded that the occurrence of
goiter in man was associated with a deficiency of environmental
iodine. It is not entirely clear what stimulated Chatin to
investigate the distribution of iodine in this way but two
events are probably significant. These are, first, the
discovery of iodine in abundance in seaweed ash by the
Frenchman Courtois in 1811 and in sponges by the Scotsman
Fyfe in 1819. Burnt sponges were known to have been used

successfully but quite empirically in the treatment of human
goiter by the ancient Greeks. The second event was the practice
initiated as early as 1820 by still another Frenchman, the
physician Coindet, of using salts of iodine therapeutically in
the treatment of goiter. Presumably these pioneer observations
led Chatin to undertake his investigations, remarkable for the
day. Certain anomalies in Chatin's data discredited his
conclusions and the iodine-deficiency theory lay almost
forgotten for several decades until it was revived triumphantly
by Marine in this country during the early years of this
century. It should nevertheless be noted that Chatin's work on
iodine and the incidence of goiter was the first demonstration
of an "area" problem involving a naturally occurring deficiency
of a trace element. It was not until the 1930s, 80 years after
Chatin's observations were first published, that it became
evident that many other area problems, involving other trace
element deficiencies and toxicities of geochemical origin, also
existed in many parts of the world. These will be considered
later.

A. Distributional Studies

During the 1920s the then new technique of emission
spectrography emerged as a means of determining the distribution
of trace elements in biological materials. This technique gave
a great stimulus to trace element research because it permitted
the simultaneous estimation of some 20 to 30 elements in low
concentrations. This is the first example, to be later repeated
several times in the history of trace element research, of the
advent of a new analytical technique stimulating a wave of
similar studies by different individuals in different locations.
This, in fact, is what is happening now with atomic absorption
spectrometry and neutron activation.

The early studies were motivated primarily by a wish to delineate the patterns of distribution of trace elements in health and disease. This type of investigation entered a new phase in the 1950s with a new motivation as a result of the development of high-energy accelerators and nuclear reactors which showed that all elements could be made radioactive and thus potential hazards to living cells. Information on the biological distribution of the stable elements became a necessary prelude to assessment of the maximum safe levels of the radionuclides and the factors affecting their distribution in the food chain from the soil to man. The most comprehensive and significant of all these spectrographic investigations of trace elements in human tissues was undoubtedly that of Isabel Tipton[8] at Tennessee, which was not published until 1963 although it was carried out some years earlier.

Several features of the spectrographic distribution studies deserve comment at this point. First, there was a tendency to argue that the failure to detect a particular element in a particular tissue implied its absence, whereas in fact it could mean simply that the method was insufficiently sensitive. Second, some trace elements could not be quantitated at all by emission spectrography. Arsenic, iodine, bromine, fluorine, mercury, and germanium are examples of such elements. This fact obviously limited the usefulness of the studies. Finally, some workers were constrained to argue teleologically from their findings, to claim that a particular concentration in a particular organ or tissue was of itself evidence of function or purpose. For instance, Birckner[9], as long ago as 1919, stated, "From its constant occurrence in the yolk of eggs, as well as in human and cow's milk, it is inferred that the element zinc exerts an important nutritive function, the nature of which is not yet understood." These proved to be prophetic words. Indeed the relatively high concentration of zinc in cow's milk was one of the factors influencing the Wisconsin workers to investigate originally the essentiality of zinc in mammalian nutrition in the early 1930s. Teleological arguments can therefore be useful stimuli to further research, however misguided the reasoning may be.

B. The Purified or Special Diet Approach

The direct approach to the problem of the nutritional significance of the trace elements by the use of diets deliberately designed to be low in the element in question was pioneered by Gabriel Bertrand in Paris and J. S. McHargue in Missouri. Both these workers carried out many of their studies during World War I and in the early twenties and both obtained highly suggestive but not entirely convincing evidence in respect to mammalian requirements for growth of zinc, copper, and manganese. They suffered from the formidable handicap, impossible to overcome at the time, of vitamin deficiencies in their purified diets, so the animals died or grew poorly even when supplemented with the trace element under study. To overcome this handicap they were forced to include a proportion of natural materials in the diets, such as yeast, meat extract, or "greens," which supplied sufficient trace elements to vitiate or partially vitiate the original deficiencies for which the basal diets were designed. Not until 20 to 30 years later, when pure natural or synthetic vitamins became available for nutritional research, did further rapid advances in the value of the purified-diet approach become possible. One of the most striking examples of the value of the latter technique is that of Scott and his collaborators at Cornell who have recently done so much to illuminate the absolute selenium requirements of rats and chicks and the relationship of these requirements to the tocopherol status of the animal.

An important aspect of the studies with purified diets
with laboratory animals is the motivation of the workers
concerned. Bertrand and McHargue and their successors were not
concerned with any economic problem in animals or with any
then known disease condition crying out for solution; they
were consumed with a desire to enlarge knowledge, to find out
what the full nutritional needs of animals were, and to define
the place of various trace elements in this wide spectrum of
needs, if any such existed. In other words, they were pure
scientists without known practical objectives.

The first major breakthroughs obtained by such means came
from the Wisconsin group led by the late E. B. Hart and the
late C. A. Elvehjem. I was privileged to work with them both
in the 1930s and would like to pay a special tribute to them
as men and as scientists. It is frequently forgotten that
their first major discovery in this area, the demonstration of
the essentiality of copper for growth and hemoglobin formation
in the rat in 1928[10], came as a by-product of their
researches on iron. For many years it had been firmly believed
that organic forms of iron and particularly "food iron" were
nutritionally superior to inorganic salts of the element for
man and laboratory species. In a series of studies which
invalidated this contention, at least for the rat, the
Wisconsin workers observed anomalies in their results with
certain natural sources of iron. This led them to suspect the
presence of another element or factor which was necessary, in
addition to iron, for satisfactory growth and hemoglobin
formation in young rats on a milk diet. This element was, of
course, copper and a third trace element was added to the list
of essential nutrients which previously had consisted only of
iron and iodine.

Within three years of this significant discovery the
Wisconsin group added a fourth trace element, manganese, to
the list of essentials[11]. They noted that mice and rats
fed a milk diet supplemented with both iron and copper were
infertile due to an impairment of ovarian activity and that
reproductive performance could be restored by supplemental
manganese. These notable findings were made possible by the
clever exploitation of a diet composed basically of cow's
milk which in its uncontaminated state is naturally deficient
in the three trace elements, iron, copper, and manganese. The
third success of this prolific group at Wisconsin, the initial
demonstration of the essentiality of zinc in mammalian nutrition
in 1934[12], came from the use of the more conventional
purified diet technique. In fact, as mentioned earlier, it
was the opposite situation to that existing with copper and
manganese, namely, the unusually high zinc concentration of
cow's milk, to which Birckner had first drawn attention, which
stimulated these workers to undertake studies with this element.

I have devoted some time to the initial investigations
leading to the addition of manganese and zinc to the list of
essential trace elements, not merely because of their conspic-
uous success with the purified or special-diet technique but
because of the tremendous stimulus that these findings gave to
trace element research at both the basic and the applied levels.
The nutritional physiology of the trace elements soon became
as fashionable and as profitable a field of study as that of
the vitamins which had long dominated the nutritional scene and
occupied so much of the brains and the resources of nutritional
science. Despite this change and despite outstanding advances
in our understanding of the needs and of the mode of action of
trace elements, it is a surprising and sobering fact that a
further 20 years elapsed before any more trace elements were

firmly added to the list of essentials and the purified-diet
approach once more yielded outstanding results. I refer, of
course, to the work of Richert and Westerfield[13] with
molybdenum and the researches of Schwarz and Mertz, first
leading to the identification of selenium as an essential
element[14] in 1957 and then to demonstrating a functional role
for chromium[15] in 1959.

The difficulties inherent in the purified-diet technique
are further illustrated by the fact that still another decade
was to elapse before any additional trace elements, notably
tin and possibly nickel, were added even tentatively to the
essential list. In this case the findings of Nielsen[16] in
respect to nickel with chicks were only made possible by the
introduction of a new level of experimental sophistication,
the plastic-isolator technique, with its further exclusion of
opportunities for environmental, particularly atmospheric,
contamination. Using this technique Schwarz and co-workers[17]
have very recently demonstrated that tin is essential for
growth in the rat and have served notice that one or more
additional essential trace elements may appear before long.

C. Naturally Occurring Area Problems

The surge of interest in trace elements which arose from
the laboratory studies just outlined were paralleled by equally
stimulating and even more economically rewarding field studies
of naturally occurring trace element deficiencies, toxicities,
and imbalances during that remarkably productive decade 1930
to 1940. The motivation for these researches was clearly
economic; field problems had to be solved if certain areas
were to become, or to remain, satisfactory for the raising of
livestock. Animals restricted to these areas failed to thrive
or to reproduce, they suffered from various debilitating

diseases, with well-marked clinical and pathological
manifestations, and in many cases mortality was high.
Scientists were called in to find the cause of these maladies
and above all to find economic means of prevention and control.

The success of these scientists in tackling applied
problems during this period can be illustrated by the following
facts. In 1931 copper deficiency in grazing cattle was demonstrated in parts of Holland and of Florida and simple control
measures were devised; in 1933 and 1934 "alkali disease" and
"blind staggers" of stock in parts of the Great Plains of the
United States were established as manifestions of chronic and
acute selenium poisoning, respectively; in 1935 cobalt deficiency was shown to be the cause of various wasting diseases
of grazing ruminants in parts of Western Australia and South
Australia; in 1937 enzootic neonatal ataxia of lambs in
Western Australia was found to be a manifestation of copper
deficiency in the ewe, completely controllable by copper
supplementation of the ewe during pregnancy; and in 1938
excessive intakes of molybdenum from the herbage were revealed
as the cause of a debilitating diarrhea affecting cattle
confined to certain restricted areas in England and which
could be controlled by massive copper therapy. A few years
later the disease hemolytic jaundice occurring in parts of
Eastern Australia, affecting both sheep and cattle, was shown
to be an expression of chronic copper poisoning brought about
either by high gross intakes of copper from the herbage of
localized areas or by normal copper intakes associated with
abnormally low pasture molybdenum levels. This last investigation proved of very great nutritional significance and
illustrates strikingly how applied studies aimed at solving
practical problems can lead to new concepts of basic scientific
interest. I refer, of course, to the concept of nutritional

balance and metabolic interrelationships among the trace
elements which are proving to be profoundly important in trace
element research and its application.

I would like to mention briefly here my own experience as
one of the earliest workers in these applied "area" problems,
which shows how dominant economic considerations were at that
time. Just after World War I the government of Western
Australia initiated a large dairy farm settlement scheme in
the southwest corner of the state. Land was cleared in blocks,
luxuriant subterranean clover pastures were developed and the
properties were stocked with dairy cattle, mostly Guernseys,
and handed over to returned soldiers and immigrants from
England. Within a few years it became apparent that the
cattle would not thrive and fertility and milk yields were
low. On many properties the calves wasted away and died
despite ample pasture of apparently satisfactory nutritional
value. "Wasting disease," as it was called locally, threatened
to completely cripple a whole industry involving the livelihood
of scores of settlers and hugh financial losses to the
government. There was a public outcry and something had to be
done.

In 1932 I returned to Western Australia from Cambridge as
a very young man with a fresh Ph.D. in nutrition and biochemistry, and considerable energy but very little else. I was
immediately told to go down to the problem area, join a very
able veterinary officer there, John Filmer, and help "solve
the problem immediately." During the five years that it took
us to discredit the iron-deficiency theory that had been
accepted as the cause of these wasting diseases in different
countries and to show that lack of cobalt in the soils and the
pastures of the affected areas was the real cause, we were
under continuous political and public pressure to provide an

economic solution to the problem. When this was achieved, there was no further interest and for many years we were unable to pursue many of the more fundamental aspects of cobalt and vitamin B_{12} metabolism in the ruminant essential to a proper understanding of the problem under study. In fact it is only in recent years that I have been able to return to this branch of nutrition with my colleagues, Dr. Somers and Dr. Gawthorne.

D. Mode of Action of the Trace Elements

In the early period just discussed, which I have elsewhere described as the "first golden era" of trace element research[18], attention was initially focused on practical means of prevention and control. Little or nothing was known of the precise metabolic roles of the trace elements or of their specific functional relationship to the clinical and pathological disturbances in the animal that accompany deficiencies and toxicoses. Outstanding advances in this area of trace element research have been made in the last decade as an outcome of collaborative studies by nutritionists, biochemists, pathologists, and enzymologists, and as a direct consequence of earlier and concurrent basic investigations in enzymology. These latter have revealed the existence of a range of metalloenzymes that participate in a remarkably wide spectrum of cellular activities affecting the structure and function of the tissues. The economic or practical motivation behind these fruitful studies has been minor. The stimulus has come largely from a need to expand knowledge for its own sake, to understand more about nutritional physiology and the specific roles that the trace elements play in living processes.

I would like to illustrate the extent of recent progress in this aspect of trace element research with a few outstanding examples involving cobalt, manganese, copper, and zinc. In

1961 Marston and associates[19] showed that a breakdown in
the utilization of proprionate, a major energy source to
ruminants, at the point of conversion of methyl-malonyl-CoA to
succinyl-CoA, was a primary metabolic defect in cobalt/
vitamin B_{12} deficiency in sheep. Subsequently my colleagues,
Dr. Somers and Dr. Gawthorne[20,21], showed that acetate
clearance rates, as well as proprionate clearance rates, were
increasingly adversely affected as cobalt/vitamin B_{12} deficiency intensified and urinary excretion of methyl malonic acid
increased significantly. Gawthorne[21] also showed that
formiminoglutamic acid (FIGLU) excretion was even more significantly increased, compared with pair-fed controls, even in
the early stages of cobalt/vitamin B_{12} deficiency. The nature
of some of the primary metabolic lesions affecting appetite
and feed utilization in cobalt deficiency in ruminants has
thus begun to emerge more than 30 years after the original
discovery that cobalt is an essential element in ruminant
nutrition and nearly 20 years after the functional relationship of cobalt to vitamin B_{12} was first demonstrated.

Skeletal abnormalities were first observed in manganese
deficiency in birds and mammals over 30 years ago and have
been studied by many workers since that time. At first it
was assumed that manganese was involved in the calcification
process per se. This belief was fostered by the fact that
bone phosphatase plays an important part in calcification and
by the finding that bone phosphatase activity is reduced in
manganese-deficient chicks and rabbits. It is now apparent
from the work of Leach[22] with chicks and of Hurley[23] and
of Everson[24] with rats and guinea pigs that a defect in
bone matrix formation rather than in calcification can be
incriminated as the cause of the skeletal abnormalities. A
severe reduction in cartilage chondroitin sulfate content,

essential to the maintenance of the structure of this tissue, has been demonstrated in manganese deficiency. Furthermore the critical sites of manganese function in chondroitin sulfate synthesis have recently been identified by Leach and co-workers[25]. These are the two enzyme systems (a) polymerase enzyme, which is responsible for the polymerization of UDP-N-acetyl-galactosamine to UDP-glucuronic acid to form the polysaccharide and (b) galactotransferase, an enzyme which incorporates galactose from UDP-galactose into the galactose-galactose-xylose trisaccharide, which serves as the linkage between the polysaccharide and the protein associated with it. A biochemical explanation for the observed effects of manganese deficiency upon the composition and histopathology of connective tissue has thus appeared and the basic biochemical defect underlying this manifestation of manganese deficiency has been identified just 30 years after the manifestation was first reported.

The critical sites of action of copper in relation to certain of the signs of deficiency of that element have been equally impressively elucidated in recent years, long after the pathological changes in the animal were first observed. Thus Mills and co-workers[26,27] have shown that the groups of nerve cells showing the morphological lesions of "swayback" or neonatal ataxia in lambs, the large motor neurones of the red nucleus and of the ventral horns of the grey matter in the spinal cord, also show the most severe biochemical lesion, a deficiency in the copper-containing metalloenzyme cytochrome oxidase[28]. The precise function of cytochrome oxidase in maintaining the functional and structural integrity of these vital components of the CNS remains to be determined.

A relationship between a biochemical defect involving another copper metalloenzyme, amine oxidase, and pathological

disturbances manifested by rupture of the major blood vessels,
and in chicks by bone abnormalities, has been even more
precisely demonstrated. In these cases the delay between the
time of the original observations of the pathological changes
in the animal and the biochemical explanation of the causes
was much shorter then in the other examples quoted earlier.
In fact, only seven years elapsed between the first reports of
aneurisms and rupture of the major blood vessels in copper-
deficient chicks by O'Dell and co-workers[29] and in
copper-deficient pigs by Carnes and co-workers[30] in 1961
and the demonstration by Hill et al.[31] that these lesions
arise from a reduction in amine oxidase activity in the aorta,
resulting in a reduced capacity for oxidatively deaminating
the epsilon amino group of the lysine residues in elastin.
Less lysine is thus converted to desmosine, resulting in fewer
cross-linkages in elastin and hence less elasticity of the
aorta. More recently Rucker, O'Dell, and others[32] have
shown that the bone defects characteristic of copper deficiency in the chick arise similarly from a reduced amine
oxidase activity with a consequent failure of incorporation
of the cross-linking structure in collagen due to impaired
oxidation of the terminal carbon atom in lysine.

II. THE FUTURE OF TRACE ELEMENT RESEARCH

The brilliantly successful researches on the mode of
action of cobalt, manganese, and copper just outlined serve
to highlight our comparative ignorance of the basic biochemical lesions which lie at the root of other trace element
deficiencies. Their very success points the way clearly to
the need for similar types of investigations with other trace
elements. Encouraging progress is already being made in these
respects with zinc and selenium. But what about the newer

trace elements, chromium, nickel, and tin? Identification of the mode of action of these elements in biochemical terms presents challenging and worthwhile problems for those scientists whose inclinations lie in trying to understand more about the basic roles of trace substances in living processes.

It seems to me also that the pure scientist has other equally challenging problems in this branch of science. What about all the other elements which occur ubiquitously in living matter? It seems very unlikely that only 10 or 11 of the scores of such trace elements that exist are essential to living organisms. It seems much more likely that the list of essentials will be lengthened as techniques improve and as the search continues. Perhaps the laboratory now being opened here in North Dakota will have the honour of extending this list and discovering further elements of physiological significance to man and animals.

Finally, I would suggest that it is not only the pure scientist who has the ball at his feet. The applied scientist with a different philosophy, whether he be in the field of human medicine and public health or of animal health and production, will have ample scope for rewarding research with the trace elements. Public health problems involving environmental loading with elements such as lead, cadmium, and mercury are already causing concern in some areas and yet we know very little indeed of the factors affecting the movements of these elements in the food chain from rocks and soils to animals and man through plants, air, and drinking water. We know still less about their possible long-term deleterious effects on man and the maximum intakes compatible with full physical and mental welfare. Furthermore, man-made changes in the environment affecting the magnitude of the exposure to trace elements are by no means confined to those resulting in the injection

of large amounts of potentially toxic elements into the
environment, important as these may be. We must recognize
also the importance of technological changes in food production,
processing, and storage which might reduce intakes of nutritionally vital elements such as iron, zinc, and chromium.
The impact of changes in agronomic practices alone involving
ever-higher-yielding crop and herbage plant varieties and ever-
higher applications of more and more concentrated fertilizers
require constant investigation and surveillance in this
respect. Applied research of this nature with a range of
trace elements could be of deep significance to the survival of
man in a changing and challenging world. The philosophy of
the pure and the applied researcher with trace elements thus
emerges as fundamentally similar - the urge to know more of
the environment in which we live. It is difficult to think of
a more worthwhile, indeed a more noble, task.

REFERENCES

[1].   Harless, E., *Arch. Anat. Physiol.*, 148, (1847).

[2].   Fredericq, L., *Arch. Zool. Exptl. et Gén.*, 7, 535 (1879).

[3].   Church, A. W., *Phil. Trans. Roy. Soc. London*, 159,
       627 (1869).

[4].   Mendel, L. B. and Bradley, H. C., *Am. J. Physiol.*, 14,
       313 (1905).

[5].   Henze, M., *Z. Physiol. Chem.*, 72, 494 (1911).

[6].   MacMunn, C. A., *Phil. Trans. Roy. Soc. London*, 177,
       267 (1885).

[7].   Chatin, A., *Compt. Rend. Acad. Sci.* 30-39, (1850-1854).

[8].   Tipton, I. H. and Cook, M. J., *Health Physics*, 9,
       103 (1963).

[9].   Birckner, V., *J. Biol. Chem.*, 38, 191 (1919).

[10]. Hart, E. B., Steenbock, H., Waddell, J., and Elvehjem, C. A.,
       J. Biol. Chem., 77, 797 (1928).

[11]. Kemmerer, A. R., Elvehjem, C. A., and Hart, E. B., J. Biol. Chem., 92, 623 (1931).

[12]. Todd, W. R., Elvehjem, C. A., and Hart, E. B., Am. J. Physiol., 107, 146 (1934).

[13]. Higgins, E. S., Richert, D. A., and Westerfeld, W. W., J. Nutr., 59, 539 (1956).

[14]. Schwarz, K. and Foltz, C. M., J. Am. Chem. Soc., 79, 3293 (1957); J. Biol. Chem., 233, 245 (1958).

[15]. Schwarz, K. and Mertz, W., Arch. Biochem. Biophys., 85, 292 (1959).

[16]. Nielsen, F. H., private communication, 1970.

[17]. Schwarz, K., Milne, D. B., and Vinyard, E., Biochem. Biophys. Res. Comm. (1970).

[18]. Underwood, E. J., Proc. First Intern. Conf. Trace Element Metab. in Animals, Aberdeen, Scotland, 1969.

[19]. Marston, H. R., Allen, S. H., and Smith, R. M., Nature, 190, 1085 (1961).

[20]. Somers, M., Austral. J. Exptl. Biol. Med. Sci., 47, 219 (1969).

[21]. Gawthorne, J. M., Austral. J. Biol. Sci., 21, 789 (1968).

[22]. Leach, R. M., Jr., Fed. Proc., 26, 118 (1967).

[23]. Hurley, L. S., Proc. 2nd Missouri Conf. on Trace Substances in Environmental Health, Columbia, Missouri, 1968, p. 41.

[24]. Tsai, H. C. C. and Everson, G. J., J. Nutr., 91, 447 (1967).

[25]. Leach, R. M., Jr., Muenster, A. M., and Wien, E. M., Arch. Biochem. Biophys., 133, 22 (1969).

[26]. Mills, C. F. and Williams, R. B., Biochem. J., 85, 629 (1962).

[27]. Fell, B. F., Mills, C. F., and Boyne, R., Res. Vet. Sci., 6, 170 (1965).

[28]. Barlow, R. M., _J. Comp. Path._, _73_, 51, 61 (1963).

[29]. O'Dell, B. L., Hardwick, B. C., Reynolds, G., and
       Savage, J. E., _Proc. Soc. Exptl. Biol. Med._, _108_, 402
       (1961).

[30]. Carnes, W. H., Shields, G. S., Cartwright, G. E.,
       and Wintrobe, M. M., _Fed. Proc._, _20_, 118 (1961).

[31]. Hill, C. H., Starcher, B., and Kim, C., _Fed. Proc._,
       _26_, 129 (1968).

[32]. Rucker, R. B., O'Dell, B. L., Parker, H. E., and
       Rogler, J. C., _Proc. 4th Ann. Conf. on Trace_
       Substances in Environmental Health (D. D. Hemphill, ed.)
       Columbia, Missouri, 1970.

Chapter 2

INTERACTIONS IN NUTRITION

D. M. Hegsted

Department of Nutrition
Harvard School of Public Health
Boston, Massachusetts

I. INTRODUCTION

In this chapter I propose to discuss "interactions" which
I believe will be very important in investigations in the
future. We have scarcely begun to deal seriously with this
problem; we need more adequate concepts and experimental
designs. It will be particularly important in the area of
trace element nutrition.

I cannot resist the opportunity to reminisce briefly since
most of the topics we are dealing with have developed since I

19

was introduced to nutrition and biochemistry. I recall as a
senior student being assigned the task of determining the lead
content of a urine sample from a patient whom the local physician suspected of having lead poisoning. The method utilizing
dithizone had just been published and I ran the urine sample
and my own urine as well as a set of lead standards. The final
extracts of the latter were arranged in ascending order in a
series of test tubes (the original photoelectric colorimeter
of Evelyn had not yet appeared on the market) and the colors
of the extracts were compared visually to the standards. I
concluded that the patient was excreting more lead than I was
and the significance of that result is not very clear to me.
I can also recall struggling with the determination of sodium
by precipitation with cobalt nitrate and potassium as the
potassium platinic chloride. The 1937 edition of Hawk and
Bergheim (and my first course in biochemistry preceded this
edition) gives the procedure for the determination of sodium
and potassium in urine. One oxidizes 100 cc of urine with
sulfuric acid and nitric acid and evaporates in a platinum
crucible to "remove as much of the sulfuric acid as possible."
Then barium, ammonia, and ammonium carbonate are added to
precipitate sulfates, phosphates, calcium, and magnesium.
After filtration, the solution is taken to dryness and the
residue weighed and it is supposed to consist of the combined
chlorides of sodium and potassium. Then this is dissolved,
the potassium is precipitated with platinum chloride, separated,
dried, and weighed. Sodium is determined by difference.

I would also point out that the experimental demonstration
in animals that magnesium was an essential nutrient occurred
in 1932 by McCollum and co-workers[1]; and the original paper
of Hart et al.[2] on the essentiality of copper was published
in 1928. When the landmark publication of Shohl[3] entitled

Mineral Metabolism appeared in 1939, only copper, manganese, and iodine were thought to be clearly identified as essential nutrients among those now commonly called the "essential trace elements." The extent of knowledge at that time concerning tissue electrolytes and minerals was remarkable considering the cumbersome methodology available. The introduction of flame photometry revolutionized the ability to look at and to interpret sodium and potassium metabolism. Newer methodologies either have or will do the same for most of the other trace elements.

I recall Karl Paul Link saying that the isolation and elucidation of the structure of the vitamins could not have happened earlier than it did, even if experimental nutrition had been more advanced. Development of the methodology for handling small amounts of materials for the determination of structure had to come first. Of course, the methods used were crude compared to those now available. The trace elements are now a frontier somewhat comparable to the vitamins in the late 1930s and much of the technology needed is readily available.

II. IODINE AND FLUORIDE

Two of the important trace elements that are not specifically discussed in the program are iodine and fluoride. The story is perhaps too well known to warrant much time. However, it is important to note that it is well over 100 years since the first iodization of salt was recommended as a preventive method for goiter. This has not yet been successfully accomplished in many parts of the world, including the United States. Repeated surveys in this country indicate highly variable use of iodized salt. It is quite clear that optional iodization is not a very effective method and requires continual education

and propaganda. It is strange that we have not yet taken legal
steps to provide for this simple public health measure. The
other aspect that requires continual consideration and is a
hindrance to the adoption of iodization is the few adverse
effects which apparently may occur when iodization is started
in some deficient areas[4]. These effects appear to be over-
emphasized by opponents and denied by proponents.

The fluoridation of public water supplies is another
proven public health method which is gaining ground only slowly
and with great difficulty. In every test it is clear that
when fluoride is provided in a deficient area, dental caries
is reduced by at least 50% and no adverse effects have yet
been demonstrated. In many ways dental caries can be considered
to be one of the most prevalent and one of the most important
problems to be solved today. It is apparent that the costs of
appropriate dental care are excessive and the needed money is
not likely to come from any source in the near future. Even
if a general legislature should provide the funds, the dentists
and technicians required are simply not available. I person-
ally feel that national legislation is required.

The other aspect of fluoride that requires additional
investigation is the relation to osteoporosis. There is
substantial evidence that high fluoride intakes retard bone
loss in the elderly[5,6] and are helpful in the treatment of
osteoporosis[7,8,9]. The study we were involved in in North
Dakota[6] indicated that in the high-fluoride area there was
approximately one half as much osteoporosis in elderly women
as in the low-fluoride areas. These kinds of investigations
need repetition in other parts of the country and the world.

III. ARSENIC

I happened to be paging through an old issue of the
Journal of Nutrition a few weeks ago and noticed a title in
1935 on the availability of arsenic. According to Dr. Coulson
and co-workers[10], shrimp which has long been known to be a
rich source of arsenic must have a special form of arsenic
since relatively little was deposited in the tissues of rats
fed shrimp compared to animals fed comparable amounts of
arsenic trioxide. Only 0.7% of the arsenic in shrimp was
stored in the tissues compared to 19% of arsenic trioxide.
Furthermore the arsenic in shrimp was mostly absorbed but
excreted in the urine. Incidentally the shrimp collected in
different places varied over tenfold in arsenic content. This
must be one kind of interaction. The best, or perhaps I
should say worst, example of this is now before us in terms
of the "iron problem." We have been adding iron to foods for
many years, we have not bothered to determine whether the iron
used was useful, and now the evidence is accumulating that
much of it is probably not useful. At best, this seems
ridiculous. It is clear, of course, that iron salts do differ
in availability, and although this has been known for many
years, it never seemed to impress anybody very much.

Without belaboring this, it is obvious that elements
occur in foods in many different forms. This may or may not
be significant depending on what happens in the gastrointestinal
tract or elsewhere in the body. That the form of iron is
important in its utilization is clear. However, it may not
be very useful to determine what forms these are since the
modification of these after they are prepared and eaten may
be a more important factor in determining their utility.

IV. BIOASSAYS

In my view it has been unfortunate, generally speaking,
that the concern with modern instrumentation and search for
easier measures of practically everything has led to a general
decline in the development and use of bioassays. Often this
search for easier ways has led us to skip a step in the
development of science. A prime example that comes readily to
mind is that of niacin. Very shortly after niacin was identified as an essential nutrient, it was shown that it could be
measured by microbiological assay. The only method available
before that was the assay with dogs, which was crude, indeed.
In any event a decent animal assay was never developed. Now
we know that much of the niacin in certain foods is in a
bound form which is unavailable to several, perhaps all,
species. The net result is that we have voluminous food
tables in which the content of "niacin" is given which may
border on nutritional rubbish. It is not certain whether it
is even worth calculating the niacin content of a diet from
these data. The situation with regard to folic acid is perhaps
even worse. Total dietary iron is similarly of doubtful
practical utility and I suppose the same will turn out to be
true of zinc, selenium, chromium, and others.

It is presumed to be crucial that when we are dealing
with bioassays we must also search for appropriate animal
models which, unless they are of interest in themselves, should
at least approach the metabolism of the human species with
regard to the particular nutrient we are concerned with. This
means, of course, that work with both animals and human beings
must be conducted so that some comparisons can be made.
Unfortunately this kind of approach often leads people to
conclude that if we have to do the work with man anyway,
studies with experimental animals may not be worthwhile.

This conclusion, however, can only be reached if we ignore the quantitive aspects of the problem.

As I have already indicated, the development of decent bioassays has had relatively little support for many years and competent application of statistics to the problems of bioassays is rare. Anyone who has tried to apply statistics to the assessment of the data available upon the nutritional requirements of man finds this a most discouraging proposition. Presumably the strength of statistics and good statistical design lies in being able to draw quantitative conclusions in complex fields where there are variables which cannot be controlled. Both statistical design and statistical treatment are most often lacking in clinical trials where it is presumably needed most. The common lack of appropriate design and analysis in animal work is even more difficult to comprehend. Most people simply do not understand how poor their data are, especially when they are trying to do quantitative assays in which one is interested not only in the mean value but also in the confidence limits of the estimated potency.

V. INTERACTION OF NUTRIENTS

What most people mean when they talk about "interaction of nutrients" is the effect of the level of one nutrient upon the availability or utilization of another. There are a legion of examples and practically everyone who has looked for them has found them. The prime example, again going far back, is the calcium-to-phosphorus ratio. This grew largely out of the observation that rickets could be produced in rats when the diet contained a very high ratio of calcium-to-phosphorus but not when these were "balanced." What we mean by balance has never been very well defined. I recall Dr. Elvehjem saying that the proper ratio was not one or two but one to two

because that was the ratio in milk. Connie forgot that the
ratio in breast milk is over two rather than one to two as in
cow's milk. The effects of varying calcium-to-phosphorus
ratios under varying conditions, expecially in growing animals,
have been investigated almost ad nauseam and these can certainly
be demonstrated when one or the other is a limiting factor in
the diet. However, in human nutrition there seems to be very
little evidence that this ratio is of any practical importance
or, if it is, when it is of importance[11]. Certainly good
nutrition can be obtained on diets varying widely in the
calcium-to-phosphorus ratio.

There is a similar voluminous literature on the effects
of a special phosphorus compound, phytate, on the availability
of calcium. Worry over this factor led the British to supplement their bread with calcium during the war. Large amounts
of phytate have been used therapeutically to inhibit calcium
absorption. Yet the general practical significance of phytate
in human nutrition continues to elude us. Presumably the
hydrolysis of phytate requires phytase, but the adaptation of
man and animals to diets high in phytate still appears to be
a mystery. Again it is clear that good nutrition in man is
achieved with diets high in whole grain cereals, high in
phytate, and low in calcium, that is, the conditions under
which phytate inhibition of calcium absorption can be demonstrated.

Many of these interactions seem to have some generalities;
that is, diets high in phosphate inhibit the utilization of
calcium, magnesium, iron, zinc, and probably all nutrients
which have relatively insoluble phosphates. The same is true
with phytate. But I would point out that this reference to
the solubility of phosphates is only a logical "explanation"
of what is often observed; it has rarely, if ever, been

actually demonstrated to be the "cause" of the poor utilization.
If we think about solubility and the relative amounts of iron
and phosphate in the diet, it is remarkable that any iron is
absorbed. However, many of us tend to think of the chemistry
of these products in simplified terms which have no reality.
Iron and many other similar metals never occur as stripped-down
ions[12]. They are always coordinated with a ligand, with
water if nothing else. Polymerization processes result in
colloidal forms or precipitates which are probably generally
less available. Hundreds of materials in the diet and gastrointestinal secretions can form ligands which prevent or modify
the olation process. These include many ions, organic acids,
amino acids, and proteins. The situation in the gut must be
exceedingly complex. If we assume that there is no direct
interaction between two materials, say calcium and iron, but
that both do react with phosphate, then it follows that there
will be some kind of secondary interaction between calcium and
iron. I would assume that practically anything that is insoluble or that precipitates in the gut might adsorb the trace
mineral on the surface and modify absorption.

I am not sure whether I should take the stance of an
apostle of despair or hope. If we are really to understand
what goes on in terms of interactions at any biological level,
we will presumably have to dissect these one by one and then
put them back together in increasingly complex systems. This
seems formidable, indeed, considering the numbers of pairs to
be studied. However, a purely empirical approach seems even
worse. Consider, if you will, the design of an experiment to
determine the effects of these interactions on the nutritional
requirement of nutrients. As a start we might say that to
determine the requirement of a single nutrient, at least five
levels ought to be investigated with perhaps five animals at

each level, or 25 animals. This is a modest study and would
probably satisfy no one. However, if we are then concerned
with two nutrients, the number becomes 25 groups or 125 animals.
If three nutrients are to be studied, we require 125 groups of
625 animals; with four nutrients, 625 groups and 3125 animals.
Multiply these kinds of numbers by whatever analytical procedures or other techniques you have to apply to evaluate the
response of the animals.

The problem is not only the massive effort that is involved
but the problem of how to handle the data. The easiest statistical approach would be to assume that there are linear dose-
response relationships but we are certain that this will
rarely, if ever, be the case. A purely empirical approach
seems even less likely to get us where we want to be than
trying to get at the basic principles.

We can at least dimly visualize the complexities of the
gut, and most interactions of minerals possibly or probably
have an explanation at this level. However, the trace elements
can be assumed to function primarily as catalysts and thus
many metabolic adaptations can be assumed to offer possibilities
for variations in requirements or functions of the trace
minerals. Here I would just point out that for many years
experimental and clinical nutritionists have viewed glucose,
sucrose, dextrin, and starch as nutritional equivalents except
for minor variations in calorie content. It is now clear that
this is not true. Even though we understand that there are
metabolic adaptations to diets in which the carbohydrate
sources are varied, we still have little "feel" for what this
really means. If I am working on some aspect of a trace
mineral, should I make the diet with glucose or sucrose, apart
from the problem of the level of the trace mineral that these
carbohydrates might contain? Similarly, in the last few years

it has become abundantly clear the dietary fat is not just fat.
The internal economy of an animal fed a diet high in saturated
fat is quite different from one fed a highly unsaturated fat.
And how much fat should one use? So again, if we begin to
think of the array of dietary fats which need investigation,
combinations with different amounts and kinds of carbohydate
and so on, we can again design unmanageable experiments very
rapidly.

These kinds of problems have had very little serious
thought. We once published an experiment[13] in which we
investigated the effects on serum cholesterol of five different
dietary fats, each fed at three different levels in the diet
in combination with two different levels of cholesterol and
studied at four different time periods. This involved 30
different diets and to cut the analytical load to a minimum we
used only two animals per group. This is the minimal number
required to yield an estimate of the variance between animals
fed the same diet. In this experiment we can test for the
effects of the main variables, dietary cholesterol level, kind
of fat, level of fat, and time. Each yielded a significant
effect on serum cholesterol. Of the six simple interactions,
four were statistically significant. Of five complex interactions, three were significant. This may be a rather trivial
example and I now believe that the rat is such a poor model
that cholesterol studies on rats scarcely warrant investigation.
Nevertheless I am convinced that this is the kind of approach
which must be used to get some economy into animal experimentation when we are dealing with complex processes.

Of course, it is also apparent that a simple analysis of
variance, which only identifies a significant interaction and
gives some idea of the magnitude of it relative to others
included in the experiment, is not adequate. We need somehow

to visualize or delineate the dose-response relationships. Although dozens of interactions can be mentioned, few, if any, have been satisfactorily quantitated. One of the earliest interactions described, presumably of very practical importance, is the relationship between thiamine requirements and dietary fat. This has been poorly quantitated and, in my opinion[14], poorly understood in spite of glib explanations in every textbook.

Another area of dietary interaction where numerous examples can be cited but where very few can be quantitated or explained is in relationships between diet and toxicology[15]. Diets high or low in fat, protein, or of differing composition modify the toxicity of hydrocarbons, insecticides, carcinogens, radiation, antioxidants, and so on. Again the data appear as empirical examples. With the great public concern in this area and particularly the increased effort that will undoubtedly be put into animal testing, it would seem clear some serious effort should be put into this field. What is the value of many of the long-term feeding trials if we can modify the outcome by selecting the proper diet before the feeding trial is set up?

I would also like to re-emphasize the point which has already been referred to by Dr. Underwood. The national food supply is changing rather rapidly, particularly in the direction of more highly processed foods and convenience foods. The first may or may not have compositions similar to more generally recognized foods; the latter impose limits on the consumer in selecting nutrient intakes. It is almost certain that we shall move toward more general fortification programs in the near future. There is danger in this since interest will be focused on the traditional nutrients, the vitamins and minerals of concern over the past 30 to 40 years. We must be aware

that unless attention is paid to other nutrients, including the
trace elements, we may be producing undesirable changes. We
must stimulate more work on the surveillance of the national
food supply in terms of all nutrients and improve our methods
for keeping track of the nutritional status of the population
with regard to all nutrients. In those areas where we are
relatively ignorant, as with the trace minerals, the problem
may be more serious than we know.

One hears the frequent complaint that biochemists are
continually involved in dissecting the cell into smaller and
smaller systems but that few are concerned with putting these
back together again so that the metabolism of organs or whole
organisms can be interpreted or predicted. Similarly,
nutritionists have of necessity worked toward more and more
simple purified diets where everything in the diet is under
control. The need for this is obvious and nowhere more evident
than in the study of trace minerals. However, we should bear
in mind that the findings under these conditions may have
little practical significance and we must not forget that an
ultimate objective is an explanation of what happens in a
more real and complex world. This explanation is what we mean
by "interaction in nutrition."

REFERENCES

[1]. Kruse, H. D., Orent, E. R., and McCollum, E. V.,
     J. Biol. Chem., 96, 519 (1932).

[2]. Hart, E. B., Steenbock, H., Waddell, J., and Elvehjem,
     C. A., J. Biol. Chem., 77, 797 (1928).

[3]. Shohl, A. T., Mineral Metabolism. Reinhold, New York,
     (1939).

[4]. Connolly, R. J., Vidor, G. I., and Stewart, J. C.,
     Lancet, 1, 500 (1970).

[5].   Leone, N. C., Stevenson, C. A., Besse, B., Hawes, L. E.,
       and Dawber, T. R., Arch. Indust. Health, 21, 326 (1960).

[6].   Bernstein, D. S., Sadowsky, N., Hegsted, D. M., Guri,
       C. D., and Stare, F. J., J. A. M. A., 198, 499 (1966).

[7].   Rich, C. and Ensinck, J., Nature, 191, 184 (1961).

[8].   Rich, R. and Ivanovich, P., Ann. Int. Med., 63,
       1069 (1965).

[9].   Bernstein, D. S. and Cohen, P., J. Clin. Endocrin.
       Metabolism, 27, 197 (1967).

[10]. Coulson, E. J., Remington, R. E., and Lynch, K. M.,
       J. Nutr., 10, 255 (1935).

[11]. Food and Agriculture Organization, Calcium Requirements.
       FAO Report Series No. 30, Rome, 1962.

[12]. Rollinson, C. L., Measures to Increase Iron in Foods
       and Diets, Proceedings of a Workshop. Food and
       Nutrition Board, National Academy of Sciences,
       Washington, D. C., 1970.

[13]. Hegsted, D. M., Gotsis, A., Stare, F. J., and
       Worcester, J., Am. J. Clin. Nutr., 7, 5 (1959).

[14]. Gershoff, S. N. and Hegsted, D. M., J. Nutr., 54,
       609 (1954).

[15]. Friedman, L., Fed. Proc., 25, 137 (1966).

Chapter 3

SPECTRAL CHARACTERISTICS OF METALS IN METALLOENZYMES*

B. L. Vallee

Biophysics Research Laboratory
Department of Biological Chemistry
Harvard Medical School
and the
Division of Medical Biology
Peter Bent Brigham Hospital
Boston, Massachusetts

I. INTRODUCTION

The biological importance of the so-called trace elements
and their essentiality to life and health have been recognized largely as a result of nutritional investigations

---

* This work was aided by Grant-in-Aid GM-15003 from the
National Institutes of Health of the Department of Health,
Education, and Welfare.

performed during the last half century on many species. It
has taken a very long time, indeed, for research on the trace
elements to become "respectable." The problem had long been
encumbered by its somewhat questionable reputation among
serious scientists in biochemistry, nutrition, and medicine.
To a large extent this may be traced perhaps to substantial
experimental difficulties which have beset the field for so
long; but it must also be admitted that overenthusiastic
claims, at times based on uncertain facts, have not been
altogether reassuring to the rank and file of biochemists
potentially interested in the field.

The dedication of a laboratory by the United States
Department of Agriculture and the University of North Dakota
is fitting tribute to the scientific maturation of the subject
and the recognition of its now established importance to human
welfare. Significant advances may justly be expected to be
the result of work to be performed here, and it is a great
pleasure to express warmest congratulations and best wishes
for a bright future.

As is well known, methodology has been critical in the
recognition of nutritional essentiality of food factors.
Apart from the indispensable biological experimentation,
advances in instrumental analysis must be credited with many
of the important advances of the last 20 years. Without
microchemistry, emission and atomic absorption spectroscopy,
or electrochemistry to monitor diets and experimental subjects,
the field might still lie fallow. Thus, the instrumental
revolution of the last two decades has given insight into the
remarkable role of trace elements in nutrition.

However, the details of the manner in which the trace
elements exercise their important biological roles are still
largely unknown. To be sure, it is appreciated that they

function in catalysis, in the synthesis and the stabilization
of the structure of proteins, and in transport, all processes
to which they entail great specificity; but little is known of
the chemical details, or the mechanisms by which these processes
take place. Clearly we need to understand not only that metals
are essential, but also in what manner they exercise their
roles; in short, how their biological specificity may be understood and described in terms of the detailed chemistry of
their interaction with macromolecules. Toward this end we
have been concerned particularly with the mechanism of action
of metals in metalloenzymes and have considered them as models
for the study of the mechanisms of action of enzymes in general.

II. CHEMICAL BASIS OF BIOLOGICAL SPECIFICITY

The chemical basis of biological specificity in general
and of enzyme action in particular are fundamental questions.
The chemical behavior of certain metalloenzymes may apparently
reflect biological specificity, since the former characteristics are not encountered in simple metal chelates studied
thus far. It should be recalled that inactivation of
nonmetalloenzymes by site-specific reagents is similarly
unique, and the underlying chemical reactions are not observed
in simple peptides or nonenzymatic proteins. Thus the inactivation of certain seryl enzymes by di-isopropylfluorophosphate,
that of sulfhydryl, tyrosyl, histidyl, or lysyl enzymes under
mild conditions, by other site-specific organic reagents has
no counterpart in other fields of chemistry. The basis of
such reactivity is currently unknown and raised questions
concerning the properties of enzymes that render certain of
their amino acid side chains so reactive chemically, since
these features of their chemistries may provide links to their
biological functions.

As a class metal ions exhibit properties and reactivities
which are distinctly different, of course, from those of amino
acid side chains of proteins. Hence some metals when involved
directly in activity can serve as excellent labels of active
enzyme sites owing to the visible color of some of their
complexes. Thus, for example, copper salts are blue, iron
salts are red or brownish and change color on oxidoreduction.
Hence it might be expected that these basic characteristics
would be preserved in biological systems while perhaps
revealing additional, characteristic features of active sites
of metalloenzymes. Such circumstances render metalloenzymes
convenient models for the study of the mechanism of enzyme
action[1].

It should be appreciated that the physicochemical properties of many of the metals which are essential to the function
of metalloenzymes, that is, largely those of the first transition series, are capable of probing their environments.
Basically physicochemical characteristics of complex metal ions
and of metalloenzymes arise from three sources: properties of
the metal altered by the ligands, properties of the ligands
altered by the metal, and specific de novo properties characteristic only of the resultant complex. Metal complex ions
are characterized by parameters such as their stability
constants, the effects of different donor groups upon their
formation, their redox potentials, spectroscopic, optical
rotatory, and magnetic properties, among others[2].

The advent of remarkably sensitive instrumental methods
for the characterization of these parameters has already begun
to have an impact on the mechanistic features of the role of
trace metals in catalysis quite akin to that of earlier
analytical instrumental developments on the assignment of
their biological roles. The conceptual innovations which

have accompanied the introduction of nuclear magnetic resonance, electron paramagnetic resonance, optical rotatory dispersion, circular dichroism, magneto circular dichroism, infrared, fluorescence, and other forms of spectroscopy of biological studies are no less profound than those which led to the advances of the previous 20 years.

Virtually all of these means have been employed to study one or another metalloenzyme, and the parameters of metalloenzymes, which can be studied by these methods are quite unusual when compared with those of complex metal ions. This has become apparent particularly from the inspection of absorption, optical rotatory dispersion, and circular dichroism, and electron paramagnetic resonance spectra of certain iron, copper, and cobalt enzymes, many of which have been examined only recently, owing to both improved equipment and availability of sufficient quantities of highly purified metalloproteins required for such physicochemical studies. Many of these spectra seem to differ from those of most model compounds[1]. It has proven difficult to assign the origin of these spectra but the findings have suggested that the coordination environment of metals in metalloenzymes reveals low symmetry, though it is not clear what factors might account for the unusual spectral properties of metalloenzymes. Moreover the spectral properties of metalloenzymes and their modification by addition of substrates, coenzymes, or inhibitors have been inferred to signal catalytic potential: these unusual physical properties might reflect biological capacity in some manner. In that case we might expect the physical properties to be influenced by conditions which alter function, as has indeed been observed[3-6]. The data basic to this discussion have been reviewed, obviating the need for their recapitulation[1,6,7].

TABLE

Spectral Parameters of Cu(II) [A]

Compound	Absorption λ, mμ (Absorptivity, M^{-1} cm^{-1})	
A.		
1. Cu(II) complex ions		
$[(Cu(NH_3)_4]^{2+}$	600 ($\sim$20)	750 ($\sim$25)
	660 ($\sim$40)	
Bis(3-phenyl-1-2,4 pentane	490 ($\sim$50)	580 ($\sim$50)
dionato) Copper(II)	520 ($\sim$25)	650 ($\sim$50)
$CuSO_4 \cdot 5H_2O$	700 ($\sim$1)	950 ($\sim$3)
	790 ($\sim$4)	
Cu(II)Gly-L-Val, pH 7.2	620 (90)	
2. Cu-Protein complexes		
Cu(II) carbonic anhydrase	760 broad (120)	
Cu(II) serum albumin	700 broad (50)	
3. Cu Proteins		
Ceruloplasmin	610 broad ($\sim$1000)	
Erythrocuprein (superoxide		
dismutase)	655 broad (280)	
Cerebrocuprein	655 broad (400)	
Plastocyanin	460 (500)	770 (1600)
	597 (4400)	
	351-532	730 (500)
	(weak bands)	
	615 (2000)	

I

and Co(II) [B] Complexes and Enzymes (6)

Ellipticity λ, mμ ($[\theta]^{25} \times 10^{-3}$)		Notes
		Tetragonal
		Twofold axis
		Tetragonal
541 (0.7)	725 (0.2)	Distorted
658 (0.2)		Tetragonal
		Unknown low symmetry
369 (−3)	615 (−10)	
532 (−4)	730 (−2)	

B. L. VALLEE

TABLE

Spectral Parameters of Cu(II) [A]

Compound	Absorption λ, mμ (Absorptivity, M^{-1} cm^{-1})	
Laccase	450 (970)	850 (700)
	608 (4000)	
Pseudomonas denitrificans blue	450 (weak)	
	594 ($\sim$3000)	800 (1000)
Pseudomonas aeroginosa blue	467 [0.003]	820 [0.0035][a]
	625 [0.051]	
	467 ($\sim$300)	621 (3000)
	521 ($\sim$200)	806 ($\sim$600)
	500 (weak)	725 (weak)
	625 ($\sim$3000)	

B.

1. Simple Co(II) complexes

$[Co(H_2O)_6]^{2+}$	510 ($\sim$5)		1200 ($\sim$2)
$[CoCl_4]^{2-}$	685 (700), complex		1700 (100), complex
$[Co(OH)_4]^{2-}$	600 ($\sim$150), complex		1400 ($\sim$50), complex
$[Co(Et_4\ dien)]Cl_2$[c]	520	660	950

<u>a/</u> [ ], oscillator strength.

<u>b/</u> Rotational strength, CGS $\times$ 10^{39}.

<u>c/</u> In organic solvents.

I

and Co(II) [B] Complexes and Enzymes (6), continued

Ellipticity λ, mμ ($[\theta]^{25} \times 10^{-3}$)		Notes
		Unknown low symmetry
		Unknown low symmetry
467 [0.4] 625 [1] 467 (-2)	820 [0.2][b/] 621 (5)	Tetrahedral distortion from planar
521 (1)	806 (1)	
		Octahedral
		Tetrahedral
		Tetrahedral
		Distortion from trigonal bi-pyramidal

TABLE

Spectral Parameters of Cu(II) [A]

Compound	Absorption λ, mμ (Absorptivity, M^{-1} cm^{-1})		
[Co(Tren Me)Cl]Cl[c]	500 (120)	625 (80) 800 (∿30) doublet 1750 (∿30)	
2. Co(II) enzymes			
Co(II) carbonic anhydrase	510 (280) 550 (380)	615 (300) 900 (30) 640 (280) 1250 (90)	
Co(II) alkaline phosphatase	510 (280) 555 (350)	610 (210) sh 640 (250)	
Co(II) carboxypeptidase	500 sh	555 (∿150) 950 (∿25) 572 (∿150)	
Co(II) yeast alcohol[d] dehydrogenase	620 (∿800) 657 (∿800) 710 (∿600)		
Co(II) neutral protease	475 sh 525 (sh)	555 (50-100)	
Co(II) yeast aldolase	490 sh	530 (150)	
Co(II) yeast enolase[e]	490 (sh)	540 (30-40) 575 (sh)	

[c] In organic solvents.

[d] Enzyme contained both cobalt and zinc.

[e] Metal-enzyme complex.

I

and Co(II) [B] Complexes and Enzymes (6), continued

Ellipticity λ, mμ ($[\theta]^{25} \times 10^{-3}$)		Notes
460 (~3) 550 (3)	610 (3)	Unknown low symmetry
470 (2) 520 (2)	575 (-0.8)	Unknown low symmetry
500 sh	538 (-0.5)	Unknown low symmetry
		Unknown low symmetry
500 sh	550 (-0.8)	Unknown low symmetry
485 (2.4)	530 (3)	Unknown low symmetry
490 sh	540 (-0.5)	Unknown low symmetry

Whereas such studies are readily performed when enzymes
contain a chromophoric metal such as iron or copper, the
presence of a metal such as zinc would at first glance obviate
such opportunities. The diamagnetism of zinc and the lack of
color of its complexes render this metal ion a poor probe in
the sense discussed here. In contrast cobalt gives rise to
characteristic spectra and is paramagnetic, qualities which
are desirable when probing the environment of active enzymatic
sites. It is fortunate that in many zinc enzymes cobalt can
be substituted for the native zinc atom(s) while the enzyme
remains active. The active site of many zinc enzymes can,
hence, be examined using a cobalt probe. The spectra of such
cobalt enzymes are quite revealing and these have been
summarized in Table I.

Cobalt alkaline phosphatase of E. coli may serve as a
brief example.

The enzyme prepared by chromatography on DEAE cellulose
contains four zinc atoms per mole of protein. Two of them are
removed rapidly by 8-hydroxyquinoline-5-sulfonic acid, and
concomitantly virtually all activity is lost. The other two
zinc atoms, apparently not involved in catalytic function,
are removed much more slowly. Similarly, the results of
restoration of zinc to the apoenzyme confirm that only two of
its zinc atoms are required for function. The binding of the
first gram atoms of cobalt by the apoprotein results in a
spectrum similar to that of octahedral complex cobalt ions
but without the induction of enzymatic activity. Addition of
a further two gram atoms of cobalt generates activity and
concomitantly leads to the development of a complex absorption
spectrum with maxima at 640 mµ (ϵ = 250 M^{-1} cm^{-1}), 610 (sh 210),
555 (350), and 510 (280). This spectrum is dissimilar from
that of either octahedral or tetrahedral complex cobalt ions;

it is suggestive of an unusual coordination environment for the metal at the active site of alkaline phosphatase[5], and bears strong resemblance to that of cobalt carbonic anhydrase[8]. The circular dichroism of cobalt phosphatase is also consistent with an unusual coordination environment, as are the alterations both of the absorption and circular dichroic spectra of the cobalt enzyme on interaction with phosphate.

Titration over the pH range from 9 to 6 progressively decreases the intensity of the spectrum associated with the cobalt atoms involved in catalytic activity. Moreover, when studied over the same pH range, the degree of restoration of the spectrum associated with these catalytically active cobalt atoms parallels closely the enzymatic activity of the cobalt enzyme[5].

Similar approaches have also been successful in completely replacing the zinc atoms of horse liver ADH either with cobalt or with cadmium resulting in enzymatically active enzymes exhibiting specific activities and spectral properties characteristic of these metals and not seen in the native enzyme[9]. Co-LADH has a broad absorption band in the near-ultraviolet region centered at 340 mμ (ε = 6500) associated with two positive and three negative circular dichroic bands between 300 mμ and 450 mμ. Absorption maxima also occur at 655 mμ (ε = 1330), 730 mμ (ε = 800), and in the near infrared between 1000 and 1800 mμ (ε = 270-540). A small negative ellipticity band is centered at 620 mμ (Figs. 1 and 2).

Cd-LADH exhibits an intense absorption band centered at 245 mμ, which may assist in identifying the ligands of the proteins binding the metal since its molar absorptivity (ε = 10,200) is close to that of 14,000 reported for the cadmium mercaptide chromophores of metallothionein.

46   B. L. VALLEE

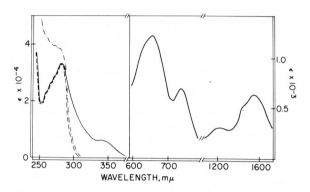

Fig. 1.　Absorption spectra of the metallodehydrogenases.
(---), Zn-LADH; (——), Co-LADH; (-·-·-·). Cd-LADH.　0.1 M tris
acetate, pH 7.0.

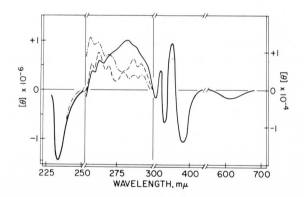

Fig. 2.　Circular dichroic spectra of the metallodehydrogenases.　(---), Zn-LADH; (——), Co-LADH; (-·-·-·), Cd-LADH.
The symbol [θ] denotes molecular ellipticity based on the
concentration and molecular weight of LADH.　0.1 M tris
acetate, pH 7.0.

The circular dichroic spectrum of Co-LADH is richer in detail than that of any other comparable cobalt enzyme studied thus far. It may be analyzed on one hand in terms of protein structure, as reflected in the intrinsic and side-chain Cotton effects of the protein, and of superimposed extrinsic Cotton effects resulting from either binding of NADH or of 1,10-phenanthroline (OP).

These metal substitutions also perturb the side-chain Cotton effects of LADH. Between 250 and 300 mμ the circular dichroic spectra of these metallodehydrogenases exhibit remarkably fine structure, characteristic of each. The circular dichroic difference spectrum of Cd-LADH vs. Zn-LADH below 270 mμ exhibits a positive ellipticity band which may well correspond to the maximum in the absorption spectrum at 245 mμ. In the region of maximum absorption due to aromatic amino acid residues, the ellipticity of the Co-LADH exceeds that of both Zn- and Cd-LADH.

The effects of the metal substitutions in LADH are reflected also in the optical properties of extrinsic chromophores, bound asymmetrically. Both the reduced coenzyme NADH and 1,10-phenanthroline (OP) bind to Zn-, Co-, and Cd-LADH while generating extrinsic Cotton effects, distinctive for each, with magnitudes which related quantitatively to binary complex formation.

Similarly, the amplitude of the circular dichroic band of the Cd-LADH-OP complex, centered at 271 mμ, markedly exceeds that of Zn-LADH-OP, while that of the Co-LADH-OP complex is considerably smaller. Thus the rotational strengths of these mixed complexes afford sensitive probes of the identity of the metal substituent at the active site.

Through work of this type it has become apparent that some of the metal present in certain metalloenzymes is critical to

the catalytic step while the rest seems to serve primarily in
protein structure[10]. It would appear that two such discrete
roles for metal atoms are maintained when cobalt or cadmium,
for example, are substituted in Zn-LADH. Both the cobalt and
cadmium enzymes bind 2 moles of OP, suggesting that, like the
native zinc enzyme, only two of the metal atoms are accessible
to this agent. Selective replacement either of the "functional"
or of the structural metal atoms with other metals, resulting
in "metal-hybrid enzymes," can now be documented by employing
the unusual absorption and circular dichroic properties
discussed, which augment the criteria available in the past.

A similar approach using the probe properties of metals
has also been employed for proteolytic enzymes. Thus far only
a rather small number of well-characterized proteolytic enzymes
are known to contain a metal in the native state and most of
these again contain zinc[2,6]. The spectral and enzymatic
characteristics of cobalt carboxypeptidase have been discussed
in detail, but analogous studies in other, similar systems
have also become possible recently.

The zinc of both thermolysin and of neutral protease can
be replaced by cobalt and other metals to yield active enzymes
and these derivatives exhibit characteristic spectra[6].

Even though the total number of cobalt enzymes examined
in this manner thus far is small, seemingly certain patterns
are becoming evident. The absorption spectra of many substituted zinc enzymes are quite similar to one another and many
have optically active bands of similar magnitude and position.
Even though it would seem premature to interpret the spectral
details, it is tempting to speculate that similarities, when
they exist, might reflect common functional characteristics.
Conceivably similarities and differences of spectra could imply
specific mechanisms.

III. SUMMARY

Not until very recently have physicochemical methods
become sufficiently discriminating to discern chemical details
of enzyme structure with a sensitivity adequate to consider
even the possibility that these might be related to catalytic
potential. The remarkable developments in physical-organic
and physical chemistry which have become increasingly applicable to macromolecules such as enzymes offer new opportunities
in this regard and give promise that recognition of the
chemistry underlying the exceptional biological activity and
specificity of enzymes may ultimately unify this vast diver-
sified area of study. The properties of various proteolytic
enzymes would seem to make them particularly suitable systems
for the investigations of this hypothesis.

REFERENCES

[1]. Vallee, B. L. and Williams, R. J. P., Proc. Nat. Acad.
      Sci. U. S., 59, 498 (1968).

[2]. Vallee, B. L. and Wacker, W. E. C., "Metalloproteins,"
      The Proteins (2nd ed.), (H. Neurath, ed.) Vol. 5,
      New York: Academic Press, 1970.

[3]. Kasper, C. B., J. Biol. Chem., 243, 3218 (1968).

[4]. Lindskog, S. and Ehrenberg, A., J. Mol. Biol., 24, 133
      (1967).

[5]. Simpson, R. T. and Vallee, B. L., Biochem., 7, 4343
      (1968).

[6]. Vallee, B. L. and Latt, S. A., Structure-Function
      Relationships of Proteolytic Enzymes (P. Desnuelle,
      H. Neurath, and M. Ottesen, eds.) Copenhagen: Munksgaard,
      1970, p. 144.

[7]. Vallee, B. L. and Riordan, J. R., Ann. Rev. Biochem.,
      38, 539 (1969).

B. L. VALLEE

[8].   Lindskog, S. and Nyman, P. O., Biochim. Biophys. Acta,
       85, 462 (1964).

[9].   Drum, D. E. and Vallee, B. L., Biochem. Biophys. Res.
       Comm., 41, 33 (1970).

[10]. Drum, D. E., Harrison, J. H., IV, Li, T.-K.,
       Bethune, J. L., and Vallee, B. L., Proc. Natl. Acad. Sci.
       U. S., 57, 1434 (1967).

Chapter 4

ROLE OF SELENIUM AS AN ESSENTIAL NUTRIENT

M. L. Scott

Department of Poultry Science and Graduate
School of Nutrition, Cornell University
Ithaca, New York

Over the thirteen years since Schwarz and Foltz first
discovered that selenium was the factor present in brewers
yeast and other materials which prevented dietary liver necrosis
in vitamin E dificient rats, numerous other studies have been
conducted which have shown that selenium is effective in
preventing some but not all of the vitamin E deficiency diseases
in laboratory and farm animals. Thus in addition to its effects
on liver necrosis in rats, selenium has been shown to prevent
exudative diathesis in vitamin E deficient chicks, myopathies
of the gizzard and heart in vitamin E deficient turkeys; to
improve reproduction in vitamin E deficient cattle and sheep;
to prevent hepatosis dietetica in vitamin E deficient pigs;

51

and to prevent white muscle disease in vitamin E deficient lambs
and calves. Until very recently, however, every deficiency
disease that responded to treatment with selenium also has been
preventable by supplementing the diet with vitamin E. It is the
purpose of this paper to describe experiments with chicks which
demonstrate that selenium is an essential nutrient for chickens,
even when they receive a complete diet including levels of
dietary vitamin E far in excess of the amounts usually found in
normal diets.

I. VITAMIN E

The chicken has been an especially useful experimental
animal for research on the mode of action of vitamin E and for
studying the factors interrelated with vitamin E in nutrition
and metabolism.

Three different vitamin E deficiency diseases are known to
occur in chickens. These are (1) vitamin E-antioxidant
interrelated diseases; (2) vitamin E-sulfur amino acid
interrelated diseases; and (3) vitamin E-selenium interrelated
diseases. In some of these, particularly the diseases which
are prevented by either vitamin E or by effective synthetic
antioxidants, vitamin E is also interrelated both nutritionally
and metabolically with linoleic acid and other polyunsaturated
fatty acids.

A. Vitamin E-Antioxidant Related Diseases

Encephalomalacia. In chickens receiving vitamin E deficient
diets containing linoleic acid, edema, small hemorrhages, and
degeneration of the Purkinje cells of the cerebellum occur at
about four to five weeks of age. When the degeneration becomes
severe, the chick shows a characteristic ataxia which has been
termed "encephalomalacia."

This disease can be prevented by supplementing the diet
with either vitamin E or certain synthetic fat-soluble
antioxidants. In the absence of synthetic antioxidants the
amount of vitamin E required to prevent encephalomalacia
depends on the level of polyunsaturated fatty acids, particularly
linoleic and arachidonic acids, in the diet. As the amount of
an effective fat-soluble synthetic antioxidant is increased in
the diet, the amount of vitamin E needed is decreased. Selenium
has no effect per se upon encephalomalacia.

B. Vitamin E-Cystine Interrelated Diseases

Nutritional Muscular Dystrophy in the Chicken. When chicks
are fed a vitamin E deficient diet containing adequate levels
of all other known nutrients except for a partial deficiency
of cystine, symptoms of nutritional muscular dystrophy occur
at about three weeks of age. Studies of this disease have been
conducted at Cornell University using vitamin E depleted chicks
and adding sufficient antioxidant (ethoxyquin, 0.0125%) to
prevent encephalomalacia, and sufficient selenium (0.1 ppm) to
prevent exudative diathesis.

Early in these studies it was found that if methionine or
cystine is added to the vitamin E deficient diet, muscular
dystrophy is prevented as long as the added sulfur amino acid
is present in the diet. Removal of the sulfur amino acid when
the chicks are three weeks of age produces a sudden onset of
muscular dystrophy within 48 hours. This procedure has been
used in several different investigations to determine the time-
sequence occurrence of events as muscular dystrophy begins to
appear and progressively increases in severity. Although the
disease is completely prevented by vitamin E, selenium alone
has no effect on nutritional muscular dystrophy.

C. Vitamin E-Selenium Interrelated Diseases in Chickens

Exudative Diathesis. A severe edema in chicks apparently
resulting from increased permeability of the capillaries,
combined with a reduced level of blood proteins, particularly
plasma albumin, has been termed "exudative diathesis." This
disease occurs only in chicks receiving diets severely
deficient in both selenium and vitamin E. Supplementation
of the basal diet with either vitamin E or selenium will
completely prevent exudative diathesis.

II. SELENIUM AS AN ESSENTIAL NUTRIENT

In the above studies and in all previous research with
selenium in the nutrition of laboratory and farm animals, the
nutritional effects of this element have always been related,
in one way or another, with vitamin E nutrition. Efforts
were undertaken, therefore, to obtain evidence as to whether
or not selenium is required in diets containing adequate
levels of all known nutrients. These experiments were conducted
with selenium-depleted chicks fed a crystalline amino acid diet
adequate in all known nutrients including high levels of
vitamin E, but severely deficient in selenium. The results
showed that a specific selenium deficiency causes poor growth,
poor feathering, and fibrotic degeneration of the pancreas.
Death usually occurs following markedly decreased absorption of
lipids including vitamin E. The pancreatic degeneration
results in a decrease in pancreatic and intestinal lipase
which causes a failure in fat digestion. Under these conditions
bile flow is almost eliminated. With the absence of bile and
of monoglycerides in the intestinal lumen, there is a failure
of micelle formation which in turn impairs the absorption of
vitamin E. Addition of bile salts to the diet did not return
fat digestion to normal levels, and only temporarily enhanced

vitamin E absorption. Addition to the basal diet of free fatty acids, monoglycerides and bile salts, improved the absorption of vitamin E and survival during the experimental period of four weeks but did not prevent the degenerative changes in the pancreas. The selenium requirement for prevention of pancreatic degeneration was found to depend on the vitamin E level in the diet. With very high dietary vitamin E levels (100 IU/kg or more) as little as 0.01 mg selenium as sodium selenite per kilogram of diet completely prevented pancreatic degeneration. However, when the vitamin E content of the diet was at more nearly normal levels (10 to 15 IU/kg), 0.02 to 0.04 mg selenium was required per kilogram of diet.

It was observed in these experiments that exudative diathesis did not occur as long as some vitamin E was being absorbed. Exudative diathesis occurred only after the absorption of vitamin E was decreased to very low levels by the pancreatic degeneration. With the use of fatty acids, monoolein and bile salts which resulted in a marked improvement in vitamin E absorption, exudative diathesis did not occur even though the pancreas under these dietary conditions continued to undergo severe atrophy and degeneration.

As a result of these studies, the following scheme is proposed to depict the interrelationship between vitamin E and selenium in the prevention of both exudative diathesis and pancreatic degeneration.

(1) When the diet contains adequate selenium, the integrity of the pancreas is preserved.

(2) With the normal production of pancreatic lipase, fat is digested, there is normal bile flow, and normal formation of bile salt-lipid micelles.

(3) Micelle formation then allows maximum absorption and good blood levels of vitamin E.

(4) Either the vitamin E or the selenium in the diet will prevent exudative diathesis, but a good blood level of vitamin E also helps to preserve the selenium in the blood and tissues, thereby reducing the dietary level of selenium required to protect the pancreas.

(5) Thus vitamin E spares the selenium requirement and, conversely, selenium enhances absorption of α-tocopherol, thereby reducing the dietary requirement for vitamin E.

Chapter 5

FACTORS THAT MODIFY THE TOXICITY OF SELENIUM

O. A. Levander

Human Nutrition Research Division
U. S. Department of Agriculture
Agricultural Research Service
Beltsville, Maryland

Selenium has long been regarded as a toxic material and indeed the substance is more toxic than arsenic[1]. In fact, Allaway has suggested that selenium may be the most toxic element in the environment on a molar basis[2]. Possible sources of exposure to excess amounts of selenium include industrial accidents, plants and animals raised on seleniferous soils, and atmospheric and water pollution. The poisonous nature of selenium requires that industrial, agricultural, and public health authorities familiarize themselves with the various aspects of the selenium problem in order to perform intelligently

in their areas of responsibility. The toxicology of selenium
has been the subject of numerous reviews[3,4,5,6].

Selenium as an industrial hazard has been recently discussed
by Glover[7]. The element is employed in the manufacture of
electrical rectifiers, in the decolorization of poor quality
green glass, in the compounding of paint pigments, and in
xerography. In spite of all these uses, relatively few workers
seem to have been affected by selenium poisoning. Glover feels
that this is because workers regard selenium with great respect,
since any small amounts accumulated under the fingernails lead
to painful nail beds. Also there are undesirable social consequences to the careless handling of selenium because of the
metallic taste and garlicky breath that can develop as a result
of selenium exposure. Glover found no evidence of excessive
mortality among selenium workers from any of the main causes of
death.

High levels of selenium in soils represent a serious
problem in agriculture since certain plants grown on such soils
can accumulate large quantities of selenium (up to thousands of
parts per million) and livestock ingesting these forages develop
a condition known as "alkali disease" or "blind staggers" which
represent two different forms of chronic selenium poisoning[3].
This hazard has been successfully controlled in the United States
by careful mapping of those areas of the Great Plains States
that are capable of producing toxic vegetation and removing such
land from agricultural use. Dangers due to seleniferous soils,
however, still remain in other countries where detailed knowledge of soil composition does not exist. A recent paper from
Venezuela, for example, reported that over half of the different
plant samples taken from various agricultural regions of the
country contained more than 3 ppm of selenium and that one fourth
of the samples contained 10 ppm of selenium[8]. Samples of

defatted seed of Lecythis ollaria (Monkey Coconut) assayed
5100 and 8100 ppm of selenium. Two naturally occurring
outbreaks of selenosis in Queensland, Australia, were described
by Knott and McCray in 1959[9]. The horses affected developed
lameness and hoof abnormalities, a condition described locally
as "change hoof disease". The similarity of these symptoms to
the well-known hoof deformities seen in alkali disease is
obvious. Brown and DeWet found a definite correlation between
the selenium content of the vegetation and the occurrence of
geeldikkop in the Karoo area of South Africa[10]. In their
extensive monograph Rosenfeld and Beath pointed out the public
health ramifications of the selenium problem by listing several
examples of human poisonings in seleniferous regions as a result
of eating locally produced foodstuffs[3]. Losses of hair and
fingernails were common symptoms of the selenosis. Water seldom
contained enough selenium to cause toxicity. Hadjimarkos has
proposed that there may be an increase in dental caries in
populations suffering from chronic selenium exposure[11], but
this claim has been questioned by others[12]. On the other
hand McLundie, Shepherd, and Mobbs did find that selenite could
increase enamel solubility in an artificial mouth[13]. Clearly
consumption of foods and feedstuffs containing high levels of
selenium presents a world-wide problem to humans and animals
alike.

During the past several months considerable concern has
been generated in the United States as a result of growing
awareness of pollution of our waterways with various heavy
metals. Mercury losses from chloralkali plants have rendered
fish in Lake Erie and Lake St. Clair unfit for consumption[14].
Arsenic found in river waters was thought to have originated
from household detergents[15]. The cause of a disease of much
suffering in Japan (itai, itai) was traced to cadmium in

irrigation waters contaminated by waste effluent from a zinc mine[16]. Although no cases of selenium pollution of waters in the United States are known at present, the occurrence of such an incident involving a silver mine in Mexico[17] demonstrates that the possibility exists. Selenium as a possible atmospheric pollutant was discussed by Hashimoto and Winchester who found that the selenium-to-sulfur weight ratio in air was a thousandfold greater than that of sea water[18] and concluded that terrestrial sources including pollution contributed to atmospheric selenium. In a later communication fuel oils were implicated as the likely source of atmospheric pollution by selenium[19].

After reading the above discussion concerning the harmful effects of selenium, it might seem unlikely that anyone would desire to add selenium intentionally to the food supply. And yet beneficial effects of trace levels of selenium have been known since 1957 when Schwarz and Foltz showed that selenium could prevent the liver necrosis of vitamin E deficient rats[20]. Moreover last year nutritional responses to selenium in the presence of adequate amounts of vitamin E were obtained in chickens[21] and rats[22]. These findings have provided considerable support for the supplementation of animal feeds in selenium-low areas to prevent naturally occurring selenium deficiency diseases in farm animals such as the sheep and cattle myopathies seen in Oregon and Washington[23], the hepatic necrosis reported in swine in Michigan[24], or the gizzard myopathies of young turkeys observed in southwestern Ohio[25]. However, the addition of selenium to feeds has not been allowed because of its reputation as a toxic material and because of its alleged carcinogenicity[26,27]. Although the carcinogenicity of selenium would seem to be refuted by the extensive work of Harr and associates[28] (in addition, an anticarcinogenic effect of selenium has been recently suggested[29]), the problem of residues of selenium in foods remains. The level of dietary selenium generally considered toxic for animals is 4 ppm[2] but Witting and Horwitt found definite toxic effects of 1.25 ppm selenium in the diet of vitamin E deficient rats[30]. Analyses of several food materials purchased locally in Maryland showed that grains, cereal products, meats, and seafoods contain 0.1 to 0.7 ppm selenium and that samples of pig, sheep, and beef kidney contain 1.4 to 1.9 ppm selenium[31]. These observations coupled with the knowledge that animals fed excess levels of selenium in the diet can accumulate 2 to 9 ppm selenium in their livers and 10 to 30 ppm selenium in their kidneys, indicate that any addition of selenium to the food chain will have to be done with caution. Allaway has presented a balanced account of the problems involved[2].

Once the issue of selenium residues in foods is settled, poultry and livestock producers will want to take a careful look at the levels of selenium they add to their animal feeds, since the optimal range of growth stimulation as a result of selenium supplementation may be quite narrow. Witting and Horwitt in their vitamin E deficient rat studies found that addition of 0.1 ppm selenium to a casein diet already containing 0.25 ppm selenium gave maximal growth stimulation but that the addition of 0.3 ppm selenium was less effective in promoting growth[30].

Since poisoning by selenium represents a potential hazard in so many diverse situations, there is a need to understand better the mechanism of action of the various factors that modify the toxicity of selenium. Research in three general areas offering promise as systems for study has been carried out in our laboratory: the antagonism of arsenic against selenium poisoning, the protective effect of linseed oil meal

in selenium toxicity, and the beneficial interaction of vitamin E
and methionine in chronic selenosis. The following review
presents a summary of this work.

I. THE ARSENIC-SELENIUM ANTAGONISM

One of the peculiarities of selenium is the fact that its
toxic effects can be decreased by yet another poisonous material,
namely, arsenic. Moxon first noted this beneficial effect of
arsenic on selenium poisoning when he found that 5 ppm of sodium
arsenite in the drinking water gave full protection against
liver damage in rats fed diets containing 15 ppm of selenium
as seleniferous wheat or as sodium selenite[32]. Later work
from his group showed this to be a unique property of arsenic
since a wide survey of other elements indicated little or no
beneficial effects against selenium poisoning[33]. However,
there appeared to be little limitation on the chemical forms of
arsenic that were active since several arsenic compounds,
including some organic arsenicals, provided protection[34,35].

Attempts to explain this antagonism of arsenic against
selenium on the metabolic level were confused by the fact that
arsenic actually inhibited the expiration of volatile methylated
selenium compounds, the major selenium detoxification pathway
in animals challenged with subacute doses of the element[36].
An important clue to the mechanism of action of arsenic in
alleviating selenium toxicity was provided by the report of
Moxon and DuBois that the livers of rats receiving a seleniferous
wheat diet and sodium arsenite in the drinking water contained
less selenium than the livers of animals fed selenium alone[33].
This was true in spite of the fact that the animals receiving
selenium plus arsenic consumed more of the seleniferous diet
than the animals receiving only selenium. In subacute dosage
experiments Ganther and Baumann showed that arsenic decreased

the retention of selenium in the liver while simultaneously
decreasing the elimination of selenium via the volatilization
pathway and increasing the excretion of selenium into the
gut[37]. Levander and Baumann[38] pursued this phenomenon
further and found that if a range of arsenic dosages was
administered to rats receiving a constant dose of selenium,
there was a negative correlation between the amounts of selenium
retained in the liver and the amounts of selenium excreted into
the gastrointestinal tract (Table I). This suggested that the
biliary pathway might be important in explaining the
arsenic-selenium antagonism[39].

In rats prepared with biliary fistulas the excretion of
selenium could be enhanced tenfold over a 3 hour period by

TABLE I

Effect of Various Dosages of Arsenite
on the Metabolism of Selenite by Rats[a]

| Dosage of Arsenite | Percent of Dose of Se-75[b] | |
mg As/kg	Liver	Gastrointestinal Contents
0.0	24.9 ± 2.5	8.7 ± 0.3
1.0	17.8 ± 2.0	11.2 ± 1.4
2.0	13.9 ± 1.4	25.4 ± 6.2
3.0	8.0 ± 0.9	36.6 ± 3.1
5.0	8.6 ± 1.0	36.7 ± 4.7

[a] Levander and Baumann[38].

[b] Distribution of radioactivity 10 hours after subcutaneous
injection of 2 mg Se/kg as Na_2SeO_3 containing about 1 μCi
^{75}Se as $H_2^{75}SeO_3$; injection of saline or stated dose of
$NaAsO_2$ preceded the selenite injection by 10 minutes.

TABLE II

Effect of Arsenite on the Biliary Excretion of Selenite[a]

| | Percent of Dose of Se-75[b] | |
	Saline only	Arsenite
Bile	4.0 ± 0.4	40.8 ± 7.2
Liver	51.3 ± 3.0	20.9 ± 3.0
Gastrointestinal contents	1.7 ± 0.3	1.5 ± 0.3
Bile volume, ml	3.0 ± 0.2	3.8 ± 0.5

[a] Levander and Baumann[39].

[b] Distribution of radioactivity 3 hours after subcutaneous injection of 0.5 mg Se/kg as $Na_2{}^{75}SeO_3$ containing about 0.5 μCi ^{75}Se as $H_2{}^{75}SeO_3$; injection of saline or 1 mg As/kg as $NaAsO_2$ followed the selenite injection by 10 minutes.

the injection of sodium arsenite soon after the selenium (Table II). Although this effect of arsenic on excretion of selenium into the bile was most marked at subacute dosage levels, a clear difference between rats receiving only selenium or selenium plus arsenic was seen at doses as low as 7 μg of selenium per rat, a dosage far removed from the known toxic levels of selenium (Table III). Various forms of arsenic were effective in stimulating the biliary excretion of selenium including some organic arsenicals used in the poultry industry as growth-promoting agents, although the inorganic arsenite was by far the most potent substance in this regard (Table IV). Attempts to increase the biliary excretion of selenium by administering other elements known to interact with sulfhydryl

TABLE III

Effect of Dosage of Selenium and Arsenic

on the Biliary Excretion of Selenium[a]

Dosage mg/kg		Percent of Dose of Se-75[b]	
Arsenite	Selenite	Bile	Liver
0	0.02	0.77 ± 0.17	36.7 ± 3.7
0.04	0.02	3.47 ± 0.89	35.9 ± 1.7
0	1.0	0.88 ± 0.08	43.9 ± 2.8
2.0	1.0	24.0 ± 4.7	11.6 ± 1.7

[a] Levander and Baumann[39].

[b] Distribution of radioactivity 1 hour after subcutaneous
injection of stated dose of selenite containing about
0.5 μCi ^{75}Se as $H_2{}^{75}SeO_3$; injection of saline or stated dose
of arsenite followed the selenite injection by 10 minutes.

groups were unsuccessful[40]. Arsenic was able to increase the
biliary excretion of selenium whether the selenium was supplied
as selenite or selenate but there was no effect of arsenic on
the biliary excretion of sulfur administered as sulfate
(Table V). Agents known to stimulate bile production such as
sodium dehydrocholate had no effect on selenium excretion into
the bile of rats injected with selenium alone (Table VI).
The amount of selenium appearing in the bile of the
arsenic-treated rats also given the choleretic agent was actually
decreased in spite of the increased volume of bile produced
(Table VII). Experiments with radioarsenic showed that selenium
increased the biliary excretion of arsenic just as arsenic
increased the biliary excretion of selenium (Table VIII). This

TABLE IV

Effect of Various Forms of Arsenic on

the Biliary Excretion of Selenium[a]

Form of Arsenic	Dosage mg As/kg	Percent of Dose of Se-75[b] Bile	Liver
None	0	0.86 ± 0.02	44.2 ± 2.0
Na 3-NO$_2$-4-OH phenylarsonate	1	2.65 ± 0.10	45.6 ± 3.5
Na 3-NO$_2$-4-OH phenylarsonate	10	5.77 ± 0.76	44.0 ± 1.6
Na arsenate	1	2.39 ± 0.53	42.0 ± 2.3
Na arsenate	5	14.9 ± 2.9	20.1 ± 1.5
Na arsenite	1	20.9 ± 2.1	15.6 ± 0.7

[a] Levander[41].

[b] Timing of injections and collections as in Table III.

suggested that arsenic might be forming a detoxification
conjugate with selenium which was preferentially eliminated
via the biliary route.

Experiments designed to determine the chemical form of
selenium in the bile of rats treated with arsenic showed that
most of the biliary selenium could be precipitated by trichloroacetic acid, whereas relatively little could be extracted into
chloroform or ether[41]. Dialysis studies revealed that only
10 to 15% of the biliary selenium was dialyzable against distilled
water. The amount of dialyzable biliary selenium could be
increased by raising the ionic strength (only 15% dialyzable
against distilled water versus 29% against 0.1 M NaCl) or the pH
(27% dialyzed against 0.1 M phosphate buffer, pH = 6.7 versus

TABLE V

Effect of Arsenite on the Biliary Excretion of Selenium Supplied either as Selenite or Selenate or Sulfur Supplied as Sulfate[a]

Forms of Selenium or Sulfur	Percent of Dose of Se-75 or S-35[b]	
	Bile	Liver
Experiment A		
Na_2SeO_3,- As	1.21 ± 0.08	42.8 ± 3.6
Na_2SeO_3,+ As	22.1 ± 2.1	15.5 ± 0.3
Na_2SeO_4,- As	1.09 ± 0.14	31.2 ± 1.7
Na_2SeO_4,+ As	12.8 ± 1.0	15.3 ± 0.9
Experiment B		
Na_2SO_4, - As	0.96 ± 0.13	----------
Na_2SO_4, + As	1.18 ± 0.29	----------

[a] Levander[41].

[b] Distribution of radioactivity 1 hour after subcutaneous injection of either 0.5 mg Se/kg containing about 0.5 μCi ^{75}Se as $H_2^{75}SeO_3$ or $H_2^{75}SeO_4$ or 0.5 mg S/kg as Na_2SO_4 containing about 1 μCi ^{35}S as $H_2^{35}SO_4$; injection of saline or 1 mg As/kg as $NaAsO_2$ followed the selenium or sulfur injection by 10 minutes.

68% against 0.1 M phosphate buffer, pH = 12.4) of the dialysis medium. Additional increments of biliary selenium could be rendered dialyzable by the incorporation of certain sulfhydryl compounds into the dialysis medium at a concentration of 10^{-3} M: control (0.1 M NaCl, pH = 7), 36.5 ± 5.8% of the selenium in bile dialyzed; control plus 2,3-dimercaptopropanol, 55.2 ± 7.3%; and control plus reduced glutathione, 72.8 ± 3.1%. These

TABLE VI

Effect of Sodium Dehydrocholate(NaDHC)

on the Biliary Excretion of Selenium[a]

| | Percent of Dose of Se-75[b] | |
	- NaDHC	+ NaDHC
Bile	1.27 ± 0.20	1.40 ± 0.25
Liver	48.2 ± 1.8	45.9 ± 2.8
Bile volume, ml	1.11 ± 0.15	2.25 ± 0.31

[a] Levander and Baumann[39].

[b] Distribution of radioactivity 1 hour after subcutaneous injection of 0.5 mg Se/kg as $Na_2{}^{75}SeO_3$ containing about 1 µCi ^{75}Se as $H_2{}^{75}SeO_3$; animals received 250 mg of NaDHC intraduodenally or saline just before the selenium injection.

TABLE VII

Effect of Sodium Dehydrocholate (NaDHC) on the Biliary

Excretion of Selenium in Rats Treated with Arsenic[a]

| | Percent of Dose of Se-75[b] | |
	- NaDHC	+ NaDHC
Bile	24.7 ± 0.9	3.4 ± 2.0
Liver	14.4 ± 0.7	35.7 ± 2.3
Bile volume, ml	1.16 ± 0.04	2.25 ± 0.06

[a] Levander and Baumann[39].

[b] Conditions as in Table VI except animals received 1 mg As/kg as $NaAsO_2$ 10 minutes after the selenite.

TABLE VIII

Effect of Selenite on the Biliary Excretion of Arsenic[a]

| | Percent of Dose of As-76[b] | |
	Saline only	Selenite
Bile	9.2 ± 1.2	18.3 ± 1.7
Liver	19.0 ± 1.5	11.0 ± 0.6
Gastrointestinal contents	1.6 ± 0.2	1.7 ± 0.2
Bile volume, ml	1.17 ± 0.07	1.22 ± 0.14

[a] Levander and Baumann[39].

[b] Distribution of radioactivity 50 minutes after subcutaneous injection of 1.0 mg As/kg as $NaAsO_2$ containing about 0.5 µCi ^{76}As as $H^{76}AsO_2$; injection of saline or 0.5 mg Se/kg preceded the arsenite injection by 10 minutes.

differences in behavior toward dialysis under various conditions suggested that the selenium in bile from arsenic-treated rats may exist in several forms, some of which may be associated with protein, although their exact nature is unknown.

At present the arsenic-selenium antagonism can only be understood in physiological terms since the precise chemical mechanism by which arsenic acts remains to be elucidated. It is possible that arsenic may increase the permeability of the liver so that selenium, which is normally held within the organ, is allowed to escape into the bile. If increased hepatic permeability were the only factor operating in the present case, however, it is difficult to comprehend why the biliary excretion of the two closely related anions selenate and sulfate was not similarly affected. Another possible explanation of

the arsenic effect is that arsenic blocks a crucial step in the
biosynthetic pathway leading to the formation of volatile
selenium compounds thus diverting selenium excretion from the
lungs to the bile. Yet the effect of arsenic is seen at low
selenium dosage levels at which the formation of volatile
selenium compounds is negligible[36], and therefore inhibition
of the volatilization pathway is not necessary for the arsenic
effect to manifest itself. Still another possible mechanism
for this effect of arsenic in selenium metabolism is the
formation of a selenoarsenic detoxification conjugate. Many
conjugated compounds are known to be excreted largely in the
bile[42] and this mechanism would account for the increased
excretion of arsenic in the selenium-treated animals as well
as the increased excretion of selenium in the arsenic-treated
rats. But there is the complicating factor of the dialysis
experiments that suggest the presence of several different forms
of selenium in the bile and thus preclude the existence of a
specific selenoarsenic detoxification complex. Clearly more
work is needed before an understanding of this fascinating
mineral antagonism can be enjoyed at the molecular level.

II. LINSEED OIL MEAL FACTOR

Workers in the field of selenium toxicity owe a great debt
to Moxon who not only discovered the arsenic-selenium antagonism
(vide supra) but who also noted for the first time the specific
ability of linseed oil meal to protect against the deleterious
effects of excess selenium intake[43]. Moxon's work was advanced
by the South Dakota group which reported that the protective
principle could be extracted from the linseed meal with hot
aqueous ethanol and concluded that some fraction of the meal
other than protein was responsible for the protective effect[44].
Levander, Young, and Meeks[45] confirmed the superiority of
linseed oil meal as opposed to casein in preventing symptoms of

chronic selenosis and also the fact[46] that rats fed seleniferous
diets containing linseed oil meal actually have considerably
higher selenium residues in the liver even though liver damage
due to selenium is much less in the linseed oil meal-fed rats
(Table IX). The latter observation suggested that the total
amount of hepatic selenium was not necessarily a valid indicator
of the status of an animal with respect to selenium toxicosis.
Therefore, a series of binding studies was carried out in the
hope that the chemical properties of the selenium in tissues
might be more useful in determining the reaction of an animal
to toxic exposure to selenium. In these experiments rats were
fed diets containing 36% casein or diets containing 18% casein
in combination with 43% linseed oil meal. Liver homogenates
prepared from these rats injected 4 hours previously with
$Na_2^{75}SeO_3$ were dialyzed against various media. A number of
chelators and sulfhydryl compounds had similar effects on the
binding of selenium by liver homogenates irregardless of whether
the casein or the casein-linseed oil meal diets were fed and
thus provided no clues as to how linseed oil meal-supplemented
rats could contain so much selenium in their livers and still
suffer so little hepatic damage (Table X). Addition of EDTA
to the dialysis medium, however, revealed a differential
response between the two homogenates in that less selenium was
lost to the EDTA medium from the homogenates of linseed oil
meal-supplemented rats as compared to homogenates of rats fed
casein as the only protein source. This difference in selenium
binding suggested that linseed oil meal or some of its metabolites might complex with the selenium and thus prevent it from
poisoning sulfhydryl or other groups in the cell susceptible
to selenium. In this way animals fed linseed oil meal could
tolerate the higher levels of selenium found in their internal
organs.

TABLE IX

Protective Effect of Linseed Oil Meal versus

Casein in Chronic Selenosis[a,b]

Protein Source		Weight Gain	Survival	Liver Damage	Selenium Content	
Casein	Linseed Oil Meal				Liver	Kidney
Percent of diet		Percent of control			$\mu g/g$ wet weight	
18	0	4.7	2/6	3.0	---------	--------
0	43	83.3	6/6	1.7	6.7 ± 0.4	17.5 ± 2.6
36	0	38.1	5/6	1.2	2.7 ± 0.3	3.8 ± 0.3
18	43	92.3	5/6	0.4	4.5 ± 0.3	8.6 ± 1.0

a/ Levander, Young, and Meeks[45].

b/ Rats fed diet containing 10 ppm selenium added as Na_2SeO_3 for 7 weeks; liver damage score based on scale normal = 0 to severe damage = 3.

TABLE X

Dialysis of Se-75 from Liver Homogenates of Rats Fed
Casein or Casein-Linseed Oil Meal Diets[a]

Dialysis Medium[b]	Percent Se-75 Dialyzable	
	36% Casein Diet	18% Casein + 43% LOM Diet
Tris·Cl buffer	52.7 ± 3.0	50.3 ± 1.2
Tris + cystein	44.2 ± 2.8	40.8 ± 1.2
Tris + reduced glutathione	76.9 ± 0.6	77.9 ± 1.0
Tris + Na$_2$EDTA	66.3 ± 1.7	52.9 ± 1.3

[a] Levander, Young, and Meeks[45].

[b] Dialysis medium always contained 0.05 M tris·Cl buffer, pH 7.4; where indicated, various chelating agents and sulfhydryl compounds were added at the level of 5×10^{-4} M.

III. METHIONINE AND ANTIOXIDANTS

There seems to exist about an equal number of papers in the literature either confirming or denying a protective effect of methionine in selenium toxicity[30,47,48,49,50]. The reason for these conflicting reports can possibly be seen in the work of Sellers, You, and Lucas who found a similar variability in their own experiments until they realized that vitamin E was essential for demonstrating an effect of methionine[51]. A reinvestigation[52] of this problem demonstrated that vitamin E was indeed necessary to show methionine protection against selenium poisoning and moreover that the degree of protection seen with a fixed level of methionine supplementation was roughly correlated with the vitamin E content of the diet (Table XI). Vitamin E alone had no protective effect. The

TABLE XI

Effect of Methionine, Vitamin E, and Methionine/Vitamin E

Supplements on the Toxicity of the Seleniferous Peanut Meal Diet[a,b]

Supplements to Diet		Weight Gain	Survival	Liver Damage	Selenium Content	
DL-methionine	dl-α-tocopheryl Acetate				Liver	Kidneys
Percent	Percent	Grams			μg/gram	μg/gram
0	0	20.8 ± 10.2	8/8	2.1 ± 0.4	6.8 ± 0.4	29.5 ± 5.7
0.5	0	35.6 ± 2.3	8/8	1.8 ± 0.3	6.7 ± 0.9	19.3 ± 3.7
0	0.05	38.1 ± 4.9	8/8	1.8 ± 0.5	6.9 ± 1.0	32.7 ± 8.9
0.5	0.01	33.3 ± 3.6	8/8	1.4 ± 0.4	5.7 ± 0.4	16.3 ± 1.6*
0.5	0.025	32.1 ± 17.8	8/8	0.9 ± 0.2*	4.5 ± 0.1*	10.1 ± 3.4*
0.5	0.05	46.1 ± 2.5	7/8	0.9 ± 0.3*	5.4 ± 0.1*	13.3 ± 2.6*

a/ Levander and Morris[52].

b/ Rats fed peanut meal diet containing 10 ppm selenium added as Na_2SeO_4 for 8 weeks; starred values (*) indicate significant differences (P<.05) from unsupplemented diet; liver damage scored on basis that normal = 0 and severe damage = 3.

type of protection obtained by feeding methionine and vitamin E
was somewhat different from that seen with linseed oil meal
since although liver damage was significantly reduced there was
little increase in growth rate. Fat-soluble antioxidants such
as N,N'-diphenyl-p-phenylenediamine (DPPD), ethoxyquin, and
butylated hydroxytoluene (BHT) all gave significant protection
against liver damage due to selenium when fed in conjunction
with methionine but methylene blue or ascorbic acid were
ineffective (Table XII). Methionine as a protective principle
could not be replaced either by another sulfur amino acid,
cysteine, or by a methyl donor such as betaine or by a
combination of both, and the methyl-group acceptor guanidoacetic acid appeared to mask the beneficial effect of the
methionine (Table XIII).

Since the amounts of selenium retained in the livers and
kidneys were less in those dietary groups that were protected
against the toxic effects of the selenium, an increased
elimination of selenium seemed to offer a likely explanation
for the beneficial effects of methionine. Two pathways could
conceivably be operating in this case: either the expiration
of volatile selenium compounds via the lungs or the urinary
excretion of trimethyl selenide (or both).
S-adenosyl-L-methionine has been shown to be the methyl donor
involved in the biosynthesis of dimethyl selenide, the major
volatile selenium metabolite produced when animals are given
subacute doses of selenium[53], so that a role of methionine
in this process seems quite reasonable. On the other hand
excretion of selenium in the urine is a more important pathway
of elimination in chronic selenium toxicity, so that an
increased formation of trimethyl selenide, which was recently
found in the urine of rats chronically poisoned with
selenium [54,55], must also be considered.

TABLE XII

Effect of Methionine Supplements with and without Various
Antioxidants on the Toxicity of the Seleniferous Peanut Meal Diet[a]

Supplements to Diet		Weight Gain	Survival	Liver Damage	Selenium Content	
					Liver	Kidneys
DL-methionine Percent	Antioxidant Percent	Grams			µg/gram	µg/gram
0	0	43.0 ± 5.8	8/8	2.1 ± 0.2	7.4 ± 0.5	32.0 ± 3.0
0.5	0	42.0 ± 8.1	8/8	1.9 ± 0.2	6.1 ± 0.5	18.1 ± 1.6*
0.5	DPPD, 0.05	35.3 ± 7.7	7/8	0.4 ± 0.2*	5.4 ± 0.2*	14.0 ± 0.8*
0.5	Ethoxyquin, 0.05	25.2 ± 7.6	8/8	0.8 ± 0.2*	4.4 ± 0.3*	15.5 ± 2.5*
0.5	BHT, 0.05	36.6 ± 7.7	8/8	1.0 ± 0.4*	5.3 ± 0.7*	18.5 ± 2.1*
0.5	Methylene blue, 0.25	28.2 ± 7.7	8/8	1.5 ± 0.5	5.6 ± 1.1	26.2 ± 2.4
0.5	Ascorbic acid, 0.50	20.1 ± 5.3*	7/8	2.3 ± 0.4	9.0 ± 3.9	27.8 ± 8.8

a/ See footnotes, Table XI.

TABLE XIII

Effect of Cysteine and Betaine Supplements on the

Toxicity of the Seleniferous Peanut Meal Diet[a]

Supplements to Diet	Weight Gain	Survival	Liver Damage	Selenium Content	
				Liver	Kidneys
	Grams		$\mu g/gram$	$\mu g/gram$	$\mu g/gram$
None	29.2 ± 10.9	8/8	2.4 ± 0.3	8.8 ± 1.4	26.8 ± 10.3
Cysteine·HCl·H$_2$O, 0.59%; and dl-α-tocopheryl acetate, 0.05%	24.6 ± 6.0	8/8	1.8 ± 0.5	7.5 ± 1.1	22.4 ± 2.6
Cysteine·HCl·H$_2$O, 0.59% Betaine·HCl, 0.51% dl-α-tocopheryl acetate, 0.05%	40.9 ± 5.5	8/8	1.6 ± 0.4	6.0 ± 0.6	26.7 ± 4.4
Betaine·HCl, 0.51% and dl-α-tocopheryl acetate, 0.05%	42.1 ± 5.7	8/8	2.0 ± 0.3	5.4 ± 0.4	22.0 ± 3.0
DL-methionine, 0.5% Guanidoacetic acid, 0.39%; and dl-α-tocopheryl acetate, 0.05%	34.6 ± 9.5	8/8	2.5 ± 0.2	6.8 ± 0.7	17.1 ± 2.4

a/ See footnotes, Table XI.

The reason for the necessity of feeding vitamin E along
with methionine to obtain a protective response could perhaps
be explained if the utilization of methyl groups for either
dimethyl or trimethyl selenide biosynthesis were impaired in
animals not getting enough vitamin E. Hove and Hardin showed
that vitamin E deficient rat liver slices had a decreased
capacity to use the methyl groups of methionine for creatine
biosynthesis from guanidoacetic acid[56]. Also vitamin E
and selenium have recently been found to accelerate the
conversion of methionine to cystine[57], which would tend to
add methyl groups to the one-carbon pool. Therefore, it seems
possible that vitamin E may function in selenium toxicity to
increase the availability of methyl groups from methionine
for selenium detoxification either via the urinary or
volatilization pathway.

IV. CONCLUDING REMARKS

The work outlined in this review illustrates that the
toxicity of selenium can be decreased by several different
factors and that each factor appears to act by its own peculiar
mechanism: arsenic stimulates the biliary excretion of selenium,
linseed oil meal increases the binding of selenium by the tissues
in a less toxic form, and methionine in concert with vitamin E
acts by enhancing either the pulmonary or urinary elimination
of selenium. Because of these varied effects on the metabolism
of selenium, it is clear that merely the total selenium content
of the diet is inadequate to judge either the harmful effects
in a selenium toxicity or the beneficial effects in an otherwise
selenium-deficient diet. Rather, the entire dietary pattern
of an animal or human must be examined before valid conclusions
can be drawn.

Although the responses seen in these studies in reducing the toxic effects of selenium are quite striking, any agricultural or medical use of these materials to counteract selenium poisoning seems quite remote at this time. Arsenic being a highly toxic material does not lend itself readily to therapeutic use. In order for linseed oil meal to be effective against selenium poisoning rather high levels must be fed in the diet which excludes this possibility on economic grounds. Methionine with vitamin E is a good protective combination against selenium but again these substances as feed additives are quite expensive and their cost probably forbids routine use at the levels required.

Any implications of these results for selenium nutrition are uncertain, but theoretically it is possible that arsenic could have a detrimental effect by increasing the loss of selenium in the bile and thus increasing the nutritional requirement of the element. Whether linseed oil meal can have a sparing effect on selenium by increasing its retention in tissues in a nutritionally active form remains to be determined. Methionine and vitamin E both decrease an animal's need for selenium so that any loss of selenium due to these materials is undoubtedly offset by their sparing effects. However, nutritionists designing experiments to elucidate the metabolic role of selenium should be aware of these possible interactions of the element with other dietary materials.

REFERENCES

[1]. Franke, K. W. and Moxon, A. L., J. Pharm. Exp. Therap., 58, 454 (1936).

[2]. Allaway, W. H., Trace Substances in Environmental Health (II) (D. D. Hemphill, ed.) Columbia, Missouri: University of Missouri Press, 1969, p. 181-206.

[3]. Rosenfeld, I. and Beath, O. A., Selenium: Geobotany,
       Biochemistry, Toxicity, and Nutrition, New York:
       Academic Press, 1964.

[4]. Moxon, A. L. and Rhian, M., Physiol. Rev., 23, 305 (1943).

[5]. Maag, D. D. and Glenn, M. W., Selenium in Biomedicine
       (O. H. Muth, ed.) Westport, Connecticut: AVI Publishers,
       1967, p. 127-140.

[6]. Cooper, W. C., Selenium in Biomedicine (O. H. Muth, ed.)
       Westport, Connecticut: AVI Publishers, 1967, p. 185-
       199.

[7]. Glover, J. R., Ind. Med. Surg., 39, 50 (1970).

[8]. Jaffe, W. G., Chavez, J. F., and de Mondragon, M. C.,
       Arch. Latinoam. Nutr., 17, 59 (1967).

[9]. Knott, S. G. and McCray, C. W. R., Australian Vet. J.,
       35, 161 (1959).

[10]. Brown, J. M. M. and DeWet, P. J., Ondestepoort J. Vet.
       Res., 34, 161 (1967).

[11]. Hadjimarkos, D. M., Arch. Envir. Health, 10, 893 (1965).

[12]. Schwarz, K., Discussion following Chapter 14. Selenium
       in Biomedicine (O. H. Muth, ed.) Westport, Connecticut:
       AVI Publishers, 1967, p. 225-226.

[13]. McLundie, A. C., Shepherd, J. B., and Mobbs, D. R. A.,
       Arch. Oral Biol., 13, 1321 (1968).

[14]. Anonymous, Chem. Eng. News, 48, 36 (1970).

[15]. Angino, E. E., Magnuson, L. M., Waugh, T. C.,
       Galle, O. K., and Bredfeldt, J., Science, 168, 389
       (1970).

[16]. Anonymous, Chem. Eng. News, 48, 16 (1970).

[17]. Williams, K. T., Lakin, H. W., and Byers, H. G.,
       U. S. Dept. Agr. Tech. Bull. No. 702, 1940, p. 1.

[18]. Hashimoto, Y. and Winchester, J. W., Environ. Sci.
       Technol., 1, 338 (1967).

[19]. Hashimoto, Y., Hwang, J. Y., and Yanagisawa, S., Environ.
       Sci. Technol., 4, 157 (1970).

[20]. Schwarz, K. and Foltz, C. M., J. Am. Chem. Soc., 79,
       3293 (1957).

[21]. Thompson, J. N. and Scott, M. L., J. Nutr., 97, 335
       (1969).

[22]. McCoy, K. E. M. and Weswig, P. H., J. Nutr., 98, 383
       (1969).

[23]. Muth, O. H., J. Am. Vet. Med. Assn., 142, 272 (1963).

[24]. Michel, R. L., Whitehair, C. K., and Keahey, K. K.,
       J. Am. Vet. Med. Assn., 155, 50 (1969).

[25]. Bruins, H. W., Ousterhout, L. E., Scott, M. L.,
       Cary, E. E., and Allaway, W. H., Feedstuffs, 38, 66
       (1966).

[26]. Nelson, A. A., Fitzhugh, O. G., and Calvery, H. O.,
       Cancer Res., 3, 230 (1943).

[27]. Tscherkes, L. A., Aptekar, S. G., and Volgarev, M. N.,
       Byul. Eksperim. Biol. Med., 53, 78 (Russian) (1961).

[28]. Harr, J. R., Bone, J. F., Tinsley, I. J., Weswig, P. H.,
       and Yamamoto, R. S., Selenium in Biomedicine (O. H. Muth,
       ed.) Westport, Connecticut: AVI Publishers, 1967,
       p. 153-178.

[29]. Shamberger, R. J., J. Nat. Cancer Inst., 44, 931 (1970).

[30]. Witting, L. A. and Horwitt, M. K., J. Nutr., 84, 351
       (1964).

[31]. Morris, V. C. and Levander, O. A., J. Nutr., 100. 1383
       (1970).

[32]. Moxon, A. L., Science, 88, 81 (1938).

[33]. Moxon, A. L. and DuBois, K. P., J. Nutr., 18, 447 (1939).

[34]. DuBois, K. P., Moxon, A. L., and Olson, O. E., J. Nutr.,
       19, 477, (1940).

[35]. Hendrick, C. M., Klug, H. L., and Olson, O. E., J. Nutr.,
       51, 131 (1953).

[36]. Olson, O. E., Schulte, B. M., Whitehead, E. I., and
       Halverson A. W., J. Agr. Food Chem., 11, 531 (1963).

[37]. Ganther, H. E. and Baumann, C. A., J. Nutr., 77, 210
       (1962).

[38]. Levander, O. A. and Baumann, C. A., Toxicol. Appl.
       Pharmacol., 9, 98 (1966).

[39]. Levander, O. A. and Baumann, C. A., Toxicol. Appl.
       Pharmacol., 9, 106 (1966).

[40]. Levander, O. A. and Argrett, L. C., Toxicol. Appl.
       Pharmacol., 14, 308 (1969)

[41]. Levander, O. A., Madison, Wisconsin: University of
       Wisconsin, 1965, (Ph. D. Thesis).

[42]. Sperber, I., Pharmacol. Revs., 11, 109 (1959).

[43]. Moxon, A. L., Madison, Wisconsin: University of
       Wisconsin, 1941, (Ph. D. Thesis).

[44]. Halverson, A. W., Hendrick, C. M., and Olson, O. E.
       J. Nutr., 56, 51 (1955).

[45]. Levander, O. A., Young, M. L., and Meeks, S. A., Toxicol.
       Appl. Pharmacol., 16, 79 (1970).

[46]. Olson, O. E. and Halverson, A. W., Proc. S. Dakota Acad.
       Sci., 33, 90 (1954).

[47]. Lewis, H. B., Schultz, J., and Gortner, R. A., Jr.,
       J. Pharmacol. Exp. Therap., 68, 292 (1940).

[48]. Olson, O. E., Carlson, C. W., and Leitis, E., Tech.
       Bull. No. 20, College Station, Brookings, South Dakota:
       South Dakota Agr. Exp. Sta., 1958.

[49]. Smith, M. I. and Stohlman, E. F., J. Pharmacol. Exp.
       Therap., 70, 270 (1940).

[50]. Klug, H. L., Harshfield, R. D., Pengra, R. M., and
       Moxon, A. L., J. Nutr., 48, 409 (1952).

[51]. Sellers, E. A., You, R. W., and Lucas, C. C., Proc. Soc. Exp. Biol. Med., 75, 118 (1950).

[52]. Levander, O. A. and Morris, V. C., J. Nutr., 100, 1111 (1970).

[53]. Ganther, H. E., Biochem., 5, 1089 (1966).

[54]. Byard, J. L., Arch. Biochem. Biophys., 130, 556 (1969).

[55]. Palmer, I. S., Fischer, D. D., Halverson, A. W., and Olson, O. E., Biochim. Biophys. Acta, 177, 336 (1969).

[56]. Hove, E. L. and Hardin, J. O., J. Pharmacol. Exp. Therap., 106, 88 (1952).

[57]. Sukharevskaya, A. M. and Shtutman, Ts. M., Vop. Pitan., 27, 13 (Chem. Abstr., 70, 18039) (1968).

Chapter 6

THE DETOXIFYING EFFECTS OF SELENIUM

INTERRELATIONS BETWEEN COMPOUNDS OF SELENIUM AND CERTAIN METALS

J. Parízek, I. Oštádalová, J. Kalouskova

A. Babický, and J. Beneš

Institute of Physiology
Czechoslovak Academy of Sciences
Prague, Czechoslovakia
and
Radioisotope Laboratories of the Institutes for
Biological Research
Czechoslovak Academy of Sciences
Prague, Czechoslovakia

I. INTRODUCTION

We would like to report on some results of experiments
concerning the interrelation between compounds of selenium and
certain metals in the organism. First, we would like to
present the evidence that certain selenium compounds are highly

efficient in protecting the organism against the toxic effects
of compounds of certain metals. There is growing evidence that
certain man-made changes in the environment are connected with
a change in exposure of large population groups to such metals
as cadmium or mercury, and that traces of these metals could
play an important role in the pathogenesis of certain diseases[1].
The protective effect of selenium could open up some new
possibilities in the prevention and/or therapy of the toxic
effects of these metals[2]. In addition, it might also be
possible that the interrelation between traces of certain metals
and selenium could help in understanding the biological role of
selenium as an essential nutrient. One of the biological functions of selenium, for example, could be the protection of the
organism against the toxicity of trace amounts of metals that
even under "normal" conditions enter the body from the environment and remain[2,3].

We would also like to call attention to another aspect
of the interrelation between the studied metals and selenium.
It seems that the exposure to traces of compounds of such
metals as mercury can decrease the biological availability of
selenium in spite of its increased retention in the organism.
Results of research suggest that this could be of particular
importance during pregnancy and lactation[2,4,5]. The aim of
further research, of course, has been to see if a long-term
exposure to traces of such metals as, for example, mercury
could evoke the symptoms of selenium deficiency and if traces
of these metals in the environment and in the organism could
play some role in the pathogenesis of those livestock diseases
known to be prevented and efficiently cured by selenium
administration[6,7].

Finally, we would like to show that in contrast to
selenite or selenomethionine the concomitant presence of traces

of mercury and certain selenium metabolites in the organism
can be very dangerous, producing a highly lethal syndrome in
experimental animals[3,8]. These results might be, perhaps, of
interest from some aspects of pathology, but in our opinion
they primarily limit the use of selenium compounds in the
prevention and/or therapy of mercury intoxication and should
be considered in general as a warning against incautious use of
selenium in the biomedical field. In addition to this, the
latter point represents yet further proof that different
compounds of the same trace element that are known to be present
in the organism can have practically opposite biological effects.
In relation to analytical problems this seems to underline the
necessity of determining not only the amount of selenium present
in biological material but also to distinguish between different
forms in which it can be present there.

Most of our work was done using compounds of metals from
the IIb group, particularly mercury. However, it can be
expected that traces of certain other metals could share some
of these effects with mercury, and from this aspect the reports
by Holló and Zlatarov[9], Rusiecki and Brzezinski[10], and
Levander and Argrett[11] concerning the interrelation between
selenium and thallium are of particular importance.

II. SELENIUM AND CADMIUM

Our first experiments in which selenium compounds were used
were directly instigated by the paper of Mason, Young, and
Brown[12], which in continuation of the work by Kar, Das, and
Mukerji[13] reported that small amounts of selenite protect
male gonads against the hemorrhagic necrosis known to be
produced by cadmium[14].

Since the first report[15] published 15 years ago in which
we were able to describe the peculiar effects of small amounts

of cadmium in the male gonad, we were able to learn that
parenteral administration of small amounts of cadmium salts
results not only in hemorrhages and necroses of the testis but
also in analogous damage in other reproductive organs.
Parenteral injection of cadmium salts to premature female
rats[16] or to adult rats in persistent oestrus[17] results in
massive hemorrhages and necroses in the ovaries. Small amounts
of cadmium given during pregnancy produce serious placental
damage connected with fetal death[18]. Toward the end of
pregnancy the effect of cadmium is accompanied by a highly
lethal, "toxemia like" syndrome affecting the mothers [19]. As
shown in our previous reports this syndrome, characterized
first by convulsions and bilateral hemorrhagic renal necrosis,
is quite specifically the effect of cadmium given during the
last few days of rat pregnancy and is strictly dependent on the
presence of the placenta in the organism[2]. This could be
interesting from several aspects of the pathology of human
pregnancy. In addition to these effects the administration of
cadmium salts to lactating rats produces damage in the mammary
gland[2].

Learning of the protective effect of selenite in cadmium
testicular necrosis, we were, of course, interested in whether
selenium compounds could also prevent these other analogous
toxic effects of cadmium related to reproduction. As could be
expected, further experiments confirmed that selenite was
highly efficient in preventing the effects of cadmium not only
in male gonads but also in the ovaries[17], placentae[20], and
mammary gland[2]. From some aspects of human pathology it seems
to be of particular interest that small amounts of selenite not
only prevented the placental damage, but also the accompanying
fetal death and the "toxemia like" syndrome produced by cadmium
during gravidity[20] (Fig. 1). (It should be noted that a
similar syndrome can be produced in pregnant rats by feeding

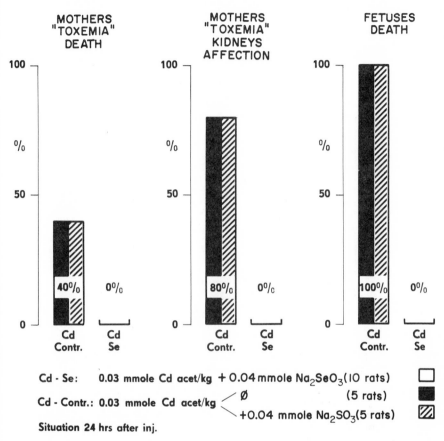

Cd - Se: 0.03 mmole Cd acet/kg + 0.04 mmole Na_2SeO_3(IO rats) ☐

Cd - Contr.: 0.03 mmole Cd acet/kg ⟨ ∅ (5 rats) ■

+0.04 mmole Na_2SO_3(5 rats) ▨

Situation 24 hrs after inj.

Fig. 1. The preventive effect of selenite in experimental "toxemia of pregnancy" induced by cadmium salts. [Experimental conditions analogous to Parízek et al., J. Reprod. Fert., 16, 506 (1968)].

them a diet rich in unsaturated fatty acids and/or its peroxides and deficient in vitamin E. The syndrome produced by this diet and described by Stamler[21] can be prevented by the administration of vitamin E but not by selenite. In contrast to this the similar syndrome produced by cadmium in our experiments can be prevented by selenite; however, vitamin E seems to be without

Group of rats	No. of rats used	Rats surviving 6 day after inj.	
		No.	%
Cd	31	3	9.7%
Cd - Se	51	51	100.0%
Cd - S	20	1	5.0%

Adult female rats

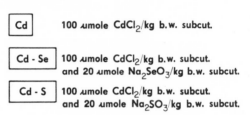

Cd   100 μmole CdCl$_2$/kg b.w. subcut.

Cd - Se   100 μmole CdCl$_2$/kg b.w. subcut.
and 20 μmole Na$_2$SeO$_3$/kg b.w. subcut.

Cd - S   100 μmole CdCl$_2$/kg b.w. subcut.
and 20 μmole Na$_2$SO$_3$/kg b.w. subcut.

Fig. 2. The effect of selenite on the survival of rats intoxicated by cadmium.

any protective effect here, and the same applies for the other effects of cadmium related to reproduction.)

In this situation it seemed to be of particular interest to learn if the protective effect of selenite was confined to the effects of cadmium related to reproduction only or if administration of selenite could also affect the nonreproductive toxicity of cadmium. As shown in our experiments in rats[20, 22,23], and by Gunn, Gould, and Anderson[24] in mice, administration of selenite very markedly affected the survival of animals intoxicated by a very large dose of cadmium. As shown in Fig. 2 analogous compounds of sulphur did not share this effect of selenite, and as shown in Fig. 3 the effect of selenite is long lasting in character.

In further experiments[2,4] we were able to show that both the reproductive and nonreproductive effects of cadmium can be prevented not only by the administration of inorganic salts of selenium but also by selenomethionine (Fig. 4).

It can be concluded, therefore, that selenium compounds seem to be able to affect the toxicity of cadmium in general and we would therefore like to suggest that small amounts of these selenium compounds should also prevent the effects of cadmium related to hypertension. We hope to be able to report on the experiments related to this problem soon.

III. SELENIUM AND MERCURY

From the aspect of the reactions responsible for the biological effects of cadmium it was of interest to learn if the interrelation with selenium was specific for salts of this metal only, or if a similar interrelation could also exist between selenium and the other metals from the IIb group, particularly mercury. Ganther and Baumann[25] described how parenteral administration of cadmium interferes with selenium metabolism, decreasing the respiratory excretion of volatile selenium compounds. Some time ago[22,26,27] we reported (Fig. 5) that mercuric compounds have a similar, and as a matter of fact, a more pronounced effect than cadmium in this respect; similar results were also obtained by Levander and Argrett[11]. As shown in Fig. 6 even quite small amounts of mercuric compounds decreased the excretion of volatile selenium compounds in animals given small amounts of selenite; and further experiments revealed that the same effect can be observed when selenium is given in the form of selenomethionine[27].

Learning that cadmium and mercury have a similar effect on selenium metabolism, we suspected that selenium compounds should affect the toxicity of both these metals in a similar

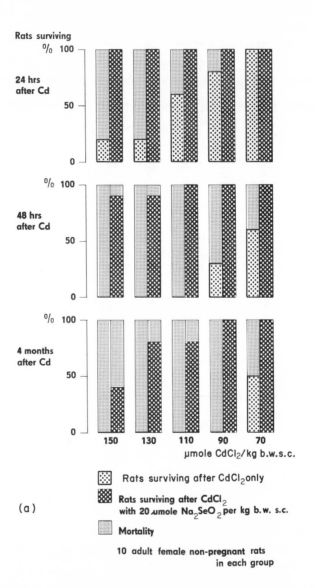

(a)

Fig. 3. The effect of selenite on the survival of rats injected with large doses of cadmium.

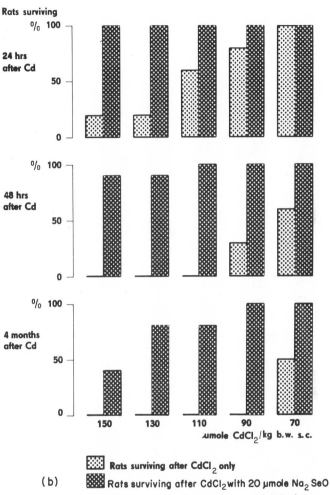

(b)

Rats surviving after CdCl$_2$ only

Rats surviving after CdCl$_2$ with 20 µmole Na$_2$ SeO

Per kg b.w. s.c.

10 adult female nonpregnant rats in each group

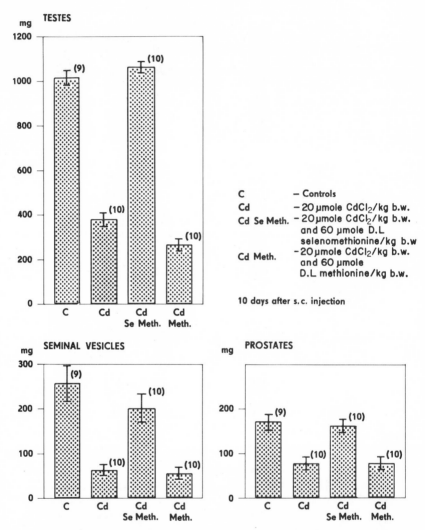

Fig. 4. Destruction of male gonads by cadmium: Protective effect of selenomethionine.

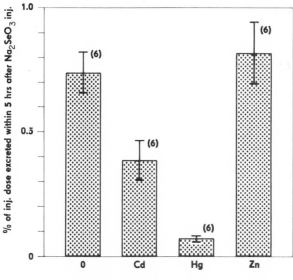

Adult female rats:
$CdCl_2$ or $HgCl_2$ or $ZnCl_2$(40 µmole/kg b.w.s.c)
Ihr before $Na_2{}^{75}SeO_3$ (2µmole/kg b.w. i.p,)

Fig. 5. The effect of cadmium, mercuric, and zinc chloride injection on the respiratory excretion of volatile selenium compounds[32].

way. In further experiments we were able to confirm this and to show[26] that small amounts of selenium compounds, when given as selenite or selenomethionine to rats intoxicated by a lethal dose of sublimate, completely protected the kidneys or intestine of these animals and ensured their survival (Figs. 7 and 8).

Further experiments revealed that in contrast to such protecting agents as BAL, the protective effect of selenite was not connected with an increased excretion of mercury but, on the contrary, with a marked decrease in mercury elimination through the urine (Fig. 9). Selenite, increasing the retention

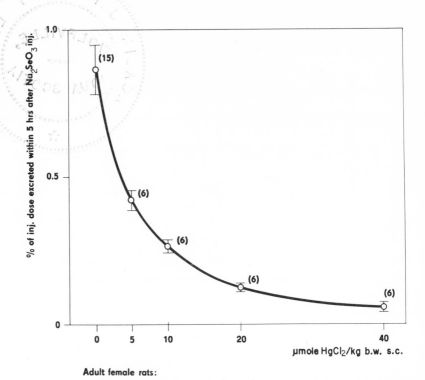

Adult female rats:
Na$_2^{75}$SeO$_3$ 0.5 µmole/kg b.w.i.p.

Fig. 6. The effect of mercuric chloride injection on the
respiratory excretion of volatile selenium compounds[32].

of mercury in the organism, changed the organ distribution of
the mercury[22]. As shown in Fig. 10 the concentration of
mercury in the kidneys and intestine of selenite-treated rats
was markedly decreased in comparison with control rats or with
animals given sulfite, and this should explain why no damage
was found in these organs. However, we should have in mind
that selenite protecting the testis against cadmium
increased[28,29] the cadmium concentration in this organ, and
the same can be observed with mercury (Fig. 10). It seems,
therefore, that the administration of selenium compounds changes
not only the organ distribution[22,30] of the metals affected

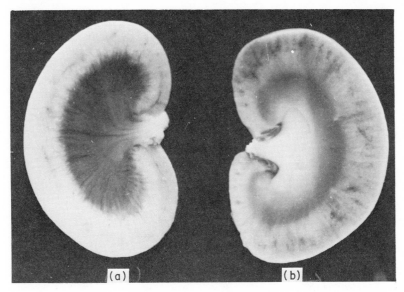

Fig. 7. Kidneys of adult female rats 26 hour after 20 μmole $HgCl_2$/kg b.w., s.c. (a) without additional treatment (a typical renal necrosis), and (b) when Na_2SeO_3 (40 μmole/kg b.w.) was given s.c. 1 hour after sublimate (full protection).

$HgCl_2$ mmole/kg	Na_2SeO_3 mmole/kg		No. of rats in each group	Rats surviving 10 day after inj.	
	simultan. with Hg^{2+}	4 hrs after Hg^{2+}		rats	%
0.02	—	—	20	0	0%
0.02	0.02	—	10	10	100%
0.02	—	0.02	10	10	100%
0.02	0.01	—	10	10	100%
0.02	—	0.01	10	10	100%
0.02	0.005	—	10	5	50%
0.02	—	0.005	10	2	20%

Fig. 8. The effect of selenite on survival of rats intoxicated by sublimate.

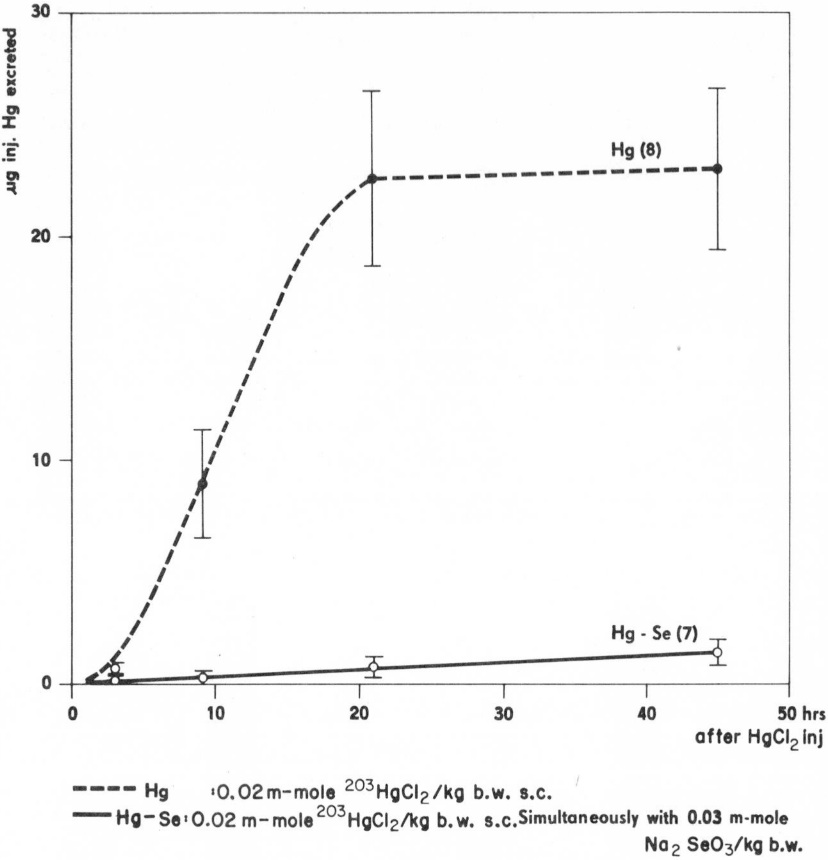

μg inj. Hg excreted
30
20
10
0
Hg (8)
Hg - Se (7)
0
10
20
30
40
50 hrs
after HgCl2 inj
Hg :0.02 m-mole 203HgCl2/kg b.w. s.c.
Hg-Se:0.02 m-mole 203HgCl2/kg b.w. s.c. Simultaneously with 0.03 m-mole
Na2 SeO3/kg b.w.

Fig. 9. The effect of selenite on the excretion of mercury by urine in sublimate intoxicated rats.

but, simultaneously, their reactivity. (This could explain why even delayed administration of selenite was effective in protecting the organism against sublimate.) The effect of selenite administration on testicular concentration of both these metals reflects the changes in blood level of these metals. One of the possible explanations for the increased testicular concentration of mercury or cadmium in selenite-treated rats

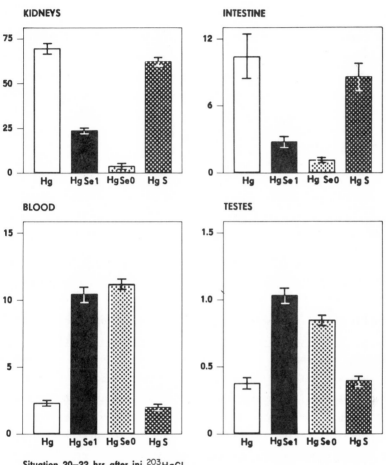

Situation 20–22 hrs after inj. ^{203}HgCl$_2$
Five adult rats in each group; results as μg inj. Hg/g
Hg – 20 μmole ^{203}HgCl$_2$/kg b.w.
Se – 30 μmole Na$_2$SeO$_3$/kg b.w.
S – 30 μmole Na$_2$SO$_3$/kg b.w.
Se0 – simultaneously with Hg
Se1 – 1 hr after Hg
S – simultaneously with Hg

Fig. 10.   The effect of selenite on the organ distribution
of mercury in sublimate intoxicated rats.

could be that selenium compounds react with cadmium or mercury,
producing compounds that, due to a known higher permeability
of testicular capillaries, could pass from the blood into the
male gonads more easily than into some other organs. It cannot
be excluded, of course, that some difference in testicular
metabolism could offer another possible explanation here.

IV.   INTERRELATIONS BETWEEN SELENIUM AND

VARIOUS GROUP IIB METALS

Figure 11 compares the effect of selenite as related to
blood concentration of cadmium, mercury, and zinc. Further
detailed analysis of this phenomenon[21] can serve as a basis
for the following conclusions.

(a) A highly increased content of mercury or cadmium can
be detected in the macromolecular fractions of blood plasma in
rats given salts of these metals and selenite. Further
experiments (in progress) should show if selenium and the
affected metals are bound together to proteins or if there is
another explanation for the increased concentration of these
metals and selenium in the macromolecular fractions (for example,
radiocolloids). In other words, further research should show
if selenite or some of its metabolites react with the metals
involved directly, or if proteins (and other substances
containing SH groups) are participating in this reaction.

(b) The administration of selenomethionine has an effect
similar to the inorganic selenium compounds; however, it does
not seem to act in this way immediately and a higher dose of
selenomethionine must be given to obtain a comparable response.
In contrast to selenite the presence of liver is an essential
prerequisite for the effect of selenomethionine.

(c) Finally, it should be mentioned that in subsequent
experiments a highly significant increase of cadmium level in

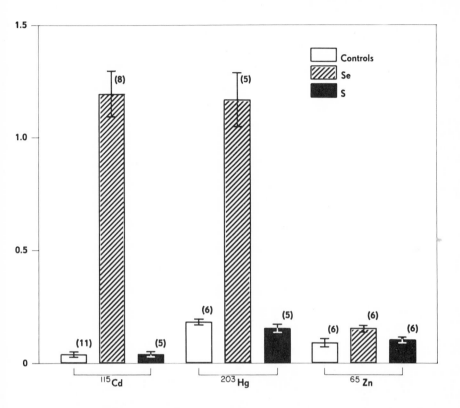

Adult female rats inj. s.c. with 20 μmole/kg b.w. $^{115}CdCl_2$or$^{203}HgCl_2$or $^{65}ZnCl$
Controls: salts of these metals only.
Se or S: 30 μmole/kg b.w. Na_2SeO_3or Na_2SO_3 inj. s.c. simultaneously with the salts
of the metals used.
Situation 5 hrs after the inj.

Fig. 11.   The effect of selenite on blood level of isotope injected[32].

blood plasma was found even when selenite was given in a very low dose, corresponding to 6 µg of selenium per rat, in one single injection. Selenium compounds also affected the blood level of cadmium when ingested.

It could therefore be concluded that a change in binding of mercury, cadmium, and perhaps some other metals could

explain the effect of selenium compounds on the toxicity and
the organ distribution of these metals. Further research is
necessary to show the exact chemical nature of the responsible
reactions, and to show if the effect of selenium compounds in
this respect could not explain at least in part the effect of
selenium as an essential nutrient. Even if further experiments
are necessary to elucidate the form in which mercury and
selenium are present in blood and blood plasma of animals given
compounds of these two elements, our data suggest that in this
form these elements cannot pass so easily across the barrier
represented by the placenta and the mammary gland.

As we were able to report on another occasion[2,3,4], the
administration of selenite to the mothers given trace amounts
of ^{203}Hg-mercuric compounds increased the retention of
^{203}Hg-mercury in pregnant or lactating rats and simultaneously
decreased the ^{203}Hg-mercury content in fetuses, milk, and
sucklings. As a result of this the mercuric content in organs
of offsprings from mothers given selenite was much lower than
in offsprings from mothers exposed to mercury only. The same
amount of sulfite did not have a similar effect. Selenite
administration did not apparently decrease the passage of
^{65}Zn-zinc from the maternal organism into offsprings.

The period of gestation and lactation seems to be of
particular interest in relation to several trace elements and
selenium is no exception. It is well known that lower selenium
levels are detected in fetal and neonatal organs in flocks
affected by selenium-responsive diseases. In this respect it
seemed to be of interest to learn how far exposure of the
maternal organism to mercuric compounds could affect not only
the excretion of selenium from the organism but also its availability for fetal and neonatal nutrition. In our first experiments in which this question was studied[3,5,32], mercuric

compounds were injected into pregnant or lactating rats given a small amount ^{75}Se-selenite, and the effect of mercury on the maternal passage of selenium was compared with that of a similar dose of zinc. In contrast to zinc salts the exposure of pregnant rats to mercuric salts increased the retention of selenium in the maternal organs decreasing simultaneously the selenium content in fetal organs. One single injection of a subtoxic dose of mercuric chloride, or in further experiments of mercuric acetate, was sufficient to increase the retention of selenium in the maternal organism, while at the same time it decreased the selenium content in fetuses and newborn animals (Fig. 12). Within certain limits the effects were dependent on the dose of mercury; however, analysis of the data suggests that even the highest dose of mercury would not completely block the transfer of selenium from the mothers into the fetuses; it cannot be excluded, therefore, that some selenium metabolite can pass unhampered from the mothers into offsprings even with the highest dose of mercury used[5]. Administration of mercuric salts also has a similar effect on the passage of selenium into milk (Fig. 13) and to sucklings. Consequently, in spite of the increased selenium content in the organism of mercury-treated lactating rats, sucklings fed by these rats contained markedly less selenium (Figs. 14 and 15).

It can be concluded, therefore, that in these acute model experiments in rats the exposure of the maternal organism to mercuric salts during pregnancy and lactation had a significant effect on the supply of selenium to the offsprings. Further experiments with chronic exposure in species with a longer period of gestation should show if the symptoms of selenium deficiency could be evoked in this way. This possibility seems to be of interest as we know that industrialization or even certain agricultural techniques (such as seed dressing or

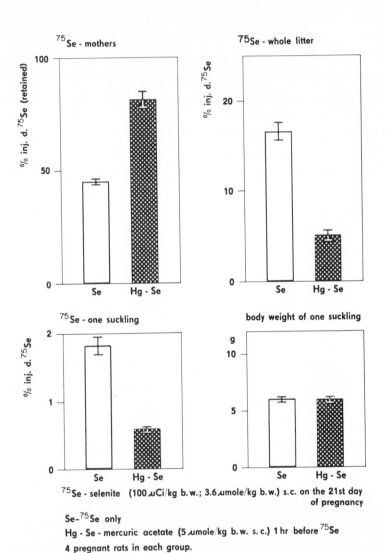

Fig. 12.   The effect of mercuric acetate given during pregnancy on the ^{75}Se content of the newborn young.   (For details see[5].

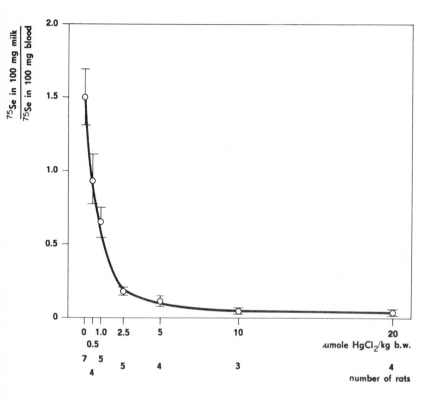

Lactating rats (11 days after delivery):
Na$_2^{75}$SeO$_3$(200 μCi/kg b.w.; 0.91 μmole/kg b.w. s.c.)
1 hr after s.c. inj. HgCl$_2$
Sucklings removed from the mothers 1 hr before the inj. of Na$_2^{75}$SeO$_3$
Milk and blood collected 24 hrs after Na$_2^{75}$SeO$_3$inj.

Fig. 13.   The effect of HgCl$_2$ on the passage of ^{75}Se into milk.

the general use of mercury-containing fungicides) can significantly increase the content of mercury in the environment.   An
increased exposure of the maternal organism (Fig. 16) to
traces of mercury (or to other similarly acting metals) could
mean that at the end of the period of nutritional dependence on

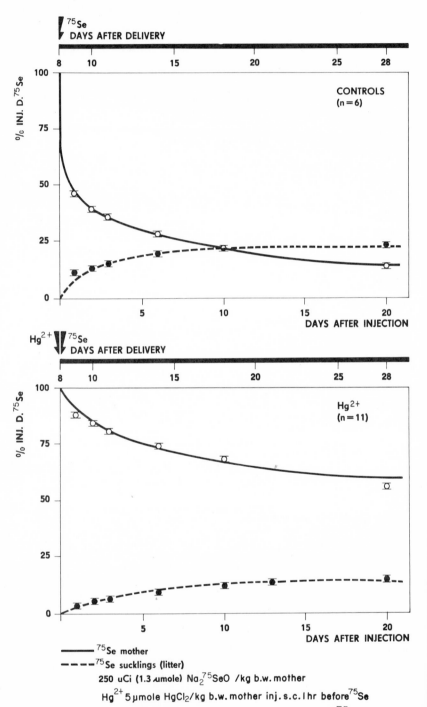

Fig. 14. The effect of $HgCl_2$ on the passage of ^{75}Se from the lactating rats into sucklings.

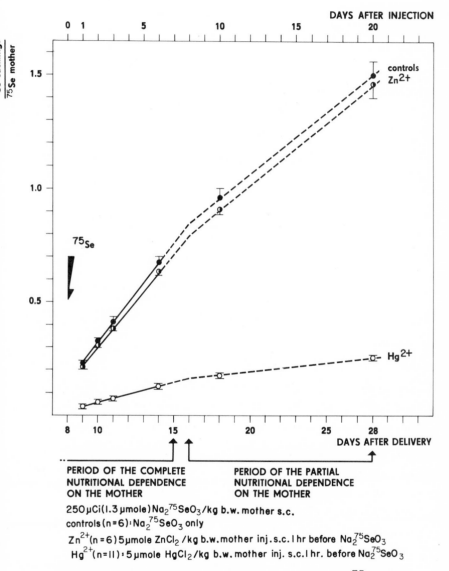

Fig. 15. The effect of $HgCl_2$ on the passage of ^{75}Se from the lactating rats into sucklings.

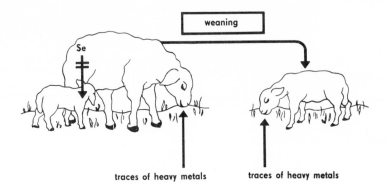

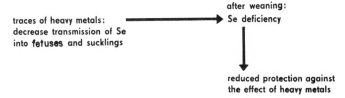

Fig. 16. Ecological consequences of metabolic interrelations between selenium and traces of certain heavy metals
during gravidity, lactation, and weaning.

the maternal organism sucklings would contain less selenium
and would in this way be deficient in the factor shown to be
able to protect them against this environmental influence.

It is clear that this effect of mercury could be compen-
sated for by an increased supply of selenium to mothers or to
newborns. However, further experiments have suggested that the
administration of selenium compounds could be surprisingly
dangerous in a situation where certain selenium metabolites
could be produced and present in an organism that would be
exposed subsequently to traces of mercury. This represents an
initially unsuspected limit to the possible use of selenium
compounds in the prevention of mercury toxicity. In addition
to this it should be noted that increasing environmental

pollution by mercury has been described recently in several
countries and a widespread use of selenium in these areas
might be connected with a hitherto unexpected danger to large
population groups.

In our first paper[26] describing the protective effect
of selenite in sublimate intoxication, we recorded the exceptional
sudden death in one of the 40 rats given selenite 1 hour after
mercuric chloride administration. Further analysis of this
phenomenon revealed that the incidence of this death, appearing
within the first few hours of the experiment, can be greatly
increased when selenite is given not after but a few hours
before mercury. In addition to this, males seem to be more
susceptible to this effect than females. The symptoms observed
in rats given selenite a few hours before mercury were quite
dissimilar to those known to be produced by sublimate but closely
resembled those described by McConnell and Portman[33] in rats
intoxicated with a very large dose of dimethylselenide.

It seems to be well established that dimethylselenide is
formed in the organism, including mammals and humans, when
given selenite or other selenium compounds, and that this
substance is rapidly excreted from the organism by respiration.
Dimethylselenide is known to be less toxic by several orders of
magnitude than most of the other selenium compounds[33]. The
biosynthesis of dimethylselenide has therefore been considered
as an important detoxifying process[6].

In spite of this very low toxicity of dimethylselenide
there were several indications of the possibility that administration of mercury could markedly increase the sensitivity of
the organism to this compound.

(a) First, most of the animals given selenite first and
mercury later died within the first few hours of the experiment. The surviving rats recovered within the next few hours

without any damage known to be produced by mercuric salts.
This suggested that a substance was involved that rapidly
disappeared from the organism.

(b) The symptoms observed in dying animals were practically
identical with those known to be produced by dimethylselenide.
Convulsions were seen frequently before death and venous
congestion, pulmonary edema, and massive pleural and pericardial
effusions were almost constant at autopsy.

(c) Finally, another point suggesting that dimethylselenide and/or some related selenium metabolites could be involved
here arises from the dependence of the lethality on the timing
of administration of selenium and mercuric compounds. As
already mentioned the biosynthesis of dimethylselenide is highly
depressed in mercury-treated rats. This means that dimethylselenide and/or related metabolites are present in the organism
when selenite is given before mercury; however, the situation is
quite different when mercury is given first and selenite later.

We therefore decided to compare the toxicity of this
selenium compound, nontoxic under normal conditions, in control
rats and in rats given a sublethal dose of sublimate. As shown
in Fig. 17 all mercury-treated animals died with the syndrome
described when exposed to the dimethylselenide in a dose
nonlethal for controls. This peculiar effect of mercury on the
toxicity of dimethylselenide does not seem to be shared by
cadmium or zinc (Fig. 18). Further experiments revealed that
the simultaneous exposure to mercuric compounds and
dimethylselenide is fatal in a high proportion of rats even when
these compounds are given in very small amounts. A good
relation was observed between the dose of mercury and this
effect.

Thus it appears (Fig. 19) that the interrelation between
selenium and mercury in the organism is very complex in

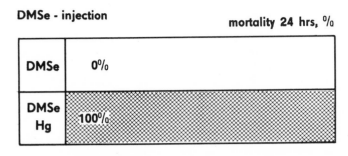

DMSe - injection   **mortality 24 hrs, %**

| DMSe | 0% |
| DMSe Hg | 100% |

DMSe - dimethylselenide   **1.4 g/kg b.w. i. p.**
   Hg−5 μmole HgCl$_2$/kg b.w.s.c.

DMSe - respiratory exposure   **mortality 3 hrs, %**

| DMSe* | 0% |
| DMSe* Hg | 100% |

DMSe* - dimethylselenide vapours   (approx. 34 mg/l air)
   Hg−20 μmole HgCl$_2$/kg b.w.s.c.

Adult female rats   10 animals in each group

Fig. 17. A highly lethal syndrome produced by simultaneous exposure to dimethylselenide and mercuric compounds.

character. Inorganic selenium compounds or selenomethionine decrease the toxicity of mercury, very probably as a result of changed mercury binding in the organism. Mercuric compounds (and certain other metals) increase the retention of selenium in the organism and decrease the amount of dimethylselenide produced. When dimethylselenide or its metabolite have already

20 μmole/kg   **mortality 24 hrs**

solvents (oil)	ZnCl$_2$	0%
	CdCl$_2$	0%
	HgCl$_2$	0%
dimethylselenide 200 μmole/kg b.w.	O	3%
	ZnCl$_2$	0%
	CdCl$_2$	7%
	HgCl$_2$	100%

100   %   0

Adult female rats (30 animals in each group)

Fig. 18. A highly lethal syndrome produced by simultaneous administration of mercuric salts and dimethylselenide.

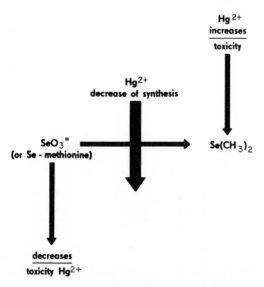

Hg^{2+}
increases
toxicity

Hg^{2+}
decrease of synthesis

SeO$_3$"
(or Se - methionine)

Se(CH$_3$)$_2$

decreases
toxicity Hg^{2+}

Fig. 19.

been formed, however, its simultaneous presence in the organism
with traces of mercury seems to be extremely dangerous.

It has not yet been decided what is the mechanism of action
of dimethylselenide and why traces of mercury increase the
sensitivity to this selenium metabolite by several orders of
magnitude. Preliminary experiments did not show a protective
effect of SH groups or tocopherol against dimethylselenide
toxicity. From the several possibilities, those which in our
opinion should be considered first are summarized in Fig. 20.

In the course of these experiments we recorded a phenomenon that might be of further importance in the study of
dimethylselenide toxicity. In our experiments on adult rats
(but not in prepubertal rats) we found a striking sex-linked
difference in the toxicity of dimethylselenide. It seems,
therefore, that there are at least two factors on which the
sensitivity of the organism to this selenium metabolite is
dependent: exposure to small amounts of mercury and sex
(Fig. 21). It seems that both these factors have an additive
effect. As a result of this males are even more susceptible
to simultaneous exposure to mercury and dimethylselenide than
females. This sexual difference can also be observed when

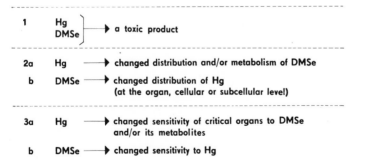

Fig. 20. Possible mechanisms responsible for the extremely
high mortality of rats simultaneously exposed to trace amounts
of dimethylselenide (DMSe) and $HgCl_2$ (Hg).

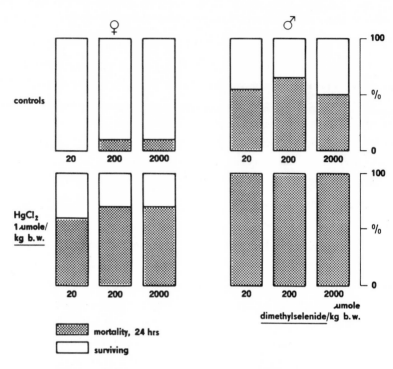

mortality, 24 hrs

surviving

Male or female rats of the same age (2 months old); 20 animals in each group

Fig. 21. Toxicity of dimethylselenide: dependence on sex and on traces of mercury.

adult males or females of the same age are given the same (per rat) very low dose of dimethylselenide and mercury (Fig. 22). It is hoped that it will soon be possible to report on the endocrine analysis of this sexual difference.

It seems at present that there are two points indicating a different mechanism by which mercury and male sex influence the toxicity of dimethylselenide. First, as shown in Fig. 23, administration of selenite was able to mask the effect of mercury even in this situation; however, the administration of

group		no of animals	mortality — 24 hrs, %
♀	DMSe	20	0%
	DMSe Hg	30	37%
♂	DMSe	20	0%
	DMSe Hg	30	87%

0   %   100

Male or female rats of the same age (3 months)
injected by the same dose per rat:
DMSe — 1 μmole dimethylselenide/rat i.p.
Hg — 0,2 μmole HgCl$_2$/rat s.c.

Fig. 22. Toxicity of dimethylselenide; dependence on sex
and traces of mercury.

the same dose of selenite did not influence the lethality of
the same dose of dimethylselenide when given to male rats
without mercury. Second, our recent experiments have shown
that the sexual difference in the toxicity of dimethylselenide
could be connected with the different metabolism of this compound
in both sexes. It should be stated here that administration
of mercuric compounds to female rats did not induce the
dimethylselenide metabolic pattern observed in males.

When a small amount of ^{75}Se-dimethylselenide is given, a
higher proportion of radioactivity is found to be retained in
the male organism during the first few critical hours
(Fig. 24). It seems of particular interest that the highest
[75]Se-selenium content was found in the male kidney, where the
[75]Se-selenium concentration was several times higher than in

J. PAŘÍZEK ET AL.

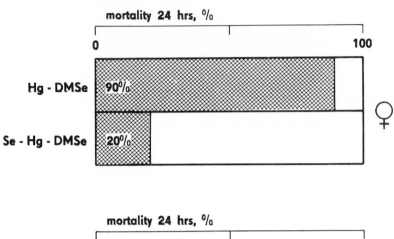

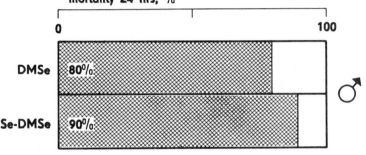

DMSe - dimethylselenide 20 μmole/kg b.w. i.p.
Hg -HgCl$_2$5μmole/kg b.w.s.c,
Se - Na$_2$SeO$_3$ 20μmole/kg b.w.s.c
      (1 hr before DMSe or DMSe + Hg)
      10 adult rats in each group

Fig. 23.   The protective effect of selenite.

the female kidney. A highly significant sex-linked difference
was also found in ^{75}Se-selenium content of the heart and some
differences also seem to be reflected in the skeletal muscle.
The sex-related difference in the retention of selenium in
animals given a small amount of dimethylselenide seems to be
confined to the first few hours (Fig. 25). Further experiments

Rats	% whole body retention	% retention in 100g b.w.	%·10⁻²/ml blood	kidney	liver	heart	%·10⁻²/g lung	spleen	adipose tissue	skeletal muscle
♂	72.1 ± 10.3	26.31 ± 4.48	12.4 ± 0.3	281.8 ± 20.0	33.5 ± 2.0	29.7 ± 2.0	21.8 ± 2.0	18.6 ± 1.0	12.0 ± 1.0	11.0 ± 0.9
♀	32.7 ± 1.9	15.4 ± 0.9	11.9 ± 0.5	56.9 ± 5.0	31.0 ± 1.0	21.5 ± 1.0	22.5 ± 2.0	17.2 ± 0.9	17.6 ± 2.0	8.2 ± 0.2
Sign.	**	**	0	**	0	**	0	0	0	•

** P <0.01   • 0.05 > P > 0.02   0 - insig.

Male and female rats 92 days old

75 Se content (expressed as percentage inj. d.⁷⁵Se) 5 hrs after 0.3 μCi/rat corresponding to 0.5 μmole/rat

⁷⁵Se - dimethylselenide i.p.. Four rats in each group

Fig. 24. Sex-linked differences in ⁷⁵Se-dimethylselenide metabolism.

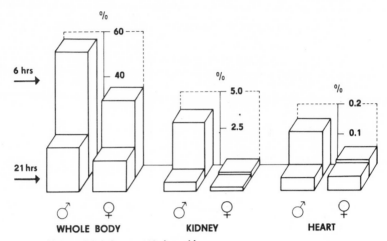

Male and female rats 110 days old
^{75}Se content (expressed as % inj. d. ^{75}Se) 6 hrs and 21 hr after 1.6 μCi/kg b.w.
corresponding to 2.4 μmole/kg b.w. ^{75}Se - dimethylselenide i.p.
Six rats in each group

Fig. 25. Sex-linked differences in ^{75}Se-dimethylselenide
metabolism.

(in progress) should show in which form selenium is present in
these organs of animals given dimethylselenide. It is also
necessary to decide if the sex-related difference could be
explained by some difference in circulation and/or retention of
dimethylselenide in the male and female organism, or if both
sexes differ in the rate of conversion of dimethylselenide into
some metabolites. In this connection it should be noted that a
surprisingly high proportion of radioactivity was found in the
urine of animals given small amounts of ^{75}Se-dimethylselenide.
In rats given 2.4 μmole/kg body weight ^{75}Se-dimethylselenide,
approximately half of the radioactivity injected (52%) was
found in the urine excreted within 24 hours after intraperitoneal injection. It cannot be excluded that trimethylselenonium ion, recently described[34-36] as a major selenium

excretory product in rat urine, is also formed from dimethylselenide. (From this aspect it must be added here that our
most recent experiments revealed that the toxicity of
trimethylselenonium ion was also dependent on sex and on the
simultaneous exposure to mercuric compounds in a manner analogous
to the toxicity of dimethylselenide.) Our experience has been
that not only dimethylselenide and trimethylselenonium ion
but also a highly toxic dimethyldiselenide can be formed in the
mammalian organism[37].

In spite of all the work that remains to be done and in
spite of the fact that all the presented data were obtained in
acute experiments, it seems that further study of the interrelation between mercury and some selenium compounds could be
of considerable importance in environmental research. Significant mercury pollution has been reported recently in several
countries. Some of these areas are rich in selenium and in
others selenium is being used in the prevention and therapy of
livestock diseases. An unexpected pathological finding has
recently been reported as resulting from exposure to mercury
under unusual conditions[38]. It seems, therefore, that
further study of the interrelation between compounds of selenium
and mercury and perhaps some other metals could be of interest
not only in relation to theoretical problems of selenium
function and toxicity but also in relation to the practical
problems of environmental research and human pathology.

REFERENCES

[1]. Schroeder, H. A., Circulation, 35, 570 (1963).

[2]. Parízek, J., Beneš, I., Oštadalová, I., Babický, A.,
Beneš, J., and Pitha, J., Mineral Metabolism in
Paediatrics. (D. Barltrop and W. L. Burland, eds.)
Oxford, England: Blackwell, 1969, p. 117.

120 J. PARÍZEK ET AL.

[3]. Parízek, J., Ostádalová, I., Kalouskova, J., and Babicky, A., Nutrition, Proceedings of the VIIIth International Congress on Nutrition, Prague, 1969, Excerpta Medica, Amsterdam, 1970.

[4]. Parízek, J., Babicky, a., Ostádalová, I., Kalouskova, J., and Pavlík, L., Radiation Biology of the Fetal and Juvenile Mammal, (M. R. Sikov and D. D. Mahlum, ed.). Oak Ridge, Tennessee: USAEC, 1969, p. 137.

[5]. Parízek, J., Ostádalová, I., Kalouskova, J., Babicky, A., Pavlík, L., and Bibr, B., J. Reprod. Fert., in press.

[6]. Rosenfeld, I. and Beath, O. A., Selenium, Geobotany, Biochemistry, Toxicity, and Nutrition, New York: Academic Press, 1964.

[7]. Muth, O. H. (ed.), Selenium in Biomedicine, Westport, Connecticut: AVI Publishers, 1967.

[8]. Parízek, J., Ostádalová, I., Kalouskova, J., Babicky, A., and Beneš, J., Cs. Gynekologie, 35, 140 (1970).

[9]. Holló, Z. M. and Zlatarov, S., Naturwissenschaften, 47, 87 (1960).

[10]. Rusiecki, W. and Brzezinski, J., Acta Polonica Pharmaceutica, 23, 69 (1966).

[11]. Levander, O. A. and Argrett, L. C., Toxicology and Appl. Pharmacology, 14, 308 (1969).

[12]. Mason, K. E., Young, J. O., and Brown, J. A., Anat. Rec., 148, 309 (1964).

[13]. Kar, A. B., Das, R. P., and Mukerji, F. N. I., Proc. Nat. Inst. Sci. India, B., 26, suppl. 40 (1960).

[14]. Parízek, J., J. Reprod. Fert., 1, 294 (1960).

[15]. Parízek, J and Zahor, Z., I. Nature (Lond.), 177, 1036 (1956).

[16]. Kar, A. B., Das, R. P., and Karkun, J. N., Acta Biol. Med. Germ., 3, 372 (1959).

[17]. Pařízek, J., Oštádalová, I., Beneš, I., and Pitha, J., J. Reprod. Fert., 17, 559 (1968).

[18]. Pařízek, J., J. Reprod. Fert., 7, 263 (1964).

[19]. Pařízek, J., J. Reprod. Fert., 9, 11 (1965).

[20]. Pařízek, J., Oštádalová, I., Beneš, I., and Babický, A. J. Reprod. Fert., 16, 507 (1968).

[21]. Stamler, F. W., Am. J. Pathol., 35, 1207 (1959).

[22]. Pařízek, J., Oštádalová, I., Beneš, I., Babický, A., and Beneš, J., Cs. Fysiol., 16, 41 (1967).

[23]. Pařízek, J., Beneš, I., Kalouskova, J., Oštádalová, I., Lener, J., Babický, A., and Beneš, J., Proc. Int. Union Physiol. Sci., 7, 337 (1968).

[24]. Gunn, S. A., Gould, T. C., and Anderson, W. A. D., Proc. Soc. Exp. Biol. Med., 128, 591 (1968).

[25]. Ganther, H. E. and Baumann, C. A., J. Nutr., 77, 210 (1962).

[26]. Pařízek, J. and Oštádalová, I., Experientia, 23, 142 (1967).

[27]. Pařízek, J., Beneš, I., Babický, A., Procházková, V., and Lener, J., Physiol. Bohemoslov., 18, 105 (1969).

[28]. Gunn, S. A. and Gould, T. C., Selenium in Biomedicine, (O. H. Muth, ed.) Westport, Connecticut: AVI Publishers, 1967, p. 395.

[29]. Gunn, S. A., Gould, T. C., and Anderson, W. A. D., J. Reprod. Fert., 15, 65 (1968).

[30]. Eybl, V., Sýkora, J., and Hrnčířová, M., Arch. Toxicol. 25, 296 (1969).

[31]. Pařízek, J., Beneš, I., Oštádalová, I., Babický, A., Beneš, J., and Lener, J., Physiol. Bohemoslov., 18, 95 (1969).

[32]. Pařízek, J., Oštádalová, I., Kalouskova, J., Babický, A., and Pavlík, L., (Proc. Czechosloslov. Physiol. Soc., July, 1969), Physiol. Bohemoslov., 18, 502 (1969).

[33]. McConnell, K. P. and Portman, O. W., J. Biol. Chem.,
       195, 277 (1952).
[34]. Byard, J. L., Arch. Biochem. Biophys., 130, 556 (1969).
[35]. Palmer, I. S., Fischer, D. D., Halverson, A. W., and
       Olson, O. E., Biochim. Biophys. Acta, 177, 336 (1969).
[36]. Palmer, I. S., Gunsalus, R. P., Halverson, A. W., and
       Olson, O. E., Biochim. Biophys. Acta, 208, 260 (1970).
[37]. Procházková, V., Beneš, J., and Pařízek, J., Physiol.
       Bohemoslov., in press.
[38]. Kurland, L. T., Faro, S. N., and Siedler, H., World
       Neurology, 1, 370 (1960).

Chapter 7

CHROMIUM METABOLISM: THE GLUCOSE TOLERANCE FACTOR

W. Mertz and E. E. Roginski

Human Nutrition Research Division
U. S. Department of Agriculture
Agricultural Research Service
Beltsville, Maryland

Although the physiological role of chromium is being
increasingly recognized, our knowledge of chromium metabolism is
incomplete. It is known that trivalent chromium acts as a
cofactor for the peripheral action of insulin[1], and that
chromium-deficient animals and some human subjects respond to
trace supplementation of this element with normalization of

their impaired glucose tolerance[2-7]. More recent studies
have demonstrated that repeated pregnancies and diabetes are
associated with lowered chromium concentrations in hair[8,9]
and that insulin-dependent diabetics metabolize chromium in a
fashion different from that of normals[10]. On the other hand,
only less than half of adult subjects tested responded to the
chromium supplement with improved glucose tolerance, the
response appeared gradually and was often observed only after
several weeks of supplementation. Attempts to obtain an
immediate response in adults by giving higher oral doses were
unsuccessful[5]. These observations are unexplained; they are
in distinct contrast to the immediate effects seen after zinc
or iron supplementation. The mechanism and even the degree of
absorption of chromium from the gastrointestinal tract is
unknown. Chromium in form of some but not other coordinate
compounds and complexes behaves like an essential nutrient. For
example, only in some form(s) does this element go across the
placenta and is available to the fetus[11].

These and other observations have led to the conclusion that
the biological activity of chromium depends strongly on the
chemical form of the complex of which the element is part. For
example, Brewers' yeast incorporates chromium salts into one or
more compounds that are much more readily available for
placental transport and other functions than are the simple
salts of the element. These fractions furthermore are of a
much greater activity than simple salts in their potentiation
of insulin in vitro. The compound(s) responsible for this
activity has not yet been chemically identified. However, it
can be described by some chemical, biochemical, and physiological
criteria, and on this basis it is termed "glucose tolerance
factor" (GTF). In the following some aspects of chromium
metabolism will be discussed in the light of this concept.

I. INTESTINAL ABSORPTION (IN VIVO)

The absorption of trivalent chromium is believed to be poor, that of the hexavalent state, somewhat better. Donaldson found an average absorption in normal subjects of 0.5% of an oral dose of $^{51}CrCl_3 \cdot 6H_2O$[12]. The absorption of chromic salts in experimental animals has been stated as <0.5[13] and 2 to 3%[14]. This low degree of absorption does not appear to be increased by chromium deficiency, and it does not appear to be dependent on the dose administered, suggesting that no appreciable homeostatic control of chromium intake exists[14]. Whereas these data are valid for ^{51}chromic chloride, they cannot be generalized. This is illustrated by a simple calculation (Table I). The most conservative measurements of chromium output

TABLE I

Absorption and Excretion of Chromium in Man

Investigator	Average/Percent of Dose in Urine	Range
A. Absorption of $CrCl_3 \cdot 6H_2O$ in Human Subjects		
Donaldson et al.	0.5 ± 0.3	0.1 - 1.2
Doisy et al.	0.69 ± 0.08	0.4 - 1.5
B. Average Dietary Chromium Intake (µg/day)		
Schroeder et al.	60	
Levine et al.	59	5 - 115
C. Calculated Absorption (µg/day) $(\frac{B \times A}{100})$		
	0.36	0.005 - 1.7
D. Total Absorption [Urinary Chromium (µg/day)]		
Pierce et al.	7.5 (5 ppb)	5.2 - 9.7
Imbus et al.	6.0 (4 ppb)	2.8 - 16.5
Tipton et al.	130	110 - 160

in urine of man have established a range of 4 to 10 µg/day.
Analyses of dietary chromium intake agree on an average of
approximately 50 µg/day[15,7]. To maintain a positive chromium
balance under these conditions with total chromium absorption
of 0.5% is obviously impossible. Since recent balance studies
with chromium in normal subjects provide no evidence for a
significant negative balance[16], it can be concluded that some
of the chromium naturally occurring in the diet is much better
available for absorption than chromic chloride.

This conclusion is borne out by experiments on intestinal
absorption and retention of two forms of chromium in rats
(Table II). A stomach tubed dose of [51]chromic chloride was
poorly absorbed by rats, so that after 4 days only a fraction
of 0.5% remained in the body. When, on the other hand, Brewers'
yeast was allowed to accumulate [51]chromic chloride, the
[51]Cr subsequently extracted from the yeast and stomach tubed
was much better retained in preliminary experiments. This

TABLE II

Absorption of [51]Chromium in the Rat[a]

Compound	Percent Retained in Body	
$CrCl_3 \cdot 6H_2O$ (N=4)	0.5	(0.4-0.9)
$CrCl_3 \cdot 6H_2O$, with milk (N=2)	0.45	(0.4,0.5)
Cr-51-GTF (N=3)	24.5	(19-28)[b]
Cr-51-GTF (N=2)	10.0	(10,10)

[a] Percent/retention 4 days after oral dose.

[b] Pregnant rats.

difference cannot be attributed to a nonspecific effect of other nutrients that may have been present in the extract, since the absorption of ^{51}chromic chloride was not enhanced by simultaneous administration of milk.

These data, although preliminary, and the above calculations suggest that the fraction of chromium available for absorption depends on the chemical form in which the element is present, and that the availability from at least one, probably more, natural sources is considerably greater than that of simple salts. These considerations emphasize the need to study not only the total concentration but also the availability of chromium in the various dietary ingredients.

II. INTESTINAL ABSORPTION (IN VITRO)

These studies were designed to investigate some characteristics of intestinal chromium transport and the influence of dietary factors thereon under controlled conditions. Their interpretation in a physiological sense is complicated because of the use of an isolated system, and because relatively simple chromium complexes and chelates were studied which may not be representative of the form(s) in which chromium from natural dietary sources is absorbed. In all of the following studies ^{51}chromium chloride was present on the mucosal side of everted sacs from the jejunum of rats fed a Torula yeast diet. The preparation was incubated in a Krebs-Ringer bicarbonate medium, pH 7.4, of which 20 ml bathed the mucosal and 0.4 ml the inverted serosal side. At the end of the incubation, aliquots were withdrawn from the media of both sides, and the sacs were cut longitudinally and thoroughly washed in cold saline. Media and pieces of the intestines were added to a measured volume of water and counted for ^{51}Cr radioactivity. The method followed

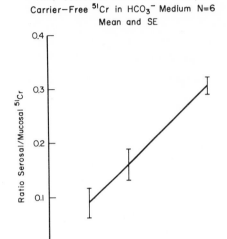

Fig. 1 Equilibration of ^{51}Cr chloride across the
intestinal wall in everted sacs. Donor animals raised on a
low-chromium, Torula yeast diet, fasted for 24 hours.

the procedure of Wilson and Wiseman[17]; details are stated
in the tables.

The transport of ^{51}Cr from mucosal to serosal side was
roughly linear throughout the incubation period of 2 hours.
It never reached equilibrium, not even after 5 hours, a time
at which the intestines can be suspected to have become
nonviable and leaky (Fig. 1). Thus it appears that chromic
chloride follows a simple diffusion process and that no active
transport is involved. This is borne out by the observation
that exogenous substrates, such as glucose or acetate, do not
influence the process, and that poisoning of energy generating
systems within the cell does not depress chromium absorption
(Table III). Contrary to observations in intact rats in which

TABLE III

Independence of Intestinal Chromium

Absorption on Substrate$^{a/}$

Addition (in 20 ml)	Number of Rats	Final Ratio ^{51}Chromium Serosal/Mucosal Side
None	9	0.34
Glucose, 20 mg	9	0.35
Acetate, 20 mg	9	0.38
Glucose	6	0.34
Glucose + DNP	6	0.40
Glucose + iodoacetate	6	0.42

$\underline{a/}$ Incubation with 0.1 µg chromium/ml for 2 hours in HCO_3^- medium.

approximately the same percentage of a given dose was absorbed, regardless of the amount administered, the isolated system of the everted sac exhibited a striking dependence on the dose levels: With increasing dose level, the rate of chromium transport diminished (Table IV). This behavior is not compatible with a simple diffusion process; it suggest a finite number of specific sites that are involved in the absorption of chromium and a mechanism similar to that of "facilitated diffusion"[18]. This hypothesis is supported by the observation that the presence of several metals in the medium, iron, manganese, calcium, and particularly titanium, appreciably depressed chromium transport (Table V). This depression was observed when the metals were present at a hundredfold excess over chromium, a ratio which is similar to or even less than that found _in vivo_. Titanium

TABLE IV

Effect of Dose on Intestinal Absorption of

$CrCl_3 \cdot 6H_2O$[a/]

Dose (μg/20 ml)	Number of Experiments	Final Ratio [51]Chromium Serosal/Mucosal Side
Carrier-free (<0.01)	6	0.35 ± 0.02
0.1	9	0.29 ± 0.04
1.0	9	0.07 ± 0.006
10.0	6	0.02 ± 0.003

[a/] Incubation for 2 hours in HCO_3^- medium.

inhibited at a tenfold excess over chromium. Since the concentration at which these elements were present was far below toxic levels, we can assume a common transport site for which they compete against chromium. It is likely that other elements, such as copper and zinc, have their own transport sites because their presence does not affect chromium transport.

The inhibition of calcium is overcome by disodium ethylenediamine tetraacetate in the medium (Table VI). The great affinity of EDTA for calcium suggests that a chelate was formed that did not compete with chromium for the absorption sites. However, a direct reaction between EDTA and chromium must also have occurred because even in the absence of calcium the presence of EDTA stimulated chromium transport, although to a lesser degree. Chromium transport is strongly stimulated by substances that form chelates with the element. A mixture of 20 amino acids nearby doubled the rate; histidine and

TABLE V

Effect of Trace Elements on Intestinal
Chromium Absorption[a]

Initial Concentration Mucosal Side (µg/20 ml)		Final Ratio [51]Chromium Serosal/Mucosal Side			
Chromium	Other	Other	Elements	Added	Phosphorus
		None	Copper	Zinc	
1	100	0.05	0.08	0.04	NS
			Manganese	Iron	
1	100	0.07	0.03	0.02	<0.005
0.1	1,000	0.29	0.05	0.03	<0.001
10	100	0.02	0.02	0.03	NS
			Vanadium	Molybdenum	
1[b]	10	0.29	0.35	0.4	NS
			Cobalt	Nickel	
1[b]	10	0.43	0.49	0.37	NS
			Selenium	Titanium	
1[b]	10	0.46	0.49	0.07	NS <0.001

[a] Incubation for 2 hours in HCO_3^- medium.

[b] Experiments in absence of calcium.

penicillamine were equally effective (Table VII). A number of
other amino acids and substances of biological importance had
intermediate effects.

All these agents have in common the tendency to form metal
chelates. Without chelation, the chromium hexa aquo complex

TABLE VI

Effect of Calcium and EDTA on

Intestinal Chromium Transport[a]

	Final Ratio [51]Chromium Serosal/Mucosal Addition	
	None	EDTA (1 mg/ml)
A. With 100 µg calcium/ml	0.03 ± 0.006	0.55 ± 0.03
B. Without calcium	0.31 ± 0.03	0.48 ± 0.04

[a] 1 µg chromium/20 ml of HCO_3^- medium.

would immediately be precipitated at the alkaline pH of the incubation medium and would therefore not be available for absorption. The ability of various potential ligands to protect against this process has been extensively studied by Rollinson,

TABLE VII

Effect of Chelating Agents on Intestinal

Chromium Absorption[a]

Addition	Number of Rats	[51]Chromium Serosal/Mucosal Side
None	27	0.35 ± 0.04
AA Mixture 200 µmoles	24	0.67 ± 0.06
None	5	0.20 ± 0.04
Histidine	5	0.58 ± 0.09
Imidazole	5	0.38 ± 0.01
DL-Penicillamine	6	0.66 ± 0.06

[a] 1 µg chromium and 20 mg addition in 20 ml HCO_3^- medium.

TABLE VIII

Different Mechanism of Action on

Intestinal Chromium Absorption

Addition	Final Ratio ^{51}Chromium Serosal/Mucosal Side	Within Tissue (cpm)
None	0.21 ± 0.04	173 ± 48
Glutamic acid	0.43 ± 0.06	218 ± 37
None	0.18 ± 0.01	123 ± 12
DL-Penicillamine	0.66 ± 0.06	26 ± 7

using equilibrium dialysis[19]. The order of effectiveness of
ligands detected in this system is similar but no identical to
the order in which they affect intestinal chromium transport[*].
Therefore it appears that keeping chromium soluble by
coordination is not the only function of these ligands and that
other mechanisms also influence chromium transport. If the
function of the ligand were only the maintenance of solubility
of chromium in the medium and if the dissociated hydrated
chromium ion diffused across the intestinal wall, the nature of
the ligand should not influence the tissue distribution of
chromium. An example given in Table VIII demonstrates, however,
that it does. Two agents, both increasing chromium transport,
caused an entirely different distribution pattern. Glutamate
increased the flux across the intestinal wall without affecting
the amount of chromium present within the tissue, whereas the
increased flux resulting from penicillamine was associated with
a significant decrease of chromium in the tissue. It is evident

---

[*] To be published separately.

from this comparison that the transport of chromium from mucosal
to serosal side is not just a simple diffusion process and that
it must consist of at least two different steps. If the first
of these were a diffusion into the mucosal cell and the second
a more specific one, transporting the intracellular chromium to
the serosal side, we could explain the observations in Table VIII
by different sites of action of the ligand: Glutamate would
increase the rate of the first step (diffusion into the cell)
with a resulting increased rate of the second step by an
increased intracellular/serosal concentration gradient.
Penicillamine, on the other hand, would primarily increase the
activity of the cell/serosa mechanism. This would increase
the flux of the first step by (lumen/mucosa) lowering the
concentration of chromium within the cell. These results,
while suggesting an intracellular site of action of some ligands,
give no information as to the form in which chromium crosses
the wall of the intestine. There is indirect evidence, to be
discussed later, that some chromium complex(es) are absorbed
intact.

III. CHROMIUM IN BLOOD

The rapid disappearance of intravenously injected chromium
chloride from the blood is shown in Fig. 2. The rate of loss is
considerably greater than that of the whole organism, so that
no radioactivity is detectable in the blood at a time when the
rest of the body still contains a considerable proportion of
the administered dose of ^{51}Cr. We have been consistently unable
to detect any biphasic behavior of the disappearance curve from
the blood such as has been demonstrated for manganese[20] or
vanadium[21]. We have suggested previously[1] that blood or
plasma chromium is not a meaningful indicator of the chromium
nutritional state of an individual, but probably only a measure

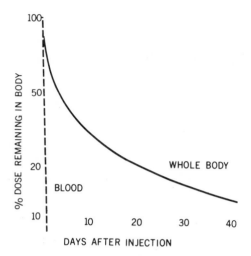

Fig. 2   Whole body radioactivity after intravenous injection of 0.1 µg/100 of ^{51}Cr (as $CrCl_3 \cdot 6H_2O$) in rats fed a low-chromium diet.   Broken line: ^{51}Cr in blood.

of recent dietary intake. K. M. Hambidge came to the same conclusion on the basis of detailed studies that failed to establish a relation between fasting plasma chromium levels and glucose tolerance[22].

The estimates of chromium concentration in the plasma of normal subjects in the fasting state have recently been revised downward. Feldman originally reported an average concentration of 29 with a range from 11 to 64 ppb[23]. Application of a more sensitive direct method using a double-beam instrument resulted in average values below 10 ppb[24]. Similar low concentrations were obtained by Hambidge with a spectrographic procedure[22]. These represent only approximately 1/100 of chromium concentration in most organs. However, it is known that certain conditions lead to an acute rise of plasma chromium in young, healthy subjects. Ingestion of glucose is followed by

two-fivefold increased concentrations within 30 to 90 minutes,
which subsequently decline again to the fasting level[25].
Possible mechanisms and nutritional significance have been
discussed in detail[1].

Attempts to duplicate these findings in rats proved to be
extremely difficult. Rats on either chromium-deficient Torula
yeast ration or commercial laboratory chows were injected with
$^{51}CrCl_3 \cdot 6H_2O$. After different periods of time, they were given
an intravenous injection of 125 mg glucose or of 100 MU of
insulin, or both, per 100 g body weight, and ^{51}Cr radioactivity
was measured in blood samples obtained from the tail before and
at intervals after the injection. The results can be summarized
as follows: Regardless of dietary status of the rats, the
insulin or glucose treatment did not influence the rate of
disappearance of ^{51}Cr when the test was performed within a few
hours after the dosing with $^{51}CrCl_3 \cdot 6H_2O$. Some degree of
response was observed in rats receiving chromium from natural
sources in the diet but only after a time of at least 3 days
had elapsed after the ^{51}Cr injection. Figure 3 demonstrates
the moderate rise of plasma radioactivity as a response to
insulin. These findings must be interpreted with great caution
because of the very low radioactivity appearing in the blood
stream. While these experiments suggested a small rise of
plasma ^{51}Cr, those performed with rats fed low-chromium
synthetic rations did not. Supplementing chromium chloride at
2 ppm in the drinking water had no effect. On the other hand
when ^{51}Cr in form of a yeast extract was administered, a very
significant rise of plasma radioactivity occurred following the
intravenous insulin challenge (Fig. 3).

These observations point out a second difference between
chromium chloride and glucose tolerance factor chromium. In
addition to a different absorption from the gastrointestinal

PLASMA ^{51}CHROMIUM AFTER INSULIN I.V.

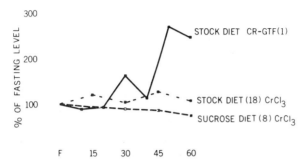

Fig. 3 Rats injected or stomach tubed with ^{51}Cr in the form indicated on figure. After more than 3 days, radioactivity in blood was determined on 20 µl before and after intravenous injection of insulin.

tract, the two chromium species, once absorbed, have a different affinity for the specific chromium pool from which the plasma increment following glucose or insulin is derived. It appears likely that the rat organism can convert some of the simple chromium salt into a form that does equilibrate with a specific pool, but only with time. The chemical nature of this chromium complex is as yet unknown.

These data suggest simple chromium salts, such as chromium chloride, disappear rapidly from the blood after they are absorbed, and that a small proportion may be built into a special organic complex. This complex becomes part of a pool from which chromium is released back into the blood following an acute rise of plasma insulin. If this specific pool were responsible for the regulation of the effectiveness of insulin in the organism,

glucose tolerance would depend on the dietary intake of glucose
tolerance factor chromium, but also on the rate of synthesis
of glucose tolerance factor from simple chromium salts.

IV. PLACENTAL TRANSPORT OF CHROMIUM

Chromium is present in the fetus and.in the newborn rat in
relatively high concentrations, but this fetal chromium pool is
not accessible to chromium chloride or acetate administered
to the mother during gestation in drinking water, by stomach
tube, or by intravenous injection[11,13]. On the other hand
the whole body chromium content of the newborn is influenced
by the concentration of chromium naturally occurring in the
diet of the mother. The young of rats fed a low-chromium
Torula yeast diet contained only half of the chromium that was
found in the young of mothers fed a natural diet of high-chromium
content[11]. This indicated clearly that there is a stringent
requirement of placental transport for specific forms of chromium
complexes, and it was subsequently shown that glucose tolerance
factor chromium prepared from yeast extracts does indeed go into
the fetus.

Table IX shows the distribution of ^{51}Cr radioactivity
in three organs of newborn rats as compared with the distribution
in their mother. The latter had been given three doses of a
[51]Cr-labeled yeast extract by stomach tube during gestation.
The concentration in all three fetal tissues investigated was
greater than in the corresponding maternal organ, but the fetal
liver had more than four times the concentration of the
maternal liver. These findings agree with those of other
investigators who have demonstrated concentrations of stable
chromium in the fetus and newborn much higher than those
found during adult life[15,26]. This demand of the fetus for
chromium cannot be met but by a specific form(s) of this

TABLE IX
^{51}Chromium Concentration in Maternal
and Newborn Tissues (N=3)[a]

(cpm/g tissue)	
Liver, maternal	48.0
Liver, fetal	187.0
Heart, maternal	29.7
Heart, fetal	45.8
Kidney, maternal	39.0
Kidney, fetal	44.5

[a] A pregnant rat received by stomach tube three doses of a
^{51}Cr-labeled yeast extract. Radioactivity was counted in
pooled organs from newborn litter and in corresponding
tissues from mother.

element in the mother's organism and diet; it may, therefore,
cause a considerable depletion of the maternal chromium stores
when the dietary supply is low. A similar situation may exist
in man. The hair chromium concentration of multiparous women
is significantly lower than that of nulliparae[8]. The question
of whether this decline in chromium levels with repeated
pregnancies is related to the progressive impairment of glucose
tolerance with increasing parity is of great importance in
nutrition research[22].

V. TISSUE DISTRIBUTION

The distribution of ^{51}Cr salts of different composition
and valence has been thoroughly investigated and has been found
to depend on the chemical nature and dose of the compound as

well as on the age of the test animal[13,27]. The distribution
of physiological doses of [51]chromium chloride in rats was
investigated by Hopkins[28]. Even with these low doses of
10 to 100 ng of chromium, there was a considerable accumulation
of chromium in the spleen, probably indicative of the removal
of colloidal chromium from the blood. A comparison of the
distribution of chromium given as chromium chloride versus that
given as glucose tolerance factor chromium from yeast extract
(Table X) reveals some interesting differences. In contrast
to the high affinity of chromium chloride for the spleen, glucose
tolerance factor chromium had no such preference. Concentration
of ^{51}Cr in the spleen ranked closely with levels in lung, heart,
intestines, pancreas, and brain, averaging close to 50% of the
concentration found in the liver. The latter organ ranked
highest in affinity to glucose tolerance factor chromium but not
to chromium chloride, followed by uterus, kidney, and bone. A
third group--muscle, ovaries, and aorta--had low concentrations
of chromium from glucose tolerance factor.

The high concentration of glucose tolerance factor chromium
in the liver as well as the high ratio of glucose tolerance
factor chromium in fetal versus maternal liver suggest that
this organ may be the site of the specific pool of biologically
important chromium in the organism. Direct evidence has not
yet been obtained for this hypothesis. However, liver is a
good source of glucose tolerance factor activity which exhibits
the biological properties of glucose tolerance factor from
yeast in its potentiation of the action of insulin in vitro
(unpublished results). Furthermore, rats raised on a natural
wheat-casein ration of high glucose tolerance factor content
contain in their livers a factor that greatly enhances glucose
tolerance of intact animals and of insulinized, eviscerated rat
preparations[29]. This factor is heat stable, as is glucose

TABLE X

Tissue Distribution of ^{51}Chromium after
Administration of ^{51}Chromium[a,b]

	^{51}Chromium-GTF		^{51}CrCl$_3 \cdot$6H$_2$O (Hopkins)
Liver	100,	100	100
Uterus	94,	101	
Kidney	84,	77	127
Bone	72,	62	
Lung	61,	53	39
Heart	59,	67	34
Intestines	56,	64	
Spleen	50,	51	222
Pancreas	49,	44	51
Brain	42,	62	39
Muscle	25,	33	
Ovaries	25,	16	226
Aorta	22,	0	

[a] In percent of concentration on liver.

[b] Data from two female rats, compared to results from reference[30].

tolerance factor; however, the relationship between these two agents is not yet clear.

VI. THE INTERACTION OF INSULIN WITH CHROMIUM

The dependence of the effect of chromium on the presence of exogenous or endogenous insulin has been demonstrated in a number of different systems[1]. These include glucose tolerance,

insulin hypoglycemia and glycogen formation in the intact rat,
and uptake and utilization of glucose for fat synthesis and
CO_2 production as well as cell entry of D-galactose in epididymal
fat tissue. The observations that chromium also increased the
effect of insulin on water permeability of isolated liver
mitochondria[30] and on the utilization of three amino acids
for protein synthesis[31] dissociated the mode of action from
glucose metabolism but left open the possibility that chromium
may be required as a cofactor for a membrane transport mechanism,
the efficiency of which becomes limiting at high but not at a
low activity. Since this model is compatible with the available
experimental data and is in contrast to the alternative hypothesis of chromium acting as a cofactor for insulin, experiments
were designed to test the validity of both[32].

It is known that the rate of glucose entry into the
epididymal fat cell is increased not only by insulin but also
by raising the concentration of glucose in the incubation
medium. When the effect of glucose tolerance factor chromium
on the glucose oxidation of epididymal fat tissue was measured
under these conditions, a different pattern emerged (Fig. 4).
Glucose tolerance factor more than doubled the slope of the
insulin response (4.2 to 8.9, P< 0.001), but it did not increase
the slope of the glucose-stimulated oxidation (6.6 to 7.3,
P> 0.1). These observations indicate that glucose tolerance
factor is not a cofactor for a membrane transport system; they
offer additional evidence for the theory of a close interaction
between it and insulin. The nature of this relation is not
clear yet. Polarographic studies[33] suggest the possibility
that chromium initiates the disulfide exchange between insulin
and membrane receptors, believed to be the first step through
which insulin increases the flux of glucose through the membrane.

Attempts to increase the activity of insulin by
reacting it *in vitro* with chromium chloride have been

EFFECT OF GTF ON CO_2 PRODUCTION STIMULATED BY:

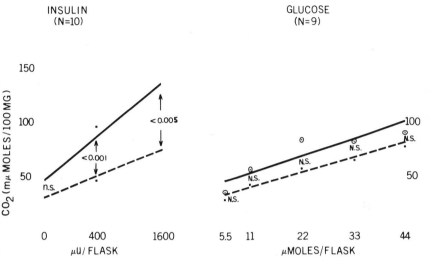

Fig. 4 Epididymal fat tissue from rats on a low-chromium Torula yeast diet was incubated for 2 hours in Krebs-Ringer phosphate medium containing 1 mg glucose and 10 mg bovine albumin/ml. Six pieces of tissue from each animal were used; three with and three without addition of glucose tolerance factor.

unsuccessful in our hands. Letting physiological concentrations of chromium stand in solution with insulin for a few hours results, if anything, in a product less effective than insulin (Table XI). This is in sharp contrast to the increased insulin activity that results from adding the hormone and chromium separately to tissue. Glucose tolerance factor, on the other hand, behaves differently in that it retains its potentiating effect even after several weeks of standing in solution with insulin.

In an effort to investigate the nature of this interaction, 7 MU of [131]iodo-insulin were left to react overnight with 7 ml

TABLE XI

Inactivation of Insulin by $CrCl_3$ In Vitro

versus Activation by GTF-Chromium

A. One MU Insulin and three levels of $CrCl_3$ after

Standing In Vitro

Glucose Uptake by Epididymal fat/100 mg
(N=12)

Control	48 ± 6
Reaction product	42 ± 5
1:10	42 ± 5
1:100	43 ± 6

B. GTF Reacted In Vitro with [131]Iodo-insulin

Insulin Peak Separated by Gel Filtration

Glucose Oxidation by Epididymal Fat
(cpm/100 mg, N=9)

No Insulin	50 µU Insulin Unreacted	50 µU Reacted	20 µU Reacted	10 µU Reacted
271	745	3433	2311	912
Increase	+587	+3136	+1973	+661
	$P<0.05$	$P<0.01$	$P<0.01$	$P<0.02$

---

of a charcoal eluate of an alcoholic extract from Brewers'
yeast grown in a chromium-supplemented medium. The solution
was put through a gel filtration column, and the resulting
fractions were counted for [131]iodine radioactivity and
subsequently lyophilized. The fractions constituting the main
[131]iodine peak were combined and concentrated in vacuo so that
1 ml contained the number of counts corresponding to 1 MU
insulin. Addition of this fraction at concentrations corresponding to 10, 20, and 50 MU insulin per flask stimulated
glucose oxidation significantly more than insulin alone

(Table XI). In order to interpret these findings, it must be realized that glucose tolerance factor in the absence of insulin does not significantly increase glucose oxidation, and that no insulin was present in these experiments other than that in the column fraction. Unless the passage through the gel imparted a much greater activity to the insulin, for which there is no evidence in the literature, we must conclude that insulin and glucose tolerance factor were present together in the ^{131}iodine peak. Because of the relatively small molecular weight of glucose tolerance factor, we would not expect that it would migrate with insulin unless a complex between the two was formed. The nature of this possible interaction is being investigated. If there is indeed such a product, it must be of much greater biological activity than insulin itself. It is not known whether this possible mechanism is also effective in vivo. The known acute rise of plasma chromium, which is possibly in the form of glucose tolerance factor, at a time when the insulin concentration also rises suggests some form of interaction within the living organism.

The time course of the interaction between chromium and insulin has been studied with chromium chloride measuring the rate of entry of D-galactose into the cells of epididymal fat tissue in vitro[34]. These experiments demonstrated that in the presence of chromium, insulin becomes effective without the lag phase that is observed when no chromium is present; they present evidence against the hypothesis that chromium increases the effect of insulin by inhibiting the destruction of the hormone by insulinase.

The time course of this effect was reinvestigated with glucose tolerance factor and a system that allows the rate of reaction of one piece of tissue to follow throughout the experiment. It has been shown[35] that insulin produces an

increase of the respiratory quotient of epididymal adipose
tissue in the Warburg apparatus. Because the magnitude of the
increase is proportional to the insulin concentration and
because it is easily measured, this procedure is used as an
assay for insulin and insulinlike activity.

When tested in this system, glucose tolerance factor, like
inorganic chromium chloride in previous experiments[34], was
ineffective in a noninsulin responsive system, such as the
epididymal fat tissue with acetate as a substrate. When glucose
was used as substrate, 200 µU of insulin produced a slight
positive change of RQ, and the presence of glucose tolerance
factor greatly increased this effect (Fig. 5). Insulin was
consistently of little effect in these experiments using
chromium-deficient tissue, and very high concentrations were
required to produce a significant effect. A representative
example of the rate of gas exchange and the effect of 400 µU
insulin with and without glucose tolerance factor is shown in
Fig. 6. The rate of gas exchange was not influenced by insulin
alone; but when glucose tolerance factor was present with the
hormone, the rate changed almost immediately after the
combination was added to the medium. Because of the total
ineffectiveness of this dose of insulin, this experiment allows
no comparison of the time-dependent action of glucose tolerance
factor and insulin versus insulin alone. By increasing the
concentration of the latter to 1600 µU/flask, a positive response
was obtained that was only slightly further increased when
glucose tolerance factor was present with insulin. Under these
conditions the resulting curves allow a valid comparison of the
time effect of these agents (Fig. 7). The addition of insulin
alone resulted in a change of the slope of the line but only
after almost 20 minutes, whereas the combination of insulin
with glucose tolerance factor changed the slope almost
immediately. This observation is interpreted in the sense that

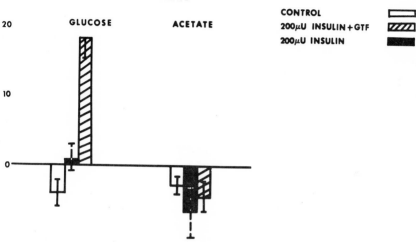

DEPENDENCE OF GTF EFFECT ON
INSULIN–RESPONSIVE SUBSTRATE

(N = 7)

Fig. 5   Six pieces of epididymal adipose tissue from
low-chromium rats were incubated for 2 hours in Krebs-Ringer
bicarbonate medium in a 95% O_2, 5% CO_2 atmosphere. After 1 hour,
saline or insulin or insulin and glucose tolerance factor
were added from side arm of Warburg vessel to main compartment.
Three pieces from each rat had glucose, the other three had
acetate as substrate (1 mg/ml).

glucose tolerance factor, like inorganic chromium, facilitates
the initial reaction of the hormone with its receptor sites in
the tissue.

VII.   CONCLUSION

The data reported or reviewed in this paper clearly
demonstrate great quantitative and qualitative differences in
the metabolism and biological effect of chromium, depending on

EFFECT OF GTF AND INSULIN ON GAS EXCHANGE
OF RAT EPIDIDYMAL FAT TISSUE

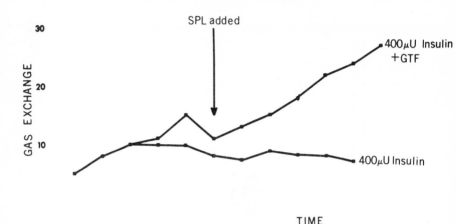

TIME

Fig. 6   Example of time course of gas exchange by epididymal
adipose tissue.   Conditions as in Fig. 5.

the form in which it is bound. When the element exists in
an organically bound form, such as is present in Brewers' yeast,
liver, kidney, wheat, and so on, it is absorbed better, has a
different tissue distribution, and is available to the fetus.
In this form chromium can be used to label physiologically
meaningful body pools, for which inorganic chromium is of little
use. In their effect on the potentiation of insulin in vitro,
both inorganic and organically bound chromium are qualitatively
similar, the latter having, however, a much greater activity
quantitatively.

All of the presently available evidence is consistent with
the hypothesis that the chromium-containing substance occurring
in Brewers' yeast and other natural sources, which is well

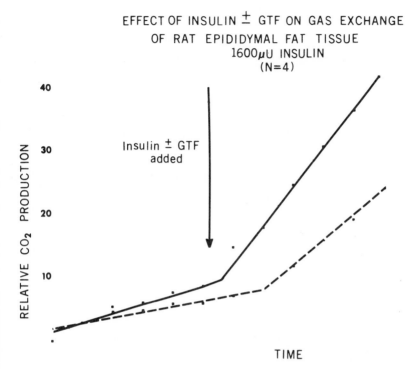

EFFECT OF INSULIN ± GTF ON GAS EXCHANGE
OF RAT EPIDIDYMAL FAT TISSUE
1600μU INSULIN
(N=4)

Fig. 7 Time course of gas exchange as influenced in
insulin alone (broken line) and insulin with glucose tolerance
factor (solid line). Conditions as in Fig. 5.

available for intestinal absorption and placental transport, is
identical with the insulin-potentiating principle. The chemical
properties, as far as determined, are identical, semipurified
preparations are active in all systems, and the biological
activity in glucose tolerance factor preparation parallels
their chromium content[1]. Finally, the dependence of the
biological action of glucose tolerance factor on the presence of
insulin is the same as that of simple chromium salts. It must
be realized, however, that conclusive proof can only come from
the identification of the chemical structure of the compound.

The problem of a classifying glucose tolerance factor in
a nutritional sense is difficult. Chromium is different from
most trace elements in that it is not, like the others, easily
built into its specific sites of action. The rat has a very
limited ability to utilize inorganic chromium salts for placental
transport. In man the effect of supplementation with chromium
chloride often takes weeks to appear, and this lag phase cannot
be overcome by higher doses. But chromium is also different
from cobalt, which has an absolute requirement for a special
organic binding. Monogastric mammals cannot synthesize
vitamin B_{12}, but there are indications that they can synthesize
the organic chromium compound, glucose tolerance factor, if only
at a limited rate. It is not known whether this synthesis occurs
within the organism itself or is a function of the intestinal
flora.

Work is now in progress to prepare sufficient quantities
of glucose tolerance factor for measuring its metabolism and its
effect on the impaired glucose tolerance in human subjects.

REFERENCES

[1]. Mertz, W., Physiol. Rev., 49, 164-231 (1969).

[2]. Mertz, W. and Schwarz, K., Am. J. Physiol., 196, 614-618
(1959).

[3]. Schroeder, H. A., J. Nutr., 88, 439-445 (1966).

[4]. Davidson, I. W. F. and Blackwell, W. L., Proc. Soc. Exptl.
Biol. Med., 127, 66-70 (1968).

[5]. Glinsmann, W. H. and Mertz, W., Metabolism, 15, 510-520
(1966).

[6]. Hopkins, L. L., Jr., Ransome-Kuti, O., and Majaj, A. S.,
Am. J. Clin. Nutr., 21, 203-211 (1968).

[7]. Levine, R. A., Streeten, D. H. P., and Doisy, R. J.,
Metabolism, 17, 114-125 (1968).

[8]. Hambidge, K. M. and Rodgerson, D. O., Am. J. Obstet.
      Gynecol., 103, 320-321 (1969).

[9]. Hambidge, K. M., Rodgerson, D. O., and O'Brien, D.,
      Diabetes, 17, 517-519 (1968).

[10]. Doisy, R. J., Streeten, D. H. P., and Chodos, R. B.,
      Proc. 2nd Annual Conf. on Trace Substances in
      Environmental Health, Columbia, Missouri: University
      of Missouri Press, 1968, p. 75-82.

[11]. Mertz, W., Roginski, E. E., Feldman, J. F., and
      Thurman, D. E., J. Nutr., 99, 363-367 (1967).

[12]. Donaldson, R. M. and Barreras, R. F., J. Lab. Clin. Med.,
      68, 484-493 (1966).

[13]. Visek, W. J., Whitney, I. B., Kuhn, U. S. G., III, and
      Comar, C. L., Proc. Soc. Exptl. Biol. Med., 84, 610-615
      (1953).

[14]. Mertz, W., Roginski, E. E., and Reba, R. C., Am. J.
      Physiol., 209, 489-494 (1965).

[15]. Schroeder, H. A., Balassa, J. J., and Tipton, I. H.,
      J. Chronic Diseases, 15, 941-964 (1962).

[16]. Tipton, I. H. and Stewart, P. L., Proc. 3rd Annual Conf.
      on Trace Substances in Environmental Health
      (D. D. Hemphill, ed.) Columbia, Missouri, 1970, p. 305-
      330.

[17]. Wilson, T. H. and Wiseman, G., J. Physiol., 123, 116
      (1954).

[18]. Park, C. R., Membrane Transport and Metabolism
      (A. Kleinzeller and A. Kotyk, eds.) New York: Academic
      Press, 1961.

[19]. Rollinson, C. L. and Rosenbloom, E. W., Coordination
      Chemistry (S. Kirschner, ed.) New York: Plenum Press,
      1969, p. 108-125.

[20]. Cotzias, G. C., Borg, D. C., and Bertinchamps, A. J.,
Metal-Binding in Medicine (J. J. Seven, ed.) Philadelphia,
Pennsylvania: Lippincott, 1960, p. 50-58.

[21]. Hopkins, L. L., Jr. and Mohr, H. H., The Newer Trace
Elements in Nutrition (W. Mertz and W. E. Cornatzer, eds.)
New York: Marcel Dekker, in press.

[22]. Hambidge, K. M., Rodgerson D. O., and O'Brien, D., The
Newer Trace Elements in Nutrition (W. Mertz and
W. E. Cornatzer, eds.) New York: Marcel Dekker, in press.

[23]. Feldman, F. J., Knoblock, E. C., and Purdy, W. C.,
Anal. Chim. Acta, 38, 489-497 (1967).

[24]. Feldman, F. J., Report at the VIIIth International
Congress of Nutrition, Prague, 1969.

[25]. Glinsmann, W. H., Feldman, F. J., and Mertz, W., Science,
152, 1243-1245 (1966).

[26]. Mikosha, A., Nauk. Zap. Stainislavs'k Med. Inst., 1959,
85-89. (Chem. Abstr., 59, 7969, 1963).

[27]. Vittorio, P. V., Wright, E. W., and Sinnott, B. E.,
Can. J. Biochem. Physiol., 40, 1677-1683 (1962).

[28]. Hopkins, L. L., Jr., Am. J. Physiol., 209, 731-735 (1965).

[29]. Mertz, W. and Schwarz, K., Am. J. Physiol., 203, 53-56
(1962).

[30]. Campbell, W. J. and Mertz, W., Am. J. Physiol., 204,
1028-1030 (1963).

[31]. Roginski, E. E. and Mertz, W., J. Nutr., 97, 525-530
(1969).

[32]. Roginski, E. E., Toepfer, E. W., Polansky, M. M., and
Mertz, W., Fed. Proc., 29, 695, Abstract, (1970).

[33]. Christian, G. D., Knoblock, E. C., Purdy, W. C., and
Mertz, W., Biochim. Biophys. Acta, 66, 420-423 (1963).

[34]. Mertz, W. and Roginski, E. E., J. Biol. Chem., 238, 868-872 (1963).

[35]. Ball, E. G., Martin, D. B., and Cooper, O. J. Biol. Chem., 234, 774-780 (1959).

Chapter 8

METABOLISM OF [51]CHROMIUM IN HUMAN SUBJECTS[1]

NORMAL, ELDERLY, AND DIABETIC SUBJECTS

R. J. Doisy, D. H. P. Streeten, M. L. Souma,

M. E. Kalafer, S. I. Rekant, and T. G. Dalakos

Departments of Biochemistry and Medicine
State University of New York
Upstate Medical Center
Syracuse, New York

I.   INTRODUCTION

Previous reports from this laboratory[1,2] have suggested that chromium deficiency may exist in the elderly population. Impaired glucose tolerances in some elderly subjects were restored to normal after supplementation of their diet with 150 µg/day of trivalent chromium. A preliminary report[2] on

155

oral ^{51}Cr absorption tests suggested no evidence of malabsorption of chromium in elderly subjects. However, it was observed that insulin-requiring diabetics appeared to absorb more chromium than did maturity-onset diabetics or normal control subjects. This report is a continuation of that study and a preliminary report on the metabolism of intravenously administered ^{51}Cr in normal and diabetic subjects.

II. MATERIALS AND METHODS

For the oral ^{51}Cr absorption tests, the subjects were 82 patients in the State University of New York, Upstate Medical Center. Twenty-four were normal individuals aged 10 to 69. Seventeen were elderly normal subjects aged 70 and over. Twenty-two were insulin-requiring diabetics, and known to develop ketosis if not given exogenous insulin. Ten were diabetics controlled by oral agents or diet, and nine were diabetics whose requirement for insulin was questionable.

For the intravenous ^{51}Cr study the normal subjects consisted of five males and two females, with an average age of 25 years and weight of 76 kg. The insulin-requiring diabetics consisted of two males and eight females, average age 34 and weight of 63 kg.

For the oral ^{51}Cr absorption tests, 100 µCi of ^{51}Cr (about 10 µg) were administered orally with breakfast. Plasma samples were obtained at 1, 2, 4, 24, 48, and 72 hours and 24 hour urine collections were made for 3 days. For the intravenous ^{51}Cr turnover studies, 50 µCi of ^{51}Cr (about 1 µg) were administered intravenously and plasma samples were obtained at 10 minutes, 1, 2, 4, and 24 hours, and daily thereafter for 14 days.

The chromium used in these studies was purchased as sodium chromate[2/] (sterile) and reduced with excess ascorbic acid[3/]

immediately before use. Initial studies demonstrated that all
radioactivity was present in the plasma, and that there were
no detectable counts associated with the red-cell fraction
after washing with saline.

Plasma and urine samples were counted in a Packard
Autogamma Scintillation Counter and corrected for decay and
background counts. All samples were counted to at least 5%
accuracy.

Standard oral glucose tolerance tests (100 g glucose)
were carried out in most subjects 14 days after administration
of the [51]Cr. Plasma samples collected during glucose tolerance
tests (and samples from the previous 13 days) were separated
by centrifugation into albumin and globulin fractions after
precipitation with saturated ammonium sulfate.

III.   RESULTS

A.   Oral [51]Chromium Absorption Tests

The plasma ^{51}Cr levels after oral administration of
chromium (expressed as percentage of the dose administered per
liter of plasma) are shown for the various groups of subjects
in Table I. The insulin-requiring diabetics display higher
plasma chromium levels than do the other three groups. The
2- and 4-hour levels for the insulin-requiring diabetics are
significantly higher (P<0.05) when compared with the other
three groups treated as a whole.

The urinary excretion of ^{51}Cr after oral administration is
shown in Table II. Again, the insulin-requiring diabetics show
significantly higher excretion (P<0.05) at 24 and 72 hours, and
total excretion over the 3 days. The elderly subjects and
maturity-onset diabetics appear to absorb and excrete amounts
of chromium similar to the normal subjects.

TABLE I

Plasma ^{51}Cr Concentration (Percent of Original Dose)

Subject		1 hour	2 hours	4 hours	24 hours	48 hours	72 hours
				Time after Administration of ^{51}Cr[a]			
Normal subjects age 21-69	x̄	0.099(11)[b]	0.082(23)	0.073(20)	0.080(11)	0.181(9)	0.139(9)
	SEM ±	0.031	0.021	0.015	0.028	0.104	0.067
Normal subjects age 70 and over	x̄	0.025(5)	0.060(16)	0.042(10)	0.030(10)	0.021(9)	0.017(7)
	SEM ±	0.009	0.010	0.009	0.005	0.005	0.006
Insulin-dependent diabetics	x̄	0.389(16)	0.398(18)	0.269(16)	0.185(14)	0.052(15)	0.125(11)
	SEM ±	0.160	0.183	0.128	0.112	0.016	0.044
Diabetics controlled by oral agent or diet values	x̄	no	0.038(9)	0.040(9)	0.024(7)	0.022(7)	0.014(4)
	SEM ±		0.009	0.008	0.005	0.004	0.003

a/ Numbers in parentheses indicate numbers of patients studied.

b/ In initial studies, plasma samples were obtained at 2 and 4 hours only.

TABLE II

Mean Urine ^{51}Cr Output (Percent of Original Dose)

Subject	Time after Administration of ^{51}Cr [a]			
	0-24 hours	24-48 hours	48-72 hours	Total
Normal subject x̄ age 21-69	0.466(24)[b]	0.158(24)	0.064(21)	0.695(21)
SEM ±	0.052	0.032	0.008	0.066
Normal subjects x̄ age 70 and over	0.364(17)	0.162(17)	0.097(17)	0.623(17)
SEM ±	0.064	0.029	0.039	0.099
Insulin dependent x̄ diabetics	0.893(22)	0.316(22)	0.210(18)	1.383(18)
SEM ±	0.131	0.080	0.063	0.169
Diabetics controlled x̄ by oral agent or diet	0.453(10)	0.107(10)	0.038(9)	0.636(9)
SEM ±	0.104	0.016	0.005	0.121

a/ Mean values which are significantly different (P<0.05) from means in normals under 70 years are underlined.

b/ Numbers in parentheses indicate numbers of patients studied.

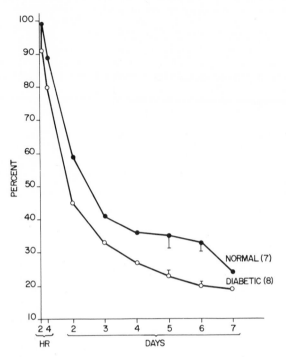

Fig. 1 Plasma ^{51}Cr levels vs. time in normal and diabetic
subjects. Percent of initial count after intravenous
administration.

B. Intravenous ^{51}Chromium Turnover Studies

The plasma levels of ^{51}Cr after intravenous administration
of 50 μCi are shown in Fig. 1. The values are expressed as
percent of the initial count rate (that is, 10 minutes and
1 hour counts for each subject were averaged and called 100%).
Days 5 and 6 are significantly lower (P<0.01) in the
insulin-requiring diabetics. Although not shown, external
counting with a probe was carried out in a number of subjects.
Although this is not a very precise procedure, it was noted in
normal subjects that increased counts over the liver and

precordial regions occurred between days 4 - 7. This is
compatible with the slower decline in plasma ^{51}Cr at that time.
The importance of this observation is not known.

The urinary excretion data for the first 24 hours are
shown in Table III and are expressed as total counts appearing
in the urine in 24 hours. The insulin-requiring diabetics have
significantly greater counts in the urine, there being no
overlap between the normal subjects and the diabetics. The
maturity-onset diabetics excrete near normal amounts of chromium.
Table IV shows the plasma ^{51}Cr counts during the glucose
tolerance tests (GTT) in normal and diabetic subjects. The

TABLE III

Urinary Excretion of ^{51}Cr during first 24 Hours (CPM × 10^6)

Normals (7)[a]	Juvenile diabetics (10)	Adult-onset diabetics (6)
2.18	3.95	2.81
1.95	2.96	2.28
1.77	2.75	2.05
1.63	2.68	1.98
1.45	2.56	1.23
1.20	2.49	1.15
1.06	2.46	1.92 ± 0.28
1.60 ± 0.15[b]	2.35	
	2.29	
	2.27	
	2.67 ± 0.15[c]	

[a] Number of subjects in parentheses.

[b] Mean ± SE.

[c] P<0.001, normal vs. juvenile diabetics.

TABLE IV

Plasma ^{51}Cr Levels during Glucose Tolerance Tests[a]

(Counts/minute/cc)

Time,min.	Normals						
	M[b]	M	M	M	M	F	F
0	99	98	85	94	101	217	184
30	94	91	82	89	101	302	156
60	93	87	88	88	97	211	335
90	88	94	82	77	98	257	182
120	83	89	80	93	98	166	194

Time,min.	Insulin-Requiring Diabetics							
	F	M	F	F	F	F	F	F
0	90	94	85	91	87	93	150	86
30	123	86	78	75	65			
60	101	51	80	66	73	74	119	66
90	88	57	78	67	64			
120	97	42	75	67	62	58	93	75

[a] GTT's carried out 14 days after administration of ^{51}Cr.

[b] M, male subjects; F, female subjects.

normal male subjects show no rise in radioactivity during the
GTT's, whereas the diabetics appear to show a fall in radioactivity. The urine appeared to be the major route of excretion
of intravenously injected chromium. Less than 1% of the dose
appeared in the stools of two healthy subjects during 5 days
following the injection.

Table V shows the plasma distribution of radioactivity in
one normal female subject. These results indicate that both

TABLE V

Plasma ^{51}Cr Distribution during Glucose Tolerance Test

(Based on Ammonium Sulfate Fractionation)

Time,min.	Total cpm/cc	Precipitate[a]	Supernate
0	184	57	127
30	156	35	121
60	335	74	261
90	182	70	112
120	194	61	133

[a] One ml of saturated ammonium sulfate was added to 1 ml of plasma and the precipitate separated by centrifugation.

the globulin and albumin fractions show changes in radioactivity after a glucose load in this subject. In addition the fasting sample is representative of all subjects studied daily throughout in terms of the relative distribution of ^{51}Cr. In contrast to the animal studies by Hopkins and Schwarz[3] the human subjects carry only 30 to 40% of the administered chromium in the globulin fraction, whereas in rats the bulk of the chromium is carried in the globulin fraction by siderophilin. The albumin/globulin ratio of ^{51}Cr was similar in diabetic and normal subjects.

IV. DISCUSSION

The oral ^{51}Cr absorption data can be interpreted in at least two ways. First, since the insulin-requiring diabetics showed increased plasma levels associated with increased urinary excretion of ^{51}Cr, there might have been increased absorption in these diabetic subjects. Unfortunately, a total balance was not established (that is, ^{51}Cr in the feces was not

measured), so the amount of chromium absorbed is not known.
(Because so little chromium is absorbed, total balance studies
were not considered meaningful.)

Second, it is possible that the diabetic subjects absorbed
the same amount of ^{51}Cr as the normal subjects but were unable
to utilize the chromium in a normal manner, which resulted in
increased plasma levels and an increased urinary excretion.

The question of dosage could be important as to whether the
amount of chromium administered is a tracer dose or a physiological dose. Approximately 10 µg of chromium were given orally.
This is one-seventh the amount that normally occurs in the diet,
and assuming 1% absorption this would mean 0.1 µg was absorbed,
probably a tracer amount.

The data based on the intravenous administration of ^{51}Cr
also demonstrate that the diabetic subjects excreted more
chromium in the urine. Since plasma ^{51}Cr levels were consistently somewhat lower throughout the period of study, this
might be interpreted as an inability to utilize the chromium.
In 24 hours the diabetics excreted 41% of the administered dose,
whereas the normal subjects excreted only 25%. The dose of
^{51}Cr administered intravenously was approximately 1 µg. There
is some evidence that this may be a physiological dose not a
tracer dose. Thus interpretation must be qualified. The
average weight of the diabetics was 63 kg, the average weight
of the control group was 76 kg; thus the diabetics might be
expected to have higher plasma levels of chromium based on their
smaller metabolic mass.

Based on the data available from our studies with chromium,
it is not possible to state with certainty whether increased
absorption or underutilization of the chromium is responsible
for the increased urinary excretion of chromium by

insulin-requiring diabetics. However, both increased absorption and underutilization of chromium seem likely in insulin-requiring diabetics. Whether this is a cause or result of the disease is not known, but the fact that abnormalities of chromium metabolism exist in insulin-requiring diabetics seems certain.

The plasma ^{51}Cr levels during glucose tolerance tests provide some preliminary data of interest even though the sex distribution of the subjects is biased. In general terms it is evident that a glucose load in diabetic subjects causes a fall in plasma ^{51}Cr in contrast to normal subjects who show no fall in plasma ^{51}Cr. GTT's were carried out 14 days after administration of the ^{51}Cr. This was done on the premise that labeled chromium is converted into glucose tolerance factor (GTF). Assuming conversion, the greater the time interval between administration of ^{51}Cr and the GTT, the greater the percentage of label that may be incorporated into the GTF pool. Only two subjects (female controls) showed any significant increase in plasma radioactivity during the glucose tolerance tests. One of these subjects was the mother of three children and might be anticipated to be chromium deficient based on the work of Hambidge and Rodgerson[4]. The control male subjects were young (that is, average age was 25) and based on the data of Schroeder, Balassa, and Tipton[5] would not be expected to be chromium deficient. Thus if they are not deficient in chromium, then presumably little or no ^{51}Cr would be incorporated into the GTF pool. It is known, however, that stable chromium does rise in the plasma of normal subjects after a glucose load[6].

Mobilization of chromium (that is, as GTF?) is a normal response to a glucose load, yet it is clear from our data that insulin-requiring diabetics did not increase the amount of ^{51}Cr in their plasma. This suggests there was no ^{51}Cr in the

pool that is mobilized after a glucose load. On the contrary
the plasma levels of ^{51}Cr fell, possibly due to increased
urinary excretion. No insulin was administered on the day of
the glucose tolerance tests and the blood glucose levels were
elevated in the fasting state and rose to the 300 to
600 mg/100 cc range, and thus diuresis presumably occurred.
Schroeder's data[7] on urinary excretion of chromium during
glucose tolerance tests in diabetics suggest a rather substantial loss of chromium in the first 2 hours after a glucose
load.

The sites of synthesis and storage of GTF are unknown, but
it is likely that two or more forms of chromium exist in plasma.
It is possible that as glucose is lost in the urine, inorganic
chromium is also lost. Normal subjects may show an increase
in stable plasma chromium due to an increase in the GTF fraction,
but all subjects may show an increased urinary excretion of
chromium, that is, both inorganic and GTF chromium.

Due to the low amount of radioactivity present in the
plasma, electrophoretic patterns for separation of the radioactivity were not feasible. However, the plasma separation into
albumin and globulin fractions with ammonium sulfate was of
interest. The amounts of ^{51}Cr in normal and diabetic plasma
fractions were not different. It is not known whether
precipitation alters the binding of the chromium to the proteins
or not. It was noted, however, that if the supernatant fraction
(that is, albumin) was saturated with excess ammonium sulfate,
the bulk of the counts (that is, 80%) did not come down with the
precipitate. This suggests that the ^{51}Cr present in this
fraction may not be associated with the albumin, but may be in
the form of a soluble compound of low molecular weight. GTF is
thought to be a low molecular weight, soluble, and dialyzable

compound[8]. Note added in proof: More recently using ultra-filtration techniques (Centriflo membrane CF 50), it was found that the ^{51}Cr associated with the plasma protein fractions is not filterable. Thus ammonium sulfate fractionation appears to disrupt or change the binding of ^{51}Cr by albumin and globulins.

In conclusion, it would appear that insulin-requiring diabetics display abnormalities in chromium metabolism. Recent reports on the metabolism of zinc in diabetic subjects suggest that similar abnormalities may exist for zinc. Diabetics excrete two- to threefold more zinc in the urine than do normal subjects. Again, whether absorption of zinc is the same or higher in diabetics is not known. It is possible that there is a kidney defect(s) associated with diabetes that leads to increased loss of trace metals in general. Further studies are necessary before this question can be answered.

---

1. Supported by U.S. Army Research and Development Command Contract No. DADA 17-68-C-8119, U.S. Public Health Service Grant No. AM 5252, and U.S. Public Health Service Grant No. RR 00229.
2. Chromotope-Na, E. R. Squibb & Sons.
3. Cevalin-Eli Lilly & Co.

REFERENCES

[1]. Levine, R. A., Streeten, D. H. P., and Doisy, R. J., Metabolism, 17, 114 (1968).

[2]. Doisy, R. J., Streeten, D. H. P., Levine, R. A., and Chodos, R. B., Trace Substances in Environmental Health II, Columbia, Missouri: University of Missouri, 1968, p. 75-81.

[3]. Hopkins, L. L., Jr. and Schwarz, K., Biochim. Biophys. Acta, 90, 484 (1964).

[4]. Hambidge, K. M. and Rodgerson, D. O., Am. J. Obstet. Gynecol., 103, 320 (1968).

[5]. Schroeder, H. A., Balassa, J. J., and Tipton, I. H., J. Chron. Dis., 15, 941 (1962).

[6]. Glinsmann, W. H., Feldman, F. J., and Mertz, W., Science, 152, 1243 (1966).

[7]. Schroeder, H. A., Am. J. Clin. Nutr., 21, 230 (1968).

[8]. Mertz, W., Physiol. Rev., 49, 165 (1969).

Chapter 9

CHROMIUM NUTRITION IN THE MOTHER AND THE GROWING CHILD

K. M. Hambidge

B. F. Stolinsky Research Laboratories
Department of Pediatrics
University of Colorado Medical Center
Denver, Colorado

The biological role of chromium and some important
metabolic functions of this essential trace element have been
established[1]. Moreover, the results of therapeutic trials
of dietary chromium supplementation [2-4] have demonstrated
that chromium deficiency can be implicated in human disease;
indeed, analyses of autopsy material[5-7] have indicated that
such a deficiency may be relatively common, especially in the
United States. Thus it appears that chromium is an essential
micronutrient of special potential interest to those concerned
with human health and nutrition.

Tipton's studies[8] demonstrated that mean tissue chromium
concentrations underwent a marked decline with increasing age,
suggesting that chromium deficiency was primarily the prerog-
ative of the middle aged and elderly. However, the young are
also at risk from suboptimal chromium nutrition, at least in a
number of special circumstances, and it is the preliminary
results of laboratory chromium investigations in the young
living subject that will provide the basis for this discussion.

The investigation of chromium nutritional status and the
detection of a deficiency state in the individual subject
present a challenging problem. Well-controlled therapeutic
trials of chromium supplementation, with serial observations
of the effects on glucose tolerance, provide a reliable test
for chromium deficiency and also a measurement of the clinical
sequelae of such a deficiency. However, this approach is
applicable only to small groups of subjects and is very tedious
for the patient; it is especially difficult with the child and
the pregnant woman. Even when such studies can be undertaken,
an initial screening device to select those subjects likely to
be chromium deficient, other than on the basis of impaired
glucose tolerance, would be invaluable. This would help to
eliminate those whose disease is caused by factors other than
chromium deficiency and would probably explain some of the
conflicting reports on the efficacy of chromium supplementation.

Thus in order to study chromium nutrition in the young
subject, it was desirable to start in the laboratory. In
contrast to studies of autopsy material, the selection of
samples readily available for analysis in the living subject
is strictly limited. These studies have been directed primarily
to the analysis of serum, hair, and urine, and an assessment of
the value of such analyses in determining the individual's
chromium status. Each of these samples and some additional

data will be discussed with particular reference to the newborn, infant, older child, and the mother during and following pregnancy.

I. INSTRUMENTATION AND ANALYTICAL METHODOLOGY

The first essential prerequisite for laboratory study is for analytical instrumentation and techniques capable of accurately measuring nanogram quantities of chromium in biological materials. Economy of sample size is also of importance for studies involving young subjects. These requirements are met with emission spectrochemical techniques, using a 1.5-meter direct reading spectrometer and a static argon dc arc chamber[9,10]. The crucial feature of this instrumentation with respect to sensitivity and precision of the analyses is the arc chamber; this was developed by William Gordon[11-13] to whom I am indebted for invaluable advice in the application of his developments to the trace analysis of biological samples.

All samples are ashed prior to analysis, primarily because the organic material adversely effects arcing characteristics. A low-temperature asher is used for the oxidation of organic material in serum, hair, and urine; this approach has proved extremely satisfactory for these samples[10], though complete removal of organic material has been much more difficult with other materials such as red cells, liver, and muscle. Recoveries of ^{51}Cr have been complete and there has been no detectable sample contamination resulting from this procedure. Moreover, the product is an ideal form for subsequent handling.

II. SERUM

In the case of serum, which is separated and stored in acid-washed polystyrene tubes, a measured volume is pipetted

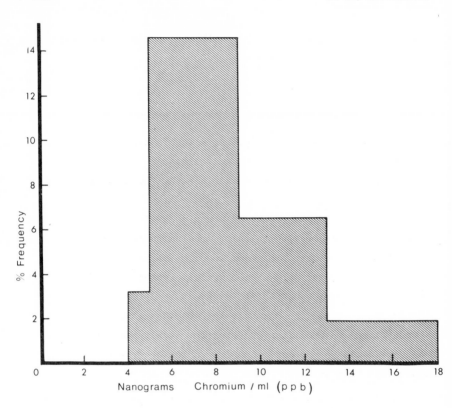

Fig. 1   Distribution of serum chromium levels in 31 normal
adults.

into a glass boat, oven dried, and then ashed in the
low-temperature asher (LTA). The ash is dissolved in situ with
100 µl 1.5 N hydrochloric acid per milliliter of original
serum; 20 µl aliquots, equivalent to 200 µl serum, are pipetted
onto the tip of three solid pointed carbon electrodes onto which
silver chloride buffer has previously been precipitated. The
electrodes are loaded into the arc chamber in batches of ten.
Each serum is analyzed in triplicate; the mean relative standard
deviation (RSD) for the serum assay is 6%.

Figure 1 illustrates the distribution of chromium concentrations obtained in the analysis of random serums from 31

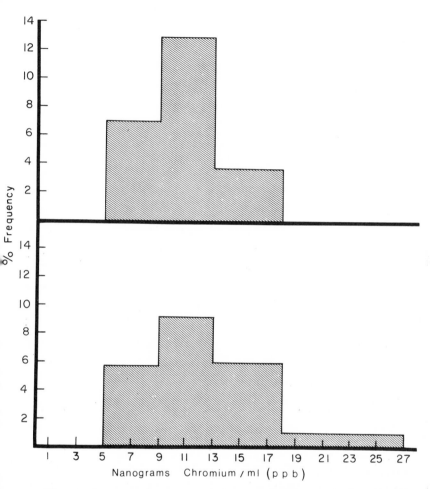

Fig. 2   Fasting serum chromium concentration - distribution
in 21 normal children (upper) and in 30 juvenile diabetics
(lower).

normal young adults.   Figure 2 illustrates the similar distri-
butions for early morning serum samples from 21 normal
children and 30 children with juvenile diabetes mellitus.
There was no correlation between serum chromium concentrations
and blood sugar levels of the diabetic children, which ranged
from 70 to 386 mg/100 ml.   No significant variations from these

serum chromium concentrations have been detected with different
age groups, pregnancy, parity, disorders of carbohydrate
metabolism, or in association with evidence of chromium
deficiency. On the basis of results from studies of both
^{51}Cr and ^{52}Cr, Mertz has concluded that serum chromium concentrations are not a valid index of chromium nutritional status[1].
Certainly these results do not conflict with this conclusion.

In contrast to solitary serum chromium estimations,
measurement of the serum chromium response to an oral glucose
load[14] is one of the most promising means of investigating
human nutrition. The absence of such a response, that is, no
increase in serum chromium levels, indicates that at least
one physiologically important pool of the body chromium may be
depleted. In my own experience the increase in serum chromium
levels most frequently coincides with the increase in plasma
immunoassayable insulin (Fig. 3). In approximately 30% of such
tests, however, there has been no correlation with plasma
insulin and the increase in serum chromium has not occurred
at any particular time interval after the glucose load.

More problematical has been the absence of any detectable
increase in serum chromium levels in less than 25% of glucose
loading tests on normal subjects with no impairment of glucose
tolerance. There are several possible theoretical explanations
other than chromium deficiency for this observation. A small
response of less that 10 to 20% increase over fasting levels
may go undetected with present analytical methodology, or an
increase may be missed between the half-hour intervals at which
blood is collected. It is also possible that a relatively
rapid removal rate of chromium from the circulation may balance
any release of glucose tolerance factor into the blood.

In particular this latter possibility has to be considered
in the pregnant woman, in whom the placenta is a potent

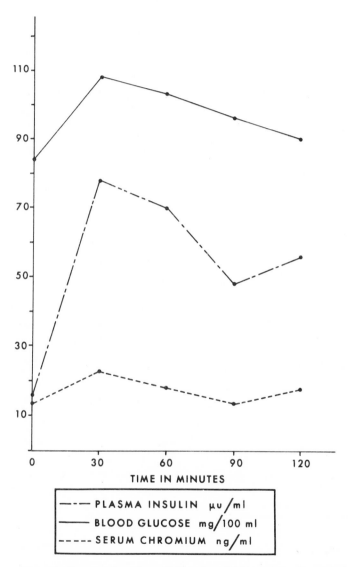

Fig. 3 Serum chromium following 100 g oral glucose load
(female 15 years).

additional factor in the removal of glucose tolerance factor
from the circulation. The serum chromium response to glucose
loading tests in young adult women is summarized in relation to
pregnancy in Table I. None of these subjects had any evidence
of impaired glucose tolerance. The left-hand column of the
table includes nonpregnant women and women of less than 36 weeks
gestation (the proportion of nonresponders in the latter group
being identical with that of the nonpregnant women). Of 16
tests on 16 different subjects, 4 tests or 25% of the total had
no detectable response. This proportion was very similar to
that of 19 subjects tested within two months postpartum, shown
in the right-hand column. In the center column are results of
tests on seven subjects during the last month of gestation.
Five of these tests, or 71% of the total, had no detectable
increase in serum chromium; though the numbers are small, this
difference is statistically significant.

The gestational diabetic merits particular attention in
view of the evidence for severe depletion of maternal chromium
reserves in pregnancy, which will be discussed later, and
because of the increased peripheral resistance to the action
of insulin that is characteristic of these patients[15]. At
this time the serum chromium response to an oral glucose load
has been studied in only twelve such subjects, seven of whom
had no detectable response. The results of one of these tests
are illustrated in Fig. 4; this particular subject had an
abnormally high insulin response in addition to impaired
glucose tolerance.

One important limitation of this test results from the
fact that the increase in serum chromium is probably mediated
directly or indirectly through the release of endogenous
insulin[14]. It is, therefore, not valid in the
insulin-dependent juvenile diabetic, whose β cells are totally

TABLE I

Serum Chromium Response to Oral Glucose Load

in Women of Child-Bearing Age with Normal Glucose Tolerance

	Less than 36 weeks gestation	36-40 weeks gestation	Less than 8 weeks postpartum	Total
Increase in serum chromium	12	2	15	29
No increase in serum chromium	4	5	4	13
Total	16	7	19	42
Percent of total with no detectable increase	25	71	21	31

(P<0.05)

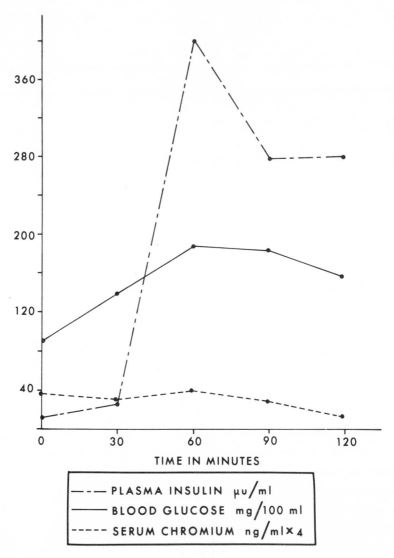

Fig. 4   Serum chromium following 100 g oral glucose load (female 22 years - 36 weeks gestation).

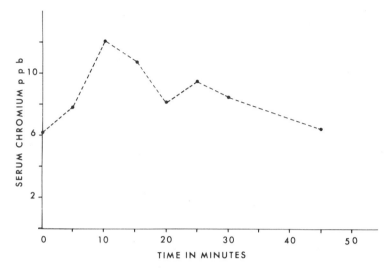

Fig. 5   Serum chromium following administration of insulin
intravenously (0.1 units/kg body weight).

depleted of insulin. Even though the response to exogenous
insulin (Fig. 5) may provide a valid alternative test, in
practice it is not so acceptable as the oral glucose load.

III.   URINE

Though the urinary excretion of chromium[16,17] has
received very little study, urine is a material of considerable
potential value in the investigation of chromium nutrition[18].
The chromium in urine is derived from the dialyzable fraction
of the serum chromium[19], which includes the biologically
active glucose tolerance factor, whereas chromium being
transported attached to transferrin is not excreted. Thus
measurement of variations in urine chromium excretion probably
provides an indirect measurement of the biologically active
component of the serum chromium.

Analysis of chromium in urine has been technically more difficult than for serum[10], and the precision of analyses less satisfactory (one relative standard deviation (RSD) for pooled urine samples is equal to 14%); although it has been impossible to measure small variations in excretion rates, major differences can be detected with confidence. The mean 24-hour urine chromium excretion for 20 young adults has been 8.4 µg, with individual results ranging from 1.6 to 21 µg/24 hours. Corresponding figures for 18 children, aged 4 to 15 years, were 5.5 (0.8 to 11.5) µg/24 hours.

Major differences from these figures have been observed in the urinary chromium excretion of two insulin-treated juvenile diabetics (Table II), whereas five others have had excretion rates within or near the normal range. These two subjects, a girl aged 9 years and a boy aged 10 years, had extremely high chromium excretion rates, which supports the conclusion[20] that chromium metabolism is abnormal in the insulin-dependent diabetic. One possible etiologic factor in this excessive loss of chromium is the effect of the exogenous insulin, which enters the circulation in an unphysiologic manner. Present data are inadequate to evaluate the effect of insulin therapy, but urine chromium excretion has been within the normal range for two children at the time of the acute clinical onset of their diabetes, prior to the commencement of insulin therapy.

IV. HAIR

The apparent remoteness of hair from metabolically important organs of the body together with the potential risk of external contamination prior to collection have been major objections to the utilization of this material for trace element studies. Certain elements, notably arsenic[21], have such a great

TABLE II
Urine Chromium Excretion
Children with Juvenile Diabetes Mellitus

| Insulin-treated | | Preinsulin therapy | |
Age (Years)	(µg Cr/24 hours)	Age (Years)	(µg Cr/24 hours)
8	10.2	8	5.4
9	41.6	14	3.2
9	3.4		
10	50.9		
13	8.9		
14	6.4		
15	12.5		

affinity for keratin that following external contact with the hair shaft they cannot be removed by usual washing procedures. As will be discussed later, however, this does not apply to chromium and as there is no metabolic turnover in the hair shaft[21] it is reasonable to assume that the chromium present in the shaft was incorporated at the time of keratinization in the hair follicle. Though the chromium in the matrix cells must be derived directly or indirectly from the rich network of blood capillaries surrounding the hair follicle, the details of this supply and its relationship to chromium uptake by other tissues require clarification. Initial investigations with ^{51}Cr in the rat have not been successful, but results of studies using inorganic chromium compounds are difficult to interpret[22]. Nevertheless it is logical to assume from these considerations that hair chromium concentrations are influenced by the body's chromium nutritional status as has been demonstrated with zinc[23].

Included among several potential advantages of hair analyses is the relatively large concentration of chromium present in this tissue. This permitted analyses of chromium in hair by less sensitive techniques[24,25] before the present analytical methodology had been developed. These earlier investigations demonstrated that parous women had very much lower chromium levels in their hair compared to nulliparous women of the same age[24]. The most probable explanation for this observation was that maternal chromium reserves had been depleted by the fetus during pregnancy; a striking depletion of maternal chromium in the liver has been reported in laboratory animals[7]. These studies also revealed that some children with juvenile diabetes mellitus had unusually low hair chromium levels, and that as a group there was a significant difference from normal children[25].

Recently hair analyses have been recommenced employing the emission spectrochemical techniques[10] already described. Hair samples routinely collected close to the scalp in the occipital region are washed sequentially in redistilled hexane, ethyl alcohol, and deionized water and then dried at 110°C. Small samples (less than 100 mg) are then introduced into ashing boats with teflon-covered forceps, accurately weighed, and ashed in a low-temperature asher. No loss of chromium has been detectable during this procedure. The ash is dissolved in situ with 20 μl 1.5 N HCl for each 5 mg of original hair; 20 μl aliquots are analyzed in triplicate, with a precision of 6% RSD. No direct comparison of recent results with the earlier atomic absorption techniques[24-26] has been possible. Though results for normal subjects have been in the same range, mean results for these children, young men, and nulliparous women have been a little lower (approximately 500 ng chromium/g hair).

Tipton, Balassa, and Schroeder[7] have found that mean autopsy tissue chromium levels were exceptionally high in the

newborn, and these recent studies have demonstrated that the
mean newborn hair chromium concentration is higher than at any
other age. In Table III chromium levels in hair collected from
15 full-term normal neonates within one week of delivery are
compared with those of their mothers collected at the same
time. The mean concentration for the newborn is two and
one-half times as great as the mean maternal concentration
(although the full effects of pregnancy on maternal concentrations probably cannot be observed so early postpartum).

TABLE III

Comparison of Newborn and Maternal

Hair Chromium Concentrations (ppb)

Newborn	Maternal	D (Newborn maternal)
1940	224	+ 1716
2000	286	+ 1714
1220	332	+ 888
1028	252	+ 776
1200	448	+ 752
884	192	+ 692
1000	320	+ 680
660	180	+ 480
850	376	+ 474
680	208	+ 472
654	224	+ 430
664	312	+ 352
612	600	+ 12
1020	1100	− 80
200	672	− 476
Mean 974	382	+ 592

Paired comparisons: - t test; P<0.001.

These results support the conclusion that the newborn
usually start life with a good reserve of chromium, but the
particularly low level in one of these newborn may be of
importance when considered in conjunction with the relatively
low chromium concentrations observed in the liver and kidney of
some individual newborn[8]. This suggests that adequate chromium
nutrition is not certain even in the very young. In the rat,
at least, chromium can only cross the placenta in the form of
the glucose tolerance factor[22]; it is feasible that an impaired
maternal ability to supply the placenta with this biologically
active organic chromium compound may result in a relatively
poor fetal supply of chromium in some individuals.

The premature infant has exaggerated postnatal nutritional
problems, particularly with respect to those nutrients, such as
iron, for which an adequate reserve acquired in utero is
necessary to avert a serious deficiency in later infancy.
Present evidence suggests that an adequate reserve of chromium
at birth is also necessary, or at least desirable. The premature
newborn would require a greater concentration of this element
to compensate for the lower total body weight to achieve the
same chromium reserve as the full-term delivery. Hair chromium
concentrations of the premature newborn (Table IV), at least
when delivered before 36 weeks gestation, have been generally
lower than those of the full-term delivery, indicating that
prematurity may result in an increased risk of chromium
deficiency in later infancy or childhood. An increase in the
chromium content of fetal bones with increasing gestational
age has been reported by Pribluda[27].

Only one hair sample from a newborn with evidence of
intrauterine growth retardation has been analyzed. The subject
was delivered at 36 weeks gestation, weighing only 1500 g; her
hair chromium concentration was extremely low (70 ppb).

TABLE IV

Hair Chromium Concentration Premature Newborn

Estimated gestational Age (weeks)	Hair chromium concentration (ppb)
32	196
32	560
33	214
33	200
34	200
34	375
35	410
35	410
36	600
36	1220

In utero the fetus is bathed in amniotic fluid and it therefore appeared theoretically possible that concentrations of trace elements in the hair could be influenced by absorption of these elements from the amniotic fluid. However, when hair samples were soaked overnight in a solution of chromium, zinc, iron, magnesium, manganese, and copper, with concentrations of these elements at least tenfold greater than those in amniotic fluid, the hair concentration of these elements was not increased with the exception of copper. The concentration of chromium in seven amniotic fluid samples are given in Table V; these results perhaps again suggest an increase in concentration with increasing gestational age.

The limited results of hair analyses available at this time indicate that the high neonatal levels are maintained during the first year of life, whereas in the second year a few high values

TABLE V

Chromium Concentrations in Amniotic Fluid

Gestation (weeks)	Chromium (ppb)
28	7
30	9
33	7
36	20
37	18
38	31
38	12
44	76

and an occasional very low value, comparable to the very low
hair zinc concentrations observed at this age, have been
recorded.

The latter is illustrated in Table VI, which details
results of hair chromium analyses on serial sections along the
length of the hair from a girl aged 18 months who had never had
a previous haircut. Hair grows at an approximate rate of
1 cm/month, and it is thus possible to calculate the chromium

TABLE VI

Hair Chromium Concentrations of Female Infant
Aged 18 Months (First Haircut)

Distance from scalp (cm)	Hair chromium (ppb)
9 - 18	940
5 - 8	576
2 - 5	330
0 - 2	144

content of the new-grown hair from many months previous by measuring the distance of the hair sample from the scalp. For example, the section of this hair from 9 to 18 cm distance from the scalp, with a concentration of 940 ppb probably represents the new-grown hair from approximately the first nine months of life. The section of this hair adjacent to the scalp, that is, that most recently grown, had a chromium concentration of only 144 ppb, which is lower than any value observed in older normal children.

The relative importance of infant nutrition in determining the rate of decline of tissue chromium levels postnatally is undetermined. Milk contains relatively little chromium, especially some infant formulas (Table VII). By comparison

TABLE VII

Chromium Content of Milk

	ng Cr/mg Ash	ng Cr/ml Milk
Human		
Subjects: a	2.1	18.5
b (mean of 4)	1.6	6.4
c (mean of 8)	2.3	7.9
d	2.0	11.2
e (mean of 2)	1.8	14.1
Mean =	2.0	11.6
Cow		
Undiluted	0.5	8.0
Infant Formula (20 cals/oz)		
Similac	0.8	5.6
Enfamil	2.2	10.5
Modilac	0.5	5.0

breast milk fares relatively well, especially on an ash-weight basis. A concentration of 10 ppb would provide approximately 1-1/2 µg/kg/day for a young infant. On a weight-to-weight basis this corresponds closely with calculated daily intakes for adults[1]; on the other hand it is likely that requirements are much greater in the growing infant. Adequate comparisons are not possible without knowing the relative availability for absorption of the ingested chromium in breast milk, infant milk formulas, and representative adult diets. Such information is not available at present.

Although certain details, some of which have already been discussed, require clarification, the relationship between hair chromium concentration and age is becoming evident (Fig. 6). Following the decline from the high concentrations of the first postnatal year, mean levels appear to remain fairly constant at approximately 500 ppb in normal subjects from 3 to 40 years of age; older age groups have not been investigated. The only

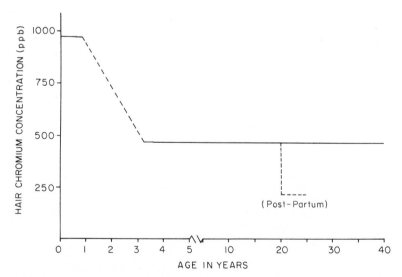

Fig. 6   Variation in hair chromium concentration with age.

"normal" circumstance in which a further marked decline in
hair chromium levels has been observed is in the postpartum
woman. This pattern of declining concentration with increasing
age is very similar to that observed in autopsy tissues[8,18].
The decline in hair levels resembles that seen in spleen and
aorta more than in liver and kidney, as the latter organs
exhibited a further decline in chromium concentration in the
second decade of life. However, comparisons in the same subjects
will be necessary before any definitive conclusions are possible.
Meanwhile it is evident that changes in hair chromium concentrations roughly parallel those in other tissues.

The results of these hair analyses have indicated certain
groups of subjects who are at the risk point from chromium
deficiency, but in practice it is also important to be able to
detect suboptimal nutrition in the individual. In order to
achieve this the ideal approach may prove to be successive
sampling of new-grown hair or serial sectioning along the length
of the hair shafts. By these means it should be possible, for
example, to determine the rate of decline in hair chromium
concentrations or the length of time over which a particularly
low hair chromium level has been present. With respect to
absolute figures, hair chromium concentrations below 200 ppb
have not been observed in normal subjects (including more than
50 children and adolescents) between the ages of 3 to 40 years
except in postpartum women. Levels below 200 ppb have been
present in certain subjects with documented impairment of
glucose tolerance, including some juvenile diabetics. The only
other children more than 3 years of age with such low levels
have been a girl aged 8 years with intestinal lymphangectasia
resulting in protein-losing enteropathy; a girl aged 15 years
with severe anorexia nervosa, who had lost nearly half her
total body weight in the preceding six months; and a boy aged
6 years with cystic fibrosis. These three patients all had

evidence of malnutrition, malabsorption, and/or hypoproteinemia; no data is available on their glucose tolerance at the time of these hair collections.

At least as a screening test the results of these studies suggest that hair analysis provides a promising approach for the detection of suboptimal chromium nutrition. If the hair chromium concentration is low, or if there are clinical features suggesting the possibility of chromium deficiency, further laboratory investigations are justified before a decision is made on dietary chromium supplementation. Examples of individual results from such evaluations are given in Table VIII. The girl aged 12 years had severe hypercholesterolemia, with complications including aortic stenosis; previous therapy had only been partially successful in reducing her serum cholesterol. Chromium supplementation was considered, but was not initiated because the results of these investigations provided no evidence of chromium deficiency; there was therefore no theoretical reason to anticipate any improvement from this approach. The second subject was a 25 year old nulliparous woman, who had a mild impairment of glucose tolerance. All of the chromium

TABLE VIII

Results of Chromium Analyses in Individual Subjects

	Female, 12 yr hypercholesterolemia	Female, 25 yr impaired glucose tolerance
Hair chromium concentration	1120 ppb	183 ppb
24 hour urine-chromium excretion	7 µg	0 µg
Increase in serum chromium following glucose load	12 ng (100%)	No increase

investigations in this case suggested that she was chromium deficient.

The one necessary criterion for any subject to have had a therapeutic trial of dietary chromium supplementation has been evidence of impaired glucose tolerance[2,14] or hypercholesterolemia[18]. However, whether these features are a sine qua non for the diagnosis of chromium deficiency remains uncertain. For example, nucleic acids contain extremely high concentrations of chromium compared with levels in other subcellular fractions[28] and it is probable that this element has a specific function in relation to DNA and RNA[1]. This observation at least suggests the possibility that chromium deficiency could have a delerterious effect on other metabolic processes before it compromises glucose and fat metabolism, especially in the rapidly growing infant or child.

V. CONCLUSIONS

These studies are at present incomplete and a more definitive discussion of chromium nutrition and malnutrition in the young must await further investigations. However, the results suggest that spectrochemical analyses of chromium in readily available samples from the living subject are of value in detecting chromium deficiency in the individual and, of greater importance, have indicated particular groups of young subjects who may be at special risk from suboptimal chromium nutrition. For example, the exceptionally low hair chromium levels in the postpartum woman and perhaps the results of serum studies in the last month of gestation indicate that pregnancy depletes maternal chromium reserves in the human as well as in laboratory animals[26]. The extent to which this represents a health hazard to the mother has not been clarified, but theoretical considerations together with the results of

initial investigations of the gestational diabetic suggest
that this depletion may have important clinical consequences.

In the child with insulin-dependent juvenile diabetes
mellitus the excessive urinary excretion of chromium observed
in some patients supports the conclusion that chromium
metabolism is abnormal[20]. The low hair chromium levels
observed in some juvenile diabetics indicate that increased
absorption[20] may not always balance excessive urinary loss.
The possible role of chromium deficiency in the later complications of juvenile diabetics including atherosclerosis and
hypercholesterolemia merits investigation.

In the infant with protein/calorie malnutrition, chromium
deficiency is one etiologic factor in the clinically important
abnormalities of carbohydrate metabolism that complicate this
disease[4]. Isolated hair analyses in older children with
diseases resulting in malnutrition in this country indicate
that chromium deficiency is a potential complication. In view
of the frequent abnormalities of carbohydrate metabolism that
occur in the newborn in early postnatal life, the exceptionally
low hair chromium concentration of the one newborn with evidence
of intrauterine malnutrition who has been studied to date is
of special interest.

The relatively poor supply of maternal glucose tolerance
factor in the case of premature deliveries, and apparently
in some full-term neonates, may compromise their chromium
nutritional status in later infancy and childhood. Finally,
it remains to be determined whether the rapid "normal" decline
in chromium levels in the first months or years of life is
entirely physiologic; it cannot be assumed that tissue chromium
concentrations within the normal adult range necessarily
indicate optimal chromium nutrition for the growing child.

ACKNOWLEDGMENTS

I wish to acknowledge in particular the collaboration of Dr. D. Baum, Dr. P. Beck, Dr. W. Droegemueller, and Mrs. C. Hambidge. Spectrochemical analyses were performed with the technical assistance of Mrs. M. Jacobs.

These studies have been supported by U.S.P.H.S. Grant No. 1-R01-Am-12432 from NIAMD; salary paid inpart by U.S.P.H.S. Grant No. RR-69.

REFERENCES

[1]. Mertz, W., Physiol. Rev., 49, 163 (1969).

[2]. Glinsmann, W. H. and Mertz, W., Metab., 15, 510 (1966).

[3]. Levine, R. A., Streeten, D. H. P., and Doisy, R. J., Metab., 17, 114 (1968).

[4]. Hopkins, L. L., Ransome-Kuti, O., and Majaj, A. S., Am. J. Clin. Nutr., 21, 203 (1968).

[5]. Tipton, I. H. and Cook, M. J., Health Phys., 9, 103 (1963).

[6]. Tipton, I. H., Schroeder, H. A., Perry, H. M., Jr., and Cook, M. J., Health Phys., 11, 403 (1965).

[7]. Schroeder, H. A., Balassa, J. J., and Tipton, I. H., J. Chron. Dis., 15, 941 (1962).

[8]. Tipton, I. H., Metal-Binding in Medicine (M. J. Seven, ed.) Lippincott, Philadelphia, 1960, p. 27.

[9]. Hambidge, K. M., Trace Substances in Environmental Health, III, Columbia Missouri, 1969, p. 371.

[10]. Hambidge, K. M., Anal. Chem., 43, 103 (1971).

[11]. Gordon, W. A., N.A.S.A., T.N. D-2598, 1965.

[12]. Gordon, W. A., N.A.S.A., T.N. D-5236, 1967.

[13]. Gordon, W. A., N.A.S.A., T.N. D-4769, 1968.

[14]. Glinsmann, W., Feldman, F., and Mertz, W., Science, 152, 1243 (1966).

[15]. Burt, R. L., Obstet. Gynec., 7, 658 (1956).

[16]. Imbus, H. R., Cholak, J., Miller, L. H., and Sterling, T.,
       Arch. Environ. Health, 6, 286 (1963).

[17]. Pierce, J. O. and Cholak, J., Arch. Environ. Health,
       13, 208 (1966).

[18]. Schroeder, H. A., Am. J. of Clin. Nutri., 21, 230 (1968).

[19]. Collins, R. J., Fromm, P. O., Collings, W. D., Am. J.
       Physiol., 201, 795 (1961).

[20]. Doisy, R. J., Streeten, D. H. P., Levine, R. A., and
       Chodos, R. B., Trace Substances in Environmental Health,
       II, Columbia Missouri, 1968, p. 75.

[21]. Rothman, S., (ed.) Physiology and Biochemistry of the
       Skin, Chicago, Illinois: Chicago University Press,
       1954, p. 641.

[22]. Mertz, W., Roginski, E. E., Feldman, F. J., and
       Thurman, D. E., J. Nutr., 99, 363 (1969).

[23]. Strain, W. H., Steadman, L. T., Lankau, C. A.,
       Berliner, W. P., and Pories, W. J., J. Lab. Clin. Med.,
       68, 244 (1966).

[24]. Hambidge, K. M. and Rodgerson, D. O., Am. J. Obstet.
       Gynec., 103, 321 (1969).

[25]. Hambidge, K. M., Rodgerson, D. O., and O'Brien, D.,
       Diabetes, 17, 517 (1968).

[26]. Hambidge, K. M., Rodgerson, D. O. and O'Brien, D.,
       Proceedings of the VIIIth International Congress on
       Nutrition, Prague, 1969, Abstract, in press.

[27]. Pribluda, L. A., Chem. Abstr., 59, 4331 (1963).

[28]. Wacker, W. E. C. and Vallee, B. L., Federation Proc.,
       18, 345 (1959).

Chapter 10

THE BIOLOGICAL ESSENTIALITY OF VANADIUM

L. L. Hopkins, Jr. and H. E. Mohr

Human Nutrition Research Division
U. S. Department of Agriculture
Agricultural Research Service
Beltsville, Maryland

I.   INTRODUCTION

Of the more than 100 elements known, only one-fifth of
these have been shown to be essential for the health and
well-being of man and the higher animals. These 20 or so
essential elements include carbon, hydrogen, oxygen, nitrogen,
and sulfur which are the elemental basis for the organic
nutrients such as the vitamins, lipids, and so forth, leaving
approximately 15 essential minerals. Although it is doubtful
that all of the elements will be found to be essential, there
are several that appear as likely candidates. One of these is
vanadium.

Several investigations over the years have indicated the
physiological importance of vanadium but none have shown its
essentiality. Although at the time it had not been established
as being physiologically essential to higher animals, some
evidence implies that it may be necessary for normal
metabolism[16]. Its presence in certain invertebrates has been
well documented[6,19]. Kalk[9] has reported that tunicates
absorbed both the anionic vanadate and cationic vanadyl ions
but that a preferential permeability was shown for the latter.

Vanadium has been found in noncarious human enamel and
dentine, and it was suggested that it may exchange with
phosphorus in the apatite tooth substances[13,17]. Geyer[5]
demonstrated that V_2O_5, administered orally or parenterally,
offered protection against caries in hamsters fed a cariogenic
diet, and Rygh[15] reported that it promoted mineralization of
teeth and bones and significantly reduced dental caries in rats
and guinea pigs. Söremark, Üllberg, and Appelgren[18] have
shown by microautoradiography that subcutaneously injected
$V_2^{48}O_5$ was highly concentrated in the areas of rapid mineralization in tooth dentine and bone in mice.

Vanadium has been found to increase greatly the oxygen
uptake of liver suspensions and to catalyze the oxidation of
phospholipids by washed liver protein[1]. The authors reported
that the oxidation took place in the fatty acid moiety of the
phospholipid molecule and that the presence of "suitable"
protein was necessary for the reaction.

The ability of this element to inhibit cholesterol
synthesis was reported by Mountain, Stockell, and Stokinger[14]
for in vivo systems and by Curran and Costello[2,4], for both
in vivo and in vitro systems. They found VO^{2+}(IV) and VO_3^-(V)
to be equally inhibitory, and concluded that the metal either

attains its active oxidation state easily or is active at any oxidation state. Vanadium salts at concentration of 5×10^{-5} M produced the inhibitor effect. Lewis[12] and Curran, Azarnoff, and Bolinger[3] showed that ingestion of vanadium or exposure to vanadium dust significantly lowered serum cholesterol levels in human subjects.

Extensive reviews on the biological aspects of vanadium have been published by Hudson[8] and Schroeder, Balassa, and Tipton[16].

An essential nutrient is one that must be available in the diet since it cannot be synthesized by the organism or cannot be synthesized at a rate great enough to maintain health. Classically, nutritionists have established essentiality by reducing the level of the nutrient in the diet below the requirement of the organism. If fed for an adequate time, deficiency symptoms appear when contrasted to the control group receiving a supplement of the nutrient in question. This is the approach we have taken in an attempt to establish whether vanadium is or is not an essential element.

II. ESSENTIALITY OF VANADIUM

Since we suspected that it would be necessary to obtain a diet containing vanadium in the parts per billion range in order to produce symptoms of a deficiency, we added certain refinements to the classical techniques in order to reduce contamination. Sex-linked cross cockerel (Rhode Island white female hen × Rhode Island red male) chicks were maintained in an environment where the air was filtered. All components within this environment were plastic so as to reduce vanadium contamination from metal and glass sources. The cages likewise were all plastic to reduce contamination.

TABLE I

Low-Vanadium Chick Diet

	g/kg
Dextrose (monohydrate)	565
Casein (vitamin free)	230
Mineral Mix (low V)	60
Solka-Floc	50
Lard (stripped)	50
Vitamin Mix	20
L-Arginine	12.5
Glycine	7.5
DL-Methionine	5.0
Vitamin D_3 (1000 ICU/kg)	20 mg

The composition of the diet used is shown in Table I and is based on casein and dextrose. It contained 10 ppb vanadium as determined by neutron activation analysis.[1] The salt-mix formulation was prepared from CP salts and is shown in Table II. Water for the chicks was obtained by running distilled water from the building source over a mixed bed resin, then distilling it in a quartz still, and storing it in plastic bottles. It contained 0.5 ppb vanadium. The chicks grew well and appeared healthy under these conditions.

The results obtained to date from two separate experiments have been a reduced feather growth within 10 days in those chicks maintained on a diet low in vanadium. The wing and tail feather growth of the chicks supplemented with 2 ppm vanadium in the drinking water was significantly greater than those from chicks receiving no supplement (Tables IV and V).

---

[1] Union Carbide Corporation, Research Center, Tuxedo, New York.

TABLE II

Low-Vanadium[a] Mineral Mix

	g/kg
$CaHPO_4$	473.33
$CaCO_3$	166.66
KCl	116.66
Na_2HPO_4	116.66
NaCl	66.66
$MgSO_4$	50.00
$MnSO_4 \cdot H_2O$	4.17
$FeC_6H_5O_7 \cdot 5H_2O$	3.33
$ZnCO_3$	2.17
$CrCl_3 \cdot 6H_2O$	0.35
$CuSO_4 \cdot 5H_2O$	0.17
KIO_3	0.17

[a] 35 ppb vanadium.

Selected tissues from these chicks were analyzed for
vanadium content (Table V). Liver and kidney samples from the
supplemented group contained approximately 100 times the vanadium
concentration found in the deficient groups. The vanadium
content of heart tissue from deficient chicks was similar to
the amount found in the liver and kidney of these same chicks.
There was a tenfold difference between the vanadium content of
heart tissue from the supplemented chicks as compared to liver
and kidney. This would indicate that the heart does not
accumulate the element in the amounts found in liver and kidney.

TABLE III

Wing-Feather Development of Chicks Fed

a Diet Low in Vanadium

Age (days)	7	14	21	27	36	43	49
Chicks/group	15	15	15	15	6	6	6
		mm[a/]					
Deficient	41	56	74	93	103	110	120
Supplemented[b/]	46	65[c/]	83[d/]	101[d/]	113[d/]	116[c/]	128

[a/] Length of primary feathers in millimeters.

[b/] 2 ppm vanadium as NH_4VO_3 in water.

[c/] $P<0.05$

[d/] $P<0.01$

TABLE IV

Tail-Feather Development of Chicks Fed

a Diet Low in Vanadium

Age (days)	14	21	27	36	43	49
Chicks/group	15	15	15	6	6	6
		mm[a/]				
Deficient	18	34	48	55	62	80
Supplemented[b/]	25	44	60[c/]	80[d/]	86[c/]	99[c/]

[a/] Length of feathers in millimeters.

[b/] 2 ppm vanadium as NH_4VO_3 in water.

[c/] $P<0.05$

[d/] $P<0.02$

TABLE V

Vanadium Content of Various Organs from

Chicks Fed a Diet Low in Vanadium[a/]

	Deficient[b/]	Supplemented[b,c/]
	(ppb)	
Liver	2.2	210
	1.7	230
	5.5	180
Kidney	4.0	590
	0.7	610
	2.3	760
Heart	1.6	14
	3.3	44
	4.2	18

[a/] Analysis by neutron activation (parts per billion
dry-weight basis).

[b/] 10 ppb vanadium in diet and 0.5 ppb in water.

[c/] 2 ppm vanadium as NH_4VO_3 in water.

These data are similar to data that will be discussed later
from Table XII where low levels of vanadium as [48]V accumulated
in liver and kidney tissue but not the heart[7].

As a result of the very interesting work of Curran[3] and
others concerning the effect of vanadium upon cholesterol
metabolism, it was of interest to observe the blood cholesterol
levels during vanadium deficiency. Table VI shows that in two
separate experiments the blood cholesterol levels were significantly lower in the deficient chicks when compared to those
supplemented with vanadium. Literature blood cholesterol values

TABLE VI

Plasma Cholesterol Levels of Chicks Fed

a Diet Low in Vanadium[a]

Experiment	Deficient (mg/100 ml)	Supplemented (mg/100 ml)	Significance
I	190 ± 12.9	225 ± 8.4	P < .05
II	161 ± 5.2	185[b] ± 5.9	P < .01

[a] 9 chicks mean ± standard error.

[b] 11 mean ± standard error.

for chicks of this age fed different, but semipurified diets, have been reported by Leveille, Sauberlich, and Shockley[10], Leveille, Tillotson, and Sauberlich[11] as 225 and 251 mg/100 ml. These data reported here indicate that vanadium-deficient chicks at four weeks of age have subnormal levels of blood cholesterol and that this element at physiological levels may play a role in cholesterol metabolism as was found by earlier investigators using pharmacological levels.

There was no significant difference in growth rate between the two groups. Similar studies have been conducted using rats but the results were inconclusive. Rats apparently have a low requirement for a number of minerals and from our data it appears that this animal was not a good model system in which to explore vanadium deficiency under the conditions imposed.

Although determining essentiality is quite important, at best it can only give clues as to the metabolic role of the nutrient. To learn more about its metabolism, [48]V of very high specific activity was injected intravenously[7]. By giving amounts of vanadium of approximately 1 ng per 100 g of body weight to rats fed a diet low in available vanadium, it was

felt that the radioactivity would distribute itself with time
into the areas of specific and physiologically meaningful pools.
Following the injection of low levels of ^{48}V, only 30%
of the radioactivity observed 10 minutes after injection
remained when the 7 hour sample of blood was taken from rats
previously fed a stock diet or a Torula yeast based diet plus
vanadium in the drinking water. Rats consuming the nonsupple-
mented torula diet containing 210 ppb vanadium retained about
twice as much as the 7 hour sampling period indicating a
homostatic mechanism that clears the vanadium when adequate
amounts are in the blood. Of interest was the individual data
from each rat which indicated that there was an actual increase
in ^{48}V in the plasma of five out of the seven rats under study
which had previously consumed the diet low in vanadium
(Table VII). These increases were observed in different rats
at the 1/2-, 1-, 2- and 4-hour intervals.

Since most of the radioactivity was found to be in the
noncellular portion of the blood, the plasma proteins were
separated using disc gel electrophoresis (Table VIII). When
plasma was taken 10 minutes after the injection of nanogram
amounts of ^{48}V and separated electrophoretically, 92% of the
gel radioactivity was not protein bound. Although a minor
amount was initially found in the transferrin region of the gel,
it was noted that within 4 hours time, the percent of total gel
radioactivity increased from 3 to 28%. The amount of unbound
^{48}V decreased proportionately. Attempts to label transferrin
by adding ^{48}V in vitro and incubated at 37°C for 4 hours were
unsuccessful (Table IX). Apparently binding to the protein
required some in vivo metabolic change.

Evidence that the ^{48}V was binding to transferrin and not
some other protein migrating near the transferrin region was

TABLE VII

The Reintroduction of [48]Vanadium into the Plasma of
Individual Young Male Rats Previously Intravenously
Injected with [48]VO_2 (Approx. 1 ng/100 grams B. W.)[a/]

Rat No.	1/6 (cpm[b/])	Hours after injection					
		1/2	1	2	4	7	24
		(Percent of 1/6 hour cpm)					
1	60	103	108	123	<u>155</u>	117	20
2	389	123	<u>126</u>	120	98	63	19
3	86	<u>115</u>	108	102	83	73	13
4	689	95	<u>96</u>	76	61	42	10
5	142	80	72	73	<u>82</u>	59	11
6	126	76	71	66	56	37	10
7	998	69	52	43	37	26	6
Ave.		94	90	86	82	60	13

[a/] Two separated experiments.

[b/] Plasma and washings from 50 µl whole blood.

obtained by injecting [59]Iron intravenously into rats (Table X).
This serum was separated identially to serum from rats that had
been injected 4 hours previously with [48]V. The transferrin
region was separated into two pieces such that a different
protein migrating in the fore or aft portion of the transferrin
region might be detected. The proportions of isotope in each
segment compared favorably between the two isotopes thus
providing evidence that transferrin was binding the metabolically
changed vanadium.

In the [48]V distribution studies tissues were sampled at
timed intervals using three different oxidation states of

TABLE VIII

Electrophoretic Separation of Protein Bound and
Free ^{48}Vanadium in Serum Following Intravenous Injection

Hour after Administration	No. Rats	Blood clearance (Percent 1/6 hour) Blood radioactivity	Percent of total gel radioactivity[a]	
			Salt front region	Transferrin region
1/6	9	100	92 ± 1.2	3 ± 0.7
1	5	77 ± 7.2	82 ± 1.4	8 ± 2.6
2	5	62 ± 1.8	80 ± 1.2	16 ± 0.4
4	6	55 ± 2.0	68 ± 1.5	28 ± 2.3

[a] Mean ± standard error.

TABLE IX

Electrophoretic Separation of Protein Bound and

Free [48]Vanadium in Serum Following Intravenous Injection

or In Vitro Addition

Hour after Administration	No. Rats	Percent of total gel radioactivity[a]	
		Salt front region	Transferrin region
Intravenous injection			
1/6	9	92 ± 1.2	3 ± 0.7
4	6	68 ± 1.5	28 ± 2.3
Addition in vitro[b]			
1/6	4	95 ± 1.0	0 ± 0
4	4	93 ± 0.8	1 ± 0.3

[a] Mean ± standard error.

[b] Incubated at 37°C.

vanadium[7]. Although there were marked differences between
tissues in their accumulation of the isotope at these very low
levels, in general there was very little effect noted within
the same tissue due to the difference in oxidation state.
There was a trend noted very early in several tissues to a more
rapid accumulation of vanadium in the +5 oxidation state
(Table XI). Most notable were the lung and sternum, where
10 minutes after injection vanadium (III) retained the least,
vanadium (IV) in between, and vanadium (V) the most. This
trend was not observed 1 hour or more after injection. Four
or more hours after injection it was observed that vanadium (V)
was lost faster, thus indicating a first-in first-out
phenomenon for vanadium (V).

TABLE X

Electrophoretic Separation of Protein Bound and Free Radioactivity in the
Sera of Rats Injected Intravenously with ^{48}Vanadium or ^{59}Iron

| | | | | Percent of protein bound radioactivity[a] | | | | |
| | | | | Transferrin region | | Pretransferrin region | | |
Isotope	No. Rats	Albumin region	Post-transferrin region	(a)	(b)	(a)	(b)	(c)
^{48}V[b]	4	2 ± 0.8	2 ± 0.8	70 ± 7.8	21 ± 6.5	3 ± 1.0	1 ± 0.3	3 ± 2.3
^{59}Fe[c]	3	0 ± 0	0 ± 0	81 ± 4.3	15 ± 3.0	2 ± 0.7	1 ± 0.3	0 ± 0.3

a/ Mean ± standard error.

b/ Serum taken 4 hours after injection of ^{48}vanadium.

c/ Serum taken 1/2 hour after injection ^{59}iron.

TABLE XI

Effect of Oxidation State upon Tissue Uptake of Intravenously
Injected ^{48}Vanadium (Approx. 1 ng/100 grams B. W.)

Tissue	Oxidation state	1/6	Hour after injection		
			1	4	24
		$\frac{\% \text{ g dose}}{\text{g tissue}}$	(Percent of 1/6 hour value)		
Lung	III	107 ± 10[a]	77	64	24
	IV	123 ± 7.3	76	66	25
	V	147 ± 16	76	53	20
Sternum	III	70 ± 2.8	96	111	80
	IV	74 ± 2.0	103	116	81
	V	81 ± 4.0	100	96	69

[a] Mean ± standard error (three to four male rats per group).

The variation in accumulation of ^{48}V in the tissues of
rats fed low levels of available dietary vanadium ranged after
4 days from 5% of the 10 minutes value in the blood to 121%
in the kidney (Table XII). Those tissues accumulating the
highest levels of ^{48}V 4 days after injection are shown in this
table and include the spleen, liver, and testes as well as the
kidney. Of interest to us from a metabolic viewpoint was the
accumulation and retention of vanadium in the liver and testes.

Analysis of testes from rats kept in a controlled
environment indicated that rats consuming an unsupplemented diet
low in vanadium had little vanadium in these organs (Table XIII).
But as demonstrated in the isotope experiments, testes accumulated the element when vanadium was available in the diet.

To learn more about the metabolism of ^{48}V, liver homogenates
from intravenously injected rats were centrifuged in order to

TABLE XII

Retention of Intravenously Injected

Trivalent [48]Vanadium (Approx. 1 ng/100 grams B. W.)

Tissue	1/6	Hours after injection			
		1	4	24	96
	(Percent dose)	(Percent of 1/6 hour value)			
Blood	19.6 ± 0.80[a]	67	52	11	5
	(Percent gram dose / gram tissue)				
Heart	97 ± 8.0	58	51	16	15
Spleen	65 ± 4.5	74	138	103	115
Liver	93 ± 11	115	177	104	99
Kidney	210 ± 18	143	177	124	121
Testis	23 ± 1.5	148	248	126	104

[a] Mean ± standard error (three to four male rats per group).

TABLE XIII

Vanadium Content of Testes from Rats

Fed a Diet Low in Vanadium[a]

Deficient (ppb)	Supplemented[b,c] (ppb)
5.6	200
1.0	250

[a] Analysis by neutron activation (parts per billion dry-weight basis).

[b] 7 ppb vanadium in diet and 0.5 ppb in water.

[c] 1 ppm vanadium as NH_4VO_3 in water.

TABLE XIV

The Relative Distribution of Radioactivity among Rat Liver[a/]

Subcellular Particles at Timed Intervales Following Intravenous

Injection of $^{48}VOCl_3$ (160 ng/100 grams B. W.)

Fraction		Hours after injection				
	1/6	1	4	24	96	192
		(Percent observed cpm)				
Nuclear	15	26	22	32	43	43
Mitochondrial	14	24	34	46	37	37
Microsomal	15	12	9	9	10	11
Supernatant	57	39	35	13	11	10

[a/] Two to six rats per group.

observe the distribution of ^{48}V among the subcellular
particles[7] as is shown in Table XIV. Initially, 10 minutes
after injection, most of the isotope was located in the supernatant fraction. With time the ^{48}V migrated into the
mitochondrial and nuclear fractions, until after 1 day post
injection approximately 40% was in each fraction. Apparently
the isotope was incorporated into these organelles since 4 days
after injection, the same distribution remained and probably
accounted for the accumulation and retention previously noted
in whole liver samples.

At these low levels, vanadium was excreted both through
the urine and feces[7]; the data are shown in Table XV. Four
days after intravenous injection almost half of the dose was
excreted through the urine and 8.6% through the feces.

TABLE XV

Excretion Routes of Intravenously Injected
Trivalent ^{48}Vanadium (Approx. 1 ng/100 grams B. W.) in Rats

Excretion route	Hours after injection			
	1	4	24	96
	(Percent dose)			
Urine	6.6 ± 1.5[a/]	18.2 ± 1.1	41.5 ± 0.58	45.5 ± 12.9
Feces	–	–	1.5 ± 0.38	8.6 ± 1.5

[a/] Mean ± standard error (three to four male rats per group).

III. SUMMARY

Over a period of many years investigations from several
laboratories have provided evidence of the biological importance
of vanadium. Today by utilizing the newer technology in animal
housing we have presented evidence that in our opinion shows
the essentiality of vanadium in the chick. The significant
symptoms observed were slower growth in both the wing and tail
feathers of chicks consuming a diet containing 10 ppb vanadium.
The analysis of tissues from these chicks indicated that they
had been depleted of vanadium down to a level of a few parts per
billion. Blood cholesterol levels of the deficient chicks were
significantly lower than in the control animals. Blood
clearance observations indicated that intravenously injected
^{48}V was possibly reintroduced into the blood 1/2 to 4 hours
after intravenous injection. A form of ^{48}V was observed that
bound to the blood protein transferrin and increased in amount
with time after injection. This change to a bound form of
vanadium took place in vivo, but not in vitro when the isotope
was incubated with serum. Timed distribution studies with low

levels of intravenously injected ^{48}V showed that the kidney,
liver, testis, and spleen accumulated and retained the isotope
for at least 4 days. In liver tissue this retention was shown
to be due to a migration of the ^{48}V into the mitochondrial and
nuclear fractions of the cell.

REFERENCES

[1].   Bernheim, F. and Bernheim, M. L. C., J. Biol. Chem.,
       127, 353-360 (1939).

[2].   Curran, G. L., J. Biol. Chem., 210, 765-770 (1964).

[3].   Curran, G. L., Azarnoff, D. L., and Bolinger, R. E.,
       J. Clin. Invest., 38, 1251-1261 (1959).

[4].   Curran, G. L. and Costello, R. L., J. Exptl. Med., 103,
       49-56 (1956).

[5].   Geyer, C. F., J. Dental Res., 32, 590-595 (1953).

[6].   Henze, M., I. Z. Physiol. Chem., 72, 494-501 (1911).

[7].   Hopkins, L. L., Jr. and Tilton, B. E., Am. J. Physiol.,
       211, 169-172 (1966).

[8].   Hudson, T. G. F., Vanadium Toxicology and Biological
       Significance. New York: Elsevier, 1964.

[9].   Kalk, M., Nature, 198, 1010-1011 (1963).

[10]. Leveille, G. A., Sauberlich, H. E., and Shockley, J. W.,
       J. Nutr., 76, 423-428 (1962).

[11]. Leveille, G. A., Tillotson, and Sauberlich, H. E.,
       J. Nutr., 81, 357-362 (1963).

[12]. Lewis, C. E., A. M. A. Arch. Ind. Health, 19, 419-425
       (1959).

[13]. Lowater, F. and Murray, M. M., Biochem. J., 31, 837-841
       (1937).

[14]. Mountain, J. T., Stockell, F. R., and Stokinger, H. E.,
       Proc. Soc. Exptl. Biol. Med., 92, 582-587 (1956).

[15]. Rygh, O., Research, London, 2, 340-346 (1949).

[16]. Schroeder, H. A., Balassa, J. J., and Tipton, I. H.,
       J. Chron. Dis., 16, 1047-1071 (1963).

[17]. Söremark, R., and Andersson, N., Acta Odontol.
       Scand., 20, 81-93 (1962).

[18]. Söremark, R., Üllberg, S., and Appelgren, L., Acta
       Odontol. Scand., 20, 225-232 (1962).

[19]. Webb, D. A., J. Exptl. Biol., 16, 499-523 (1939).

Chapter 11

STUDIES ON THE ESSENTIALITY OF NICKEL

F. H. Nielsen

Human Nutrition Laboratory
Agricultural Research Service
U. S. Department of Agriculture
Grand Forks, North Dakota

This presentation will be different than the ones given previously as the literature will be reviewed extensively. It appears that nickel may be emerging as an essential trace element, and thus its present status as such should be presented to those interested in trace element nutrition.

I. REVIEW OF THE LITERATURE

The literature has an overwhelming amount of indirect evidence which infers that nickel can have an important physiological role or roles in living organisms. Nickel was first found to be present in plants and animals in the 1920s[1,2]. It has been found in air, water, and soils[3-6]. Schroeder, Balassa, and Tipton[7] have listed a number of foodstuffs that they have analyzed for nickel. From this report and others[8-13] it appears that nickel is high in such foods as rice, rice products, legumes, oats, and most vegetables, and in such drinks as tea, cocoa, cider, and coffee. On the other hand, nickel is quite low in red meats, cottonseed, corn meal, apples, unsaturated oils, milk, and milk products.

Nickel is present in animals; however, the amount of nickel in different tissues and species varies greatly. Human blood and its components have been measured for nickel many times and the results range from the average value of 2.5 µg to 35 µg/100 ml for blood[14-23], 0.22 µg to 5.53 µg/100 ml for serum[22,24-28] and 0.20 µg to 2.3 µg/100 ml for plasma[29-31]. The latter analyses with improved methods tend to be lower and are probably more valid.

In other human tissues[7,32-34], nickel seems to be present in higher amounts in the lung, pancreas, adrenal glands, brain, teeth, bone, kidney, heart, aorta, and skin. Relatively small amounts are found in the testes, ovaries, intestine, blood, and muscle. Several tissues are of special interest. Nerve tissue contains nickel, and it has been reported that brain contains 0.43 ppm and nickel is located in all areas. A significantly greater amount is located in the substantia nigra[35]. Brain proteins have been shown to contain 2.9 ppm nickel[36]. The aorta reportedly contains as high as 6 ppm nickel and this level decreases in atherosclerosis[37,38]. Yagovdik[39-41] has indicated that nickel occurs in skin in concentrations as high as 0.38 ppm and decreases with age. There appears to be more in some skin, such as that from the thigh, than in other areas, such as that from the abdomen. Nickel has been found in bone ash at the 108 to 111 ppm level, with highest amounts usually in 0- to 20-year-old age group[42]. Scientists in the Soviet Union have analyzed human embryos in

various stages of development for trace elements, including
nickel[32,43-48]. It appears to be present in embryo blood
in highest concentrations at 12-25 weeks of age and decreases
until birth, with the newborn still having higher levels than
infants. In tissues other than blood, nickel increases from
12-25. weeks of age until birth in the liver and spleen and
decreases in the kidney, pancreas, thyroid, and thymus.

Because nickel is found with such consistency in active
metabolizing areas such as the embryo, it probably has a
biological role. Therefore the effect of supplemental nickel
on plants and animals which could possibly indicate an important
physiological role will be discussed. First, it must be pointed
out that a nickel deficiency severe enough to show that nickel
is essential for life has not been reported in the literature.
Nonetheless, nickel supplementation has resulted in improved
growth or yields with asparagus, lettuce[49], peas, oats[50],
grapes[51], rice[52], cotton[53], and potatoes]54,55]. Nickel
supplementation apparently increases vitamin P and C production
in several vegetables[56-62] and increases carotene, carotenoids,
and chlorophyll in corn[63] and sugar beets[64]. There are
reports that nickel is required for growth of some forms of
lower life including E. coli, T. pyriformis, C. sporogenes[65],
blue marine algae[66], C. cerebella fungus[67], and C.
vulgaris[68]. Other effects of nickel supplementation include
increased sporulation by B. coagulans[69] and increased growth
and vitamin B_{12} production by propionic acid bacteria[70-72].

Reports on the beneficial effects of nickel for higher
animals are not quite as extensive. Nickel may help alleviate
cobalt deficiency or bush sickness in sheep, but it can not
replace cobalt completely[73,74]. Schroeder, Balassa, and
Vinton[75] have found that adding 5 ppm of nickel to the
drinking water of rats fed approximately 100 ppb nickel in the

diet results in a decrease of tumors in females but, on the
other hand, the mortality rates in males are increased. These
meager data do not strongly infer an important specific biological role for nickel in higher animals, so perhaps nickel
metabolism should be examined in other ways. The alteration of
nickel distribution in some pathological conditions may be one
method. Certainly nickel is not the only trace element deranged
or altered in distribution in these cases, but is one and thus
may be playing a role in the etiology of the disorder.

Pathological conditions that result in an increase in
nickel in some tissue include the following: Increased amounts
of nickel are found in the blood and neoplastic tissues of
people with cancer[76,77]. It has been reported that nickel
increases in the blood in leukemia and at the terminal stage
is triple the normal value[78]. Other reports state that in
cancer of the uterus, nickel increases in the blood, neoplastic
tissues, and in all organs analyzed[79]; and in cancer of the
stomach, patients have increased nickel in the blood and
liver[80]. Some skin disorders often have a derangement of
nickel distribution[81-84]. Analyses indicate that people with
psoriasis, photodermatitis, radiodermatitis, and several forms
of eczema including seborrheic, microbe, medical, occupational,
and true have increased nickel levels in the blood and often
in the skin. Myocardial infarction usually results in an
increase in the concentration of nickel in the serum[28,85,86].
Acute myocardial ischemia induced in dogs results in an increased
nickel concentration in the myocardium[87]. It has been
suggested that measurements of serum nickel may be useful in
the diagnosis of myocardial infarction[28,88]. Finally, nickel
may increase in the blood in gastrogenic iron deficiency[77],
infectious toxic anemia[77], thyrotoxicosis[89,90], gastric
ulcers[91], cardiac form of rheumatic disease[92], and Botkin's

disease[93]. In the chronic phase of this last disorder, nickel has been correlated with high serum bilirubin.

Following are some disorders in which nickel decreases in some tissue: It apparently decreases in the blood in several forms of anemia[94-97]. These include hemorrhagic, grave alimentary, vitamin B_{12} deficiency, and Addison-Biermer anemias. There are reports that nickel decreases in atherosclerotic aorta and in the atherosclerotic foci in the advanced stage[37,38], in several organs of babies that have died of bronchopneumonia[98], in the blood, liver, and spleen of dogs with radiation sickness[99], and in the blood of pemphigus patients[100].

It is difficult to speculate on the possible implications of these changes, but perhaps nickel does have a role in the prevention or production of some diseases. However, changes in nickel distribution tell little about which metabolic pathways are being changed or affected by the absence or presence of nickel. Thus a discussion on the pathways or compounds on which nickel does show some action is presented here. Two of the more likely areas in which nickel will probably be shown to have a physiological role are in hormonal action and/or membrane phenomena. Therefore these will be discussed first. Other possible roles, such as enzyme activation or a structural role, will also be presented. Finally, the effect of nickel on vitamin, lipid, nucleic acid, carbohydrate, protein, and mineral metabolism will be discussed in conjunction with the above, or separately. It should be pointed out that most of these effects discussed will be those of nickel injected as a compound such as $NiCl_2$, or have been done in vitro, therefore, could be just pharmacological actions. Still, it is felt that these actions can sometimes indicate a possible physiological role.

One of the earliest effects to be studied was the relation
of nickel to diabetes and the hormone insulin[101-104].
Bertrand and Macheboeuf in the 1920s found that the pancreas
is richer in nickel and cobalt than many other organs. This
resulted in their study of the action of these elements on the
hypoglucemic action of insulin. They found that nickel
administered after insulin did not modify the velocity of the
hypoglucemic action of insulin, but intensified and prolonged
that action so that the end result was an increased hypoglucemic
activity. Their studies were with dogs and rabbits. A later
report also indicated nickel reinforced and sustained the
hypoglucemic action of insulin[105]. Injected nickel apparently
can lower the sugar curve in dogs with alimentary glycemia[106]
and reduce adrenaline glycemia[105,107]. Dixit and Lazarow[108]
found that in vitro, nickel ions enhanced glucose uptake, its
oxidation to carbon dioxide, and its incorporation into fat
pad lipids, thus simulating the action of insulin. Furthermore
nickel increased glucose incorporation into glycogen.

In addition to the depressant effect of nickel on adrenaline
glycemia just mentioned, nickel can alter other actions of
adrenaline. Nickel weakens the hypertensive action, thus
reducing the effect of adrenaline (and also, histamine) on
blood pressure[109,110]. It decreases the vasomotor action of
adrenaline and histamine, thus heart action is not increased
as greatly by these compounds in the presence of nickel[111].
The level of nickel and level of adrenaline and noradrenaline
in blood has been correlated[112], and in vitro nickel helps
in the respiration or oxidation of adrenaline[113].

Another effect on hormonal action may be in water balance.
Nickel may increase the ability of muscle to take up water[114].
Nickel gives an antidiuretic action[115] and when added to
pituitary extract prolongs antidiuresis[116,117].

Nickel also has been shown to double the excretion of corticoids in the urine[118].

Nickel may have a role in melanin or pigment formation in various organisms. Japanese scientists have looked extensively at this, especially groups headed by H. Kikkawa and K. Abe. Kikkawa, Ogita, and Fujito noted that pigments derived from tyrosine and associated with nickel were white[119], and that nickel was found in white pigments derived from tryptophan in insects[120]. They then measured various trace metals in several species of animals with different colors. Following are some of their, and other groups, results. Eyes of a white mutant of Drosophila contain a larger amount of nickel and less iron, copper, and cobalt than do normal eyes[120]. White eggs from silkworms contain more nickel than do colored eggs[121]. In the integument of the silkworm, white is associated with nickel, red with molybdenum, and yellow with titanium[122]. Red goldfish accumulated more molybdenum and less nickel than do white goldfish[123]. More nickel is taken into the body and liver of the white mouse, more cobalt into the black[124]. Finally, ashes of albumins and globulins from livers of white mice contain more nickel than cobalt and copper; black, vice versa[125]. It was suggested that the receptor molecules of these metals are gene controlled. In a later paper Kikkawa, Ogita, Abe, and Doi[126] stated that some of the changes they reported in trace metal content with color may be erroneous; nonetheless, there appeared to be a relationship between white color and nickel[126]. In addition to these studies, it has been found that the reaction between o-quinone and tyrosine in melanin formation can be catalyzed by nickel[127], and that nickel can activate the first stage of melaninogenesis of dopa by tyrosinase[128].

Nickel may also have a role in three other interrelated
areas, those of nerve impulse transmission, membrane permability,
and muscle contraction. Experiments have been performed studying
the effect of nickel on the Ranvier node, the part of the
myelinated nerve fiber that does not have the myelin
sheath[129-131]. The action potential at this node can be
stopped by novacaine, or procaine, and it has been suggested,
by acting against the binding of calcium to phospholipids,
thus disturbing the orientation of the lipid and protein
molecules. Nickel can overcome this action perhaps by replacing
calcium in the binding of the phospholipid and reorientating
it properly to the protein present. It has been proposed that
nickel could also possibly play the part of calcium in the
liberation of the mediator in the mechanism of transmitter
release in the frog neuromuscular junction[132]. Nickel
apparently can replace calcium in the spread of excitation at
the sarcolema and transverse tubular system but not in the
activation of actomyosin ATPase in muscle excitation-contraction
coupling[133]. In calcium-free media, nickel is efficient in
restoring tonic contraction to the teniae coli of guinea
pigs[134], and can restore potassium-induced contracture of
skeletal muscle[135]. In addition to calcium the metabolism
of other ions, such as potassium and sodium, may be affected
in nerve and muscle tissue by nickel. Donskikh and
Babskii[136,137] state that it can accelerate the decrease of
sodium permeability and/or increase potassium permeability in
membranes after the myocardium has been stimulated. Khodorov
and Belyaev[138-140] have found that in the presence of nickel,
the Ranvier node has a slowing of the inactivation of sodium
permeability and an increase in potassium permeability. This
effect on permeability may explain the observation that nickel
increases the critical level of membrane potential in the

Ranvier node and lengthens the plateau phase of transmembrane action potential of ventricular muscle fibers[141].

Since the level of nickel can change in blood in some pathological conditions, nickel may have some role related to blood, its components, and related systems. In 1948 it was stated that nickel is indispensable for hematopoiesis[142]. Although it is doubtful if at present there is any support for this, there are reports that nickel has a temporary stimulating effect on hematopoiesis and it synergizes with vitamin B_{12} in this respect[143-145]. Apparently nickel has no effect on the production of hemoglobin, but does have a favorable or slightly stimulatory effect on the production of erythrocytes, leukocytes, and reticulocytes. Other reports indicate that nickel can enhance the adhesiveness of polymorphonuclear neutrophils in vitro[146], and in inflammation can reactivate the clumping of leukocytes that have been separated by EDTA[147]. In addition to inducing the clumping and phagocytosis of leukocytes[148] nickel can induce the aggregation of human thrombocytes in vitro[149].

Another possible role for nickel may be one of maintaining structure. In 1959 Wacker and Vallee[150] found a number of metals consistently present in their RNA preparations. Nickel was one of these, and it was found regularly in concentrations several orders of magnitude higher in the RNA than in the native material from which the RNA was isolated. This is the first report of nickel being associated with a specific biological compound. Since then, nickel has been shown to be consistently present in tobacco mosaic virus and its component RNA[151], to stabilize phage T5 against heat inactivation[152], and to increase the melting point of calf thymus DNA[153] and to stabilize it against heat denaturation[154]. In yeast RNA, nickel has been found at the 130 ppm level[155]. When RNA is

irradiated, the nickel level decreases, in some preparations
up to 68.7%. RNase acts faster on the resultant irradiated
RNA [156]. These results strongly suggest that nickel can
indeed have a structural role in the nucleic acids.

Nickel may also have a structural role in proteins,
especially enzymes. King[157] reported that the growth of bovine
pancreatic ribonuclease depends on the presence of a metal in
the crystallization medium. He found that nickel normally
gave the modification in the protein necessary for crystal
growth. He also observed that crystals made in nickel solution
became quite fragile upon soaking in a nickel-free solution.
In addition to a structural role, there have been many reports
of nickel activation, inhibition, and no effect on many enzyme
systems. Most of these studies have been done in vitro and,
of course, the concentration of nickel in the medium could
determine the effect nickel has on the system. There are
reports of activation, inhibition, and no effect on the same
type of enzyme, the variance probably being due to the level
of nickel used, the level or presence of other ions or cofactors,
or the source of the enzyme. It should be noted that when
nickel does have an effect on an enzyme, there are always some
other trace metals that have a similar effect. Nickel has not
been shown to be a specific activator of some enzyme.
Nonetheless, nickel has been shown to activate the following
enzymes: arginase[158-162], cholinesterase[163], DNAse[164],
esterase[165], NAD specific isocitric dehydrogenase[166],
phospholipase A[167], acetyl coenzyme A synthetase[168],
trypsin[169], tyrosinase[170], carboxylase[171], phosphoglu-
comutase[172], pyruvate dehydrogenase[173], glucosulfatase[174],
carboxypeptidase[175], histidine decarboxylase[176],
phytase[177], and aspartase[178]. Nickel has been shown to
inhibit the following enzymes: histidine deaminase[179,180],

estrogen sulfotransferase[181], isocitric dehydrogenase[182], aldolase[183], RNase[184], enolase[185], urease[186,187], ascorbic acid oxidase[188], creatine kinase[189], alanine aminotransferase[190], glutamic dehydrogenase[190], triose phosphate dehydrogenase[191], and glucose isomerase[192]. Not all enzymes affected are listed, but it is evident that nickel is not an indifferent ion in in vitro enzyme studies, and thus may have some effect in vivo.

The effect of nickel in carbohydrate metabolism has been discussed with insulin, nucleic acid metabolism with a possible structural role, and protein metabolism with a structural or enzyme role. In vitamin metabolism the possible interaction between nickel and vitamin B_{12} and cobalt has been indicated. This and the report that vitamin B_1 is stimulated by nickel as indicated by increased glycogen and galactose formation in the liver[193] are the extent of what was found in the literature on the interaction of vitamins and nickel in animals.

Nickel may have a role in lipid metabolism as cholesterol is reduced in the blood of rats fed 5 ppm nickel when compared to controls fed 100 ppb nickel[194]. Also liver mitochondrial preparations from rats fed supplemental nickel may exhibit an increased cholesterol oxidation when compared to that of control[195].

Finally, nickel may interact with other ions. Cobalt, calcium, potassium, and sodium have been discussed. However, there are other interactions that should be mentioned. The application of molybdenum to the soil and foliage made the Satsuma mandarin tree more vigorous and lessened injury due to excess nickel which suggests an antagonism between molybdenum and nickel[196,197]. The same relationship is true with the two metals in flax[198]. In oats, nickel toxicity is reduced

by aluminum[199] and iron[200,201]. In the C̲. cephalonica
larvae[202], N̲. crassa[203], and A̲. niger[204], magnesium and
iron can overcome nickel toxicity. Strontium ions reduce the
inhibitory effect of nickel ions for the fission of Paramecium
caudatoum[205]. Finally, cows on rations high in nickel have
an increased excretion of nickel in the feces and a reduction
of its retention when supplemented with higher levels of
copper[206].

Nickel toxicity has been studied quite extensively, but
since this presentation is stressing essentiality, toxicity
will be discussed lightly here. Nickel carbonyl poisoning has
been studied in depth by Sunderman and co-workers[207-220].
This compound, which is a component of cigarette smoke, is a
carcinogen. It is blamed for the high incidence of cancer in
the respiratory tract in early workers in nickel factories[221,
222]. Nickel as a metal in dust also has been implicated as a
carcinogen[223,224], and as an agent that can cause
skin-sensitizing dermatitis[225,226]. Nickel given as a soluble
compound, such as $NiCl_2$, in the diet is quite nontoxic to
mammals[227,228]. Over 1000 ppm have to be added to the diet
in short-term studies before adverse effects are seen in the
chick and mouse[229,230].

Thus the review of the literature should indicate why
nickel is an intriguing element. It is an element that occurs
in living organisms with consistency, it has biological
activity in vitro, its distribution is altered in pathological
conditions, and it can affect several metabolic pathways. In
other words it appears to be a dynamic trace element with an
important physiological role, and yet it still has not been
found to be essential for life in animals.

II. EXPERIMENTS

My efforts the past 3 years have been concerned with the
production of evidence that nickel is essential to animals.
Initially efforts to obtain a nickel deficiency in rats were
made and were unsuccessful. However, it was realized from these
experiments that getting a nickel deficiency in an animal was
going to be difficult and some new approaches were needed. It
was then the decision to use chicks was made. Chicks often
seem to have a higher requirement for specific minerals than
many other animals, and they often show more gross deficiency
symptoms in mineral studies, especially in the leg area.

One of the major problems with producing a nickel deficiency
is preparing a diet low in nickel. Nickel is a very ubiquitous
element when one is working in the parts per billion range.
The conventional method of using purified proteins, carbohydrates, vitamins, and minerals does not appear to be a good
method for obtaining nickel-deficient diets. The supplementation of reagent grade minerals still adds much contamination as
some chemicals contain upwards to 20,000 ppb nickel. Therefore
attempts to concoct a diet made of natural feedstuffs that are
low in nickel and that contain most vitamins and minerals in
amounts so no major addition of chemicals would be necessary
have been made. Four experiments with chicks have been
conducted, all with slightly different diets. The basic
ingredients have been the same as those in Table I in all
diets but the amounts have been varied, trying to find a
combination that would give good growth and deficiency symptoms.
The main ingredients are dried skim milk, corn meal, and corn
oil. The diet presented, which was used in Experiment 4, gave
a growth rate of approximately 220 grams in 4 weeks, and
according to colorimetric analysis[231] contains 40 ppb, or

TABLE I

Basal Chick Diet Low in Nickel

(<40 Ni)

Ingredient	Diet
Skim milk, dry powder[a]	665.0
Corn meal, yellow degerminated enriched[b]	226.0
Solka floc[c]	30.0
Corn oil	50.0
Arginine	10.0
Glycine	8.0
Vitamin mix[d]	0.7
Choline chloride	0.3
Mineral mix[e]	10.0
Total	1000.0

[a] General Biochemicals, Chagrin Falls, Ohio

[b] The Quaker Oats Co., Chicago, Illinois.

[c] Brown Co., New York, New York.

[d] The vitamin mix contained: in milligrams, vitamin A palmitate (250,000 IU/g), 8.0; vitamin D_3 (200,000 ICU/g), 4.0; tocopherol acetate (250 IU/g), 40.0; menadione, 0.6; niacin, 15.0; pyridoxine·HCl, 2.0; folic acid, 1.0; biotin, 0.1; vitamin B_{12} (0.1% triturate in mannitol), 5.0; neomycin sulfate, 25.0; thiamine, 1.0; dextrose, 598.3.

[e] The mineral mix contained: in grams, ZnO, 0.0500; KI, 0.0005; $CuSO_4$, 0.0075; $MnSO_4 \cdot 5H_2O$, 0.2400; iron sponge (dissolved in HCl), 0.0350; dextrose 0.6670; corn meal, 9.000.

Iron sponge and $MnSO_4 \cdot 5H_2O$ "Specpure", Jarrell-Ash Co., Waltham, Massachusetts.

less, nickel on an air-dried basis. Control chicks were given the same diet supplemented with 3-5 ppm nickel as nickel chloride. The diets and quartz distilled water were provided ad libitum to a heavy breed of chicks (New Hampshire Red (Experiment 3), Sex-Linked Cross (Experiment 4), White Rock (Experiment 1,2)).

In all experiments the chicks have been housed in all-plastic, controlled environment systems[232] so that nickel present in conventional housing, dust, and air would not be available to them. In the last two experiments, rigid plastic isolators were employed. These isolators were all plastic in the inside, and so were the cages, filters, feeding, and watering accessories. The heat sources for the chicks were plastic-covered heating pads which kept the temperature close to 34 degrees at one end of an inside cage. The first two experiments have been presented elsewhere[233], and thus they will not be discussed here, except for an isotope study performed in one.

In all experiments, after 4 weeks, the gross appearance of the chicks was affected by the amount of nickel in the diet. One difference was most nickel-deficient chicks showed a brighter orange-yellow color in the legs, while the nickel-supplemented chicks showed some form of a paler brown-yellow color. Color in chick legs often is associated with carotenoids, and Kikkawa, Ogita and Fujito[234] have reported that white color in anthocyanins and carotenoids in plants is associated with nickel. Therefore there may be some relation between nickel, carotenoid production, and color in the chick. Perhaps mention of the fact that in pemphigus patients, pigmentation occurs and this has been correlated with a decrease in nickel in the blood (100) should be made here.

Another difference was found in leg structure. A slight
swelling of the hock and some thickening of the leg, especially
near the joint area was noted in the nickel-deficient chicks
when compared to those supplemented with nickel. This change
was never severe, and thus its significance is somewhat unclear.
In the literature review it was noted that nickel could replace
calcium in some metabolic pathways, such as muscle contraction
and nerve transmission. In addition, nickel can replace calcium
in activating complement[235], it can inactivate the calcifying
mechanism in rachitic bone cartilage slices[236], and high
levels of nickel can result in a change in calcium content in
plants[237]. Thus perhaps calcium and nickel are interacting in
some way in bone formation and this results in the slight changes
seen in leg structure.

Many of the chicks fed the nickel-deficient diet appeared
to have a slight dermatitis on their shank skin, especially near
the metatarsal joints. When compared to chicks fed supplemental
nickel, the skin had a rougher appearance. The scales did not
overlap well and appeared to protrude slightly from the surface
of the leg. Reports that nickel can affect skin metabolism are
extensive. The affinity of nickel for epithelial tissues has
been shown[238], and nickel dermatitis is common in nickel
refineries[226]. Raben and Antonev[225] found that nickel
accumulates in the follicular apparatus of the dermis. These
effects are more due to high levels of nickel, or nickel metal,
but they still show that nickel can alter the metabolism of skin,
and therefore the lack of nickel may cause some disturbance in
the shank skin of the chicks.

In the last two experiments approximately 10% of the
nickel-deficient chicks died suddenly. Upon autopsy, no
apparent reason was found for the deaths. This did not occur
in the nickel-supplemented groups.

At 4 weeks the chicks were dissected to remove various
tissues. It was noted that many of the livers of the
nickel-supplemented chicks were more friable or had more
tendency to tear upon removal. Often the livers of the
nickel-deficient chicks appeared slightly paler in color.
Gross analyses were made on the livers and other tissues.
The data in Table II give the ether-extractable lipid content
of the livers on a fresh and dry basis in the last two experiments. In both experiments the lipid content was significantly
reduced in the nickel-deficient chicks. In the first of these
experiments, on the fresh basis, the value was 1.92% compared
to 4.24% for the controls. In this experiment a significant
weight difference was obtained 205 g versus 171 g. No weight
differences were obtained in any other of the three experiments,

TABLE II

Ether-Extractable Lipid Content of Livers

Group	Fat fresh basis (percent)	Fat dry basis (percent)	Average chick weight (grams)
Experiment 3			
Nickel low	1.92[a]	6.92[a]	171[a]
Nickel high	4.24	13.69	205
Experiment 4			
Nickel low	1.73[a]	5.62[a]	212
Nickel high	2.71	8.69	214

[a] Significantly less (P<0.01) than comparable nickel high
group.

but this may be a symptom of nickel deficiency as experiments
with quail show that nickel deficiency may result in a reduced
growth rate[239]. In the last experiment the lipid content of
the liver was also significantly reduced in deficient chicks,
being 1.73% compared to 2.71% for the controls. Table III
gives other tissues which show some change in ether-extractable
lipid. These include the aorta and perhaps the kidney and heart.
Table IV shows that the ether-extractable lipid content of bone,
muscle, lung, and gizzard is not altered in nickel deficiency.
In the shank skin it appears that the ether-extractable lipid
is higher in the nickel-deficient chicks than in the controls.

TABLE III

Ether-Extractable Lipid Content of Aorta, Heart, and Kidney

Tissue	Experiment	Nickel supplemented (ppm)	Fat fresh basis (percent)	Fat dry basis (percent)
Aorta	3	0	5.38	22.08
Aorta	3	3	7.72	30.47
Aorta	4	0	10.91	33.54
Aorta	4	3	14.98	40.99
Kidney	3	0	2.11	9.36
Kidney	3	3	2.25	9.96
Kidney	4	0	2.12	7.97
Kidney	4	3	2.43	9.33
Heart	3	0	1.29	6.12
Heart	3	3	2.40	11.32
Heart	4	0	5.72	24.71
Heart	4	3	5.92	25.23

TABLE IV

Ether-Extractable Lipid Content of

Bone, Muscle, Lung, Gizzard, and Skin

Tissue	Experiment	Nickel supplemented (ppm)	Fat fresh basis (percent)	Fat dry basis (percent)
Bone	3	0	7.80	16.67
Bone	3	3	7.85	16.95
Muscle	3	0	1.40	6.10
Muscle	3	3	1.38	6.16
Lung	4	0	1.70	7.95
Lung	4	3	1.79	8.32
Gizzard	3	0	1.04	4.36
Gizzard	3	3	0.90	3.88
Gizzard	4	0	2.88	9.99
Gizzard	4	3	3.13	10.25
Skin	3	0	3.26	8.89
Skin	3	3	2.68	7.70
Skin	4	0	3.89	10.12
Skin	4	3	3.65	9.26

Because chicks fed low levels of nickel have less ether-extract-able lipid in their livers, hearts, aortas, and kidneys when compared to those from chicks fed nickel at a level that can occur in commercial feeds, it is speculated that nickel has a role in lipid metabolism in the chick. Serum cholesterol has been measured, and an example is given in Table V. No signifi-cant changes have been found, but usually the average value for the nickel-supplemented chicks is 10% to 20% lower than that of the nickel-deficient chicks. This is just the opposite of the direction of change in the ether-extractable lipid in the

TABLE V

Plasma Cholesterol,[a] Experiment 3

Nickel low (mg/100 ml)	Nickel high (mg/100 ml)
131 ± 6	117 ± 7

[a] Values are not significantly different from each other.

liver, heart, aorta, and kidney, but is the same as that in the shank skin. It does correspond to the observation of Schroeder that cholesterol is reduced in the blood of rats supplemented with nickel[194].

Table VI data indicate that the nickel-deficient chicks usually have a higher ash value in the tissues analyzed on a dry basis. For example, in these two experiments the deficient liver contained 4.70% and 4.57% ash; the supplemented contains 4.39% and 4.33%. In nickel-deficient brain, ash was 5.42% compared to 4.76% for the controls. In heart, the deficient contained 4.44% compared to 4.21% for controls, and so on, with similar differences in the aorta, skin, and lung. When these changes are expressed on the fat-free, dry basis, however, they are not as evident because of the changes in the lipid content in these tissues. A calcium-nickel interaction may also here have a bearing on these results.

In an earlier experiment[233] some deficient and control chicks were intubated with approximately 25 μCi of [63]nickel at the end of 3 1/2 weeks, and a number of tissues were removed for [63]nickel analysis. The results were quite variable, and the number of chicks per time-period group never exceeded 3, so the analysis of variance did not show many significant

TABLE VI

Ash Content of Tissues

Tissue	Experiment	Nickel supplement (ppm)	Ash fresh basis (percent)	Ash dry basis (percent)	Ash fat-free dry basis (percent)
Liver	3	0	1.39	4.70	5.05
Liver	3	3	1.34	4.39	5.09
Liver	4	0	1.38	4.57	4.80
Liver	4	3	1.35	4.33	4.75
Brain	4	0	1.11	5.42	
Brain	4	3	0.99	4.76	
Heart	3	0	0.93	4.44	4.64
Heart	3	3	0.90	4.21	4.86
Heart	4	0	1.01	4.29	5.54
Heart	4	3	0.96	4.05	5.36
Aorta	4	0	0.71	2.46	3.66
Aorta	4	3	0.59	1.85	3.00
Skin	3	0	0.71	1.91	2.09
Skin	3	3	0.40	1.15	1.25
Skin	4	0	0.91	2.39	2.66
Skin	4	3	0.83	2.07	2.38
Lung	3	0	1.25	6.49	
Lung	3	3	1.20	5.89	
Lung	4	0	1.22	5.71	6.23
Lung	4	3	1.07	5.04	5.49
Kidney	3	0	1.20	5.34	5.98
Kidney	3	3	1.24	5.39	6.38
Kidney	4	0	1.28	4.86	5.23
Kidney	4	3	1.33	5.25	5.79
Muscle	3	0	1.00	4.48	4.76
Muscle	3	3	0.91	4.14	4.41
Gizzard	3	0	0.87	3.64	3.78
Gizzard	3	3	0.84	3.61	3.82
Gizzard	4	0	0.98	3.31	3.65
Gizzard	4	3	0.94	3.15	3.55

differences. However, from Tables VII and VIII (results are given in percent of administered dose) it appears that bone and its related tissue, liver, and kidney took up relatively large amounts of [63]nickel. Other tissues, such as blood and muscle, retained relatively small amounts of the isotope. In fact it was barely detectable 24 hours after administration. In some tissues from the nickel-deficient chicks, including bone

TABLE VII

[63]Nickel Distribution in Selected Tissues, Experiment 2

Tissue	Hours post administration	Administered dose	
		Ni low	Ni high
		(percent)	
Bone	6	0.296[a]	0.128[a]
	24	0.101	0.076
	48	0.098[a]	0.041[a]
Primary spongiosa	6	0.134	0.072
	24	0.034	0.023
	48	0.029	0.024
Liver	6	0.103[a]	0.042[a]
	24	0.062	0.039
	48	0.069	0.035
Muscle	6	0.018	0.017
	24	0.003	0.004
	48	0.003	0.003
Blood, whole	6	0.041	0.035
	24	0.004	0.005
	48	0.002	0.002

[a] Values for the same tissue and in the same time period are significantly different (P<0.10) from each other.

TABLE VIII

[63]Nickel Distribution in Selected Tissues, Experiment 2

Tissue	Hours post administration	Administered dose	
		Ni low	Ni high
Kidney	6	0.609	0.292
	24	0.291	0.173
	48	0.193	0.141
Spleen	6	0.044[a]	0.023[a]
	24	0.021	0.020
	48	0.017	0.010
Aorta	6	0.157[a]	0.053[a]
	24	0.026	0.016
	48	0.021	0.025
Feather	6	0.032	0.035
	24	0.040	0.049
	48	0.064	0.046
Gizzard lining	6	0.102[a]	0.196[a]
	24	0.008[a]	0.016[a]
	48	0.006	0.005

[a] Values for the same tissue and in the same time period are significantly different ($P < 0.10$) from each other.

at the 6- and 48-hour, and liver, spleen, and aorta at the 6-hour time periods, there was a significantly increased uptake of [63]nickel when compared to those from chicks fed supplemental nickel. The only tissue that showed a greater amount of [63]nickel retention in the nickel-supplemented group was the gizzard lining. Interestingly tissues that showed fat changes, such as the liver and aorta, and those that had some appearance change, such as the bone, showed significant differences in

^{63}nickel retention at some time period. A specific biological function for nickel may be indicated in these tissues because of these separate observations.

It should be pointed out that in all four experiments thus far, there has been some form of stress on these chicks. These stresses were as follows. Experiment 1, lack of heat and crowded conditions; Experiment 2, lack of heat, crowded conditions, and salmonella infection; Experiment 3, high humidity and diarrhea; Experiment 4, hot, humid, and crowded conditions. In attempts to repeat this work these must be kept in mind, as it has been indicated in the literature review, nickel may be playing a role synergistic with some hormone.

In conclusion, it appears from the literature that nickel is a dynamic trace element with a possible essential role in animals. This statement has been further substantiated by the experimental data presented which show that low levels of nickel in the diet can cause changes in the chick. These changes include a different shade of yellow in the shank skin; slightly swollen hocks; slightly thickened legs; a dermatitis on the shank skin; a change in the texture and color of the liver; a reduction in ether-extractable lipid in the liver, heart, aorta, and kidney; an increase in the ash in many tissues on a dry basis; a difference in the manner in which ^{63}nickel is handled; and, perhaps, occasional death and growth retardation.

However, the nickel deficiency described is at best borderline. Further improvements in diets and methods are needed. My current efforts are in this area, and it is hoped that a deficiency severe enough so that it is completely obvious that nickel is needed for optimum performance, health, and life in animals will be obtained.

ACKNOWLEDGMENT

The author expresses his appreciation to Mrs. Darla Higgs and Mr. Harold Mohr for their technical assistance and to Mrs. Genevieve Thomas for performing the statisical analyses in the experiments.

REFERENCES

[1]. Berg, R., Biochem. Z., 165, 461 (1925).

[2]. Bertrand, G. and Macheboeuf, M., Compt. Rend., 180, 1380 (1925).

[3]. Malyuga, D. P., Trav. Lab. Biogeochim. Acad. Sci. U. R. S. S., 5, 91 (1939).

[4]. Guelbenzu, M. D., Anales Real Acad. Farm., 17, 237 (1951).

[5]. Turekian, K. K. and Kleinkopf, M. D., Bull. Geol. Soc. Am., 67, 1129 (1956).

[6]. Hettche, H. O., Air Water Pollution, 8, 185 (1964).

[7]. Schroeder, H. A., Balassa, J. J., and Tipton, I. H., J. Chron. Dis., 15, 51 (1962).

[8]. Archibald, J. G., J. Dairy Sci., 32, 877 (1949).

[9]. Heinzelman, D. C. and O'Connor, R. T., J. Am. Oil Chem. Soc., 28, 373 (1951).

[10]. Taktakishvili, S. D., Vopr. Pitaniya, 22, 73 (1963).

[11]. Los, L. I., Pyatnitskaya, L. K., and Samsonova, A. S., Vopr. Pitaniya, 25, 84 (1966).

[12]. Petrova, R. and Radenkov, S., Gradinar. Lozar. Nauka, 6, 115 (1969).

[13]. Burke, K. E. and Albright, C. H., J. Ass. Offic. Anal. Chem., 53, 531 (1970).

[14]. Leonov, V. A., Mikroelementy v Sel'sk. Khoz. i Med. Sbornik, 1956, 559 (1956).

[15].   Cluett, M. L. and Yoe, J. H., Anal. Chem., 29, 1265
        (1957).
[16].   Usov, I. N., Trudy Beloruss. Nauch.-Issled. Inst.
        Perelivan. Krovi, 6, 180 (1957).
[17].   Pavlova, A. K., Vestnik Akad. Nauk Belorus. S. S. R.,
        3, 83 (1956).
[18].   Voldko, L. V. and Pristupa, C. V., Vestsi Akad. Navuk
        Belarusk. S. S. R., Ser. Biyal. Navuk, 1962, 107 (1962).
[19].   Korobenkova, M. M., Dokl. Akad. Nauk Belorussk.
        S. S. R., 6, 527 (1962).
[20].   Imbus, H. R., Cholak, J., Miller, L. H., and
        Sterling, T., Arch. Environ. Health, 6, 286 (1963).
[21].   Butt, E. M., Nusbaum, R. E., Gilmour, T. C.,
        Didio, S. L., and Mariano, S., Arch. Environ. Health,
        8, 52 (1964).
[22].   Lifshits, V. M., Tr. Voronezhsk. Gos. Med. Inst., 49,
        110 (1962).
[23].   Schaller, K. H., Kuehner, A., and Lehnert, G., Blut.,
        17, 155 (1968).
[24].   Zhernakova, T. V., Lab Delo, 1967, 184 (1967).
[25].   Sunderman, F. W., Jr., Clin. Chem., 13, 115 (1967).
[26].   Mertz, D. P., Koschnick, R., Wilk, G., and
        Pfeilsticker, K., Z. Klin. Chem. Klin. Biochem., 6,
        171 (1968).
[27].   Timakin, N. P., Petrakovskaya, E. A., Bagdasarova, L. B.,
        Malyutina, G. N., Zak, R. Y., and Rudchenko, V. A.,
        Vop. Teor. Klim. Gematol., Tomsk. Med. Inst., 1967, 114
        (1967).
[28].   Sunderman, F. W., Jr., 4th Ann. Conf. on Trace
        Substances in Environmental Health, Columbia, Missouri,
        1970, p. 352.
[29].   Paixão, L. M. and Yoe, J. H., Clin. Chim. Acta, 4, 507
        (1959).

[30]. Lifshits, V. M., Vopr. Med. Khim., 9, 610 (1963).

[31]. Lifshits, V. M., Lab Delo, 1965, 655 (1965).

[32]. Takaoka, K., Folia Endocrinol. Japon., 30, 499 (1954).

[33]. Perry, H. M., Jr., Tipton, I. H., Schroeder, H. A., and Cook, M. J., J. Lab. Clin. Med., 60, 245 (1962).

[34]. Tipton, I. H. and Cook, M. J., Health Phys., 9, 103 (1963).

[35]. Glavatskikh, G. I. and Ermakov, V. V., Biol. Rol Mikroelementov v Organizme Cheloveka i Zhivotn. Vost. Sibiri i Dal'nego Vostoka, Akad. Nauk S. S. S. R., Sibirsk. Otd., Komis. Po Izuch. Mikorelementov, Buryatsk. Kompleksn. Nauchn.-Issled. Inst., Tr. Konf., Ulan-Ude, 1962, 32 (1962).

[36]. Dmitriev, V. F., Gazarkh, L. A., and Shipitsyn, S. A., Mikroelementy v Pochvakh. Vodakh. i Organizmakh Vost. Sibiri i Dal'nego Vostoka i Ikh Rol v Zhizni Rast., Zhivotnykh i Cheloveka, Akad. Nauk S. S. S. R., Sibirsk. Otd., Tr. Pervoi Konf., Ulan-Ude, 1960, 99 (1960).

[37]. Bala, Y. M., Plotko, S. A., and Furmenko, G. I., Ter. Arkh., 39, 105 (1967).

[38]. Avtandilov, G. G., Arkh. Patol., 29, 40 (1967).

[39]. Yagovdik, N. Z., Dokl. Akad. Nauk Beloruss. S. S. R., 3, 77 (1959).

[40]. Yagovdik, N. Z., Dokl. Akad. Nauk Belorussk. S. S. R., 7, 350 (1963).

[41]. Yagovdik, N. Z., Vestsi Akad. Navuk Belarusk. S. S. R., Ser. Biyal. Navuk, 1964, 93 (1964).

[42]. Nusbaum, R. E., Butt, E. M., Gilmour, T. C., and Didio, S. L., Arch. Environ. Health, 10, 227 (1965).

[43]. Leonov, V. A., Vestsi Akad. Navuk Belarusk. S. S. R., Ser. Biyal. Navuk, 1956, 151 (1956).

[44]. Leonov, V. A. and Sakovich, L. T., Vestsi. Akad. Navuk
      Belarusk. S. S. R., Ser. Biyal Navuk, 1957, 101 (1957).

[45]. Sakovich, L. T., Sbornik Nauchn. Rabot., Minsk. Med.
      Inst., 19, 259 (1957).

[46]. Leonov, V. A., Dokl. Akad. Nauk Belorussk. S. S. R.,
      6, 457 (1962).

[47]. Mikosha, A., Nauk Zap. Stanislavs'k Med. Inst., 1959,
      85 (1959).

[48]. Krasnoshlykov, G. Y., Tr. 5-i Nauchn. Sessii.
      Aktyubinsk. Med. Inst., 1965, 73 (1965).

[49]. Arnon, D. I., Am. J. Botany, 25, 322 (1938).

[50]. Kashin, V. K., Mikroelem. Sib., 6, 78 (1968).

[51]. Dobrolyubskiĭ, O. K., Vinodelie i Vinogradarstvo
      S. S. S. R., 17, 19 (1957).

[52]. Otsuka, K., Nippon Dojo-Hiryogaku Zasshi, 33, 465 (1962).

[53]. Markman, A. L. and Kruglova, E. K., Tr. Tashkent.
      Politekh. Inst., 42, 59 (1968).

[54]. Lapa, V. G., Romanchuk, P. S., Skuratovskaya, M. Z.,
      and Levina, N. I., Pochv. Usloviya i Effektivnost.
      Udobr., 1963, 131 (1963).

[55]. Lapa, V. G. and Romanchuk, P. S., Mikroelem. Sel. Khoz.
      Med., Akad. Nauk Ukr. S. S. R., Respub. Mezhvedom. Sb.,
      1966, 126 (1966).

[56]. Lo, T. Y. and Wu, C. H., J. Chinese Chem. Soc., 10, 58
      (1943).

[57]. Lo, T. Y. and Chen, S. M., Proc. Inst. Food Tech.,
      1945, 154 (1945).

[58]. Lo, T. Y. and Chen, S. M., Food Res., 11, 159 (1946).

[59]. Lo, T. Y. and Chen, S. M., Chinese J. Nutr., 1, 5 (1946).

[60]. Lo, T. Y. and Chen, S. M., Chinese J. Nutr., 1, 29
      (1946).

[61]. Lo, T. Y. and Chen, S. M., Sci. Rec. (China), 2, 81
      (1947).

[62]. Lo, T. Y. and Chen, S. M., Sci. Rec. (China), 2, 84
       (1947).

[63]. Efimov, M. V., Kashin, V. K., and Bakhanova, G. S.,
       Mikroelem. Biosfere Ikh Primen. Sel. Khoz. Med. Sib.
       Dal'nego Vostoka, Dokl. Sib. Konf., 2nd, 1964, 289
       (1964).

[64]. Lipskaya, G. A., Vestsi Akad. Navuk Belarusk. S. S. R.,
       Ser. Biyal. Navuk, 1962, 53 (1962).

[65]. Van Heyningen, W. E., Brit. J. Exptl. Pathol., 36,
       373 (1955).

[66]. Kinne-Diettrich, E. M., Kiel. Meeresforsch., 11, 34
       (1955).

[67]. Wazny, J., Acta Soc. Botan. Polon., 32, 575 (1963).

[68]. Bertrand, D. and de Wolf, A., C. R. Acad. Sci., Paris,
       Ser. D, 265, 1053 (1967).

[69]. Amaha, M., Ordal, Z. J., and Touba, A., J. Bacteriol.,
       72, 34 (1956).

[70]. Vorob'eva, L. I., Dokl. Akad. Nauk S. S. S. R., 145,
       1381 (1962).

[71]. Popova, Y., Chaga, S., and Beshkova, M., Nauchni. Tr.,
       Nauchnoizsled. Inst. Konservna Prom., Plovdiv, 1, 147
       (1963).

[72]. Kotala, L. and Luba, J., Acta Polon. Pharm., 22, 419
       (1965).

[73]. Rigg, T., 10th Ann. Rept. Dept. Sci. Ind. Research,
       New Zealand, 1936, 30 (1936).

[74]. Filmer, J. F. and Underwood, E. J., Aust. Vet. J., 13,
       57 (1937).

[75]. Schroeder, H. A., Balassa, J. J., and Vinton, W. H., Jr.,
       J. Nutr., 83, 239 (1964).

[76]. Gul'ko, I. S., Voprosy Onkol., 7, 46 (1961).

[77]. Lifshits, V. M., Nekotorye Vopr. Kardiol., Mikroelementy,
       Voronezh, Sb., 1964, 88 (1964).

[78]. Leonov, V. A. and Ustinovich, A. K., Dokl. Akad. Nauk
Belorussk. S. S. R., 10, 219 (1966).

[79]. Gul'ko, I. S., Vestsi Akad. Navuk Belarusk. S. S. R.,
Ser. Biyal. Navuk, 1960, 117 (1960).

[80]. Rybnikov, V. I. and Volkova, L. A., Med. Radiol., 15,
52 (1970).

[81]. Gaul, L. E. and Staud, A. H., Arch. Dermatol. Syphilol.,
30, 697 (1934).

[82]. Yagovdik, N. Z., Sbornik Nauch. Rabot. Belorus.
Nauchn.-Issled. Kozhno-Venerol. Inst., 6, 303 (1959).

[83]. Prokopchuk, A. Y., Sosnovskii, A. T., Vagovdik, N. Z.,
and Orlova, Z. I., Vestsi Akad. Navuk Belarusk. S. S. R.,
Ser. Biyal. Navuk, 1964, 92 (1964).

[84]. Leonov, V. A. and Yagovdik, N. Z., Mikroelementy v
Sel'sk Khoz. i Med. Sb., 1963, 577 (1963).

[85]. D'Alonzo, C. A., Pell, S., and Fleming, A. J., J.
Occupational Med., 5, 71 (1963).

[86]. D'Alonzo, C. A. and Pell, S., Arch. Environ. Health, 6,
381 (1963).

[87]. Ryabova, V. V., Tr., Voronezh. Gos. Med. Inst., 58,
94 (1967).

[88]. Scheel, L. D., Am. Ind. Hyg. Assoc. J., 26, 585 (1965).

[89]. Hesse, E., Carpus, I., and Zeppmeisel, L., Arch. Exptl.
Path. Pharmakol., 176, 283 (1934).

[90]. Burov, V. V., Mater. Povolzh. Konf. Fiziol., Farmakol.,
Biokhim. Uchastiem Morfol. Klin., 4th, Saratov, 1, 120
(1966).

[91]. Pristupa, C. V., Zdravookhr. Belorussii, 1962, 28 (1962).

[92]. Pauk, A. I., Vestsi Akad. Navuk Belarusk. S. S. R.,
Ser. Biyal. Navuk, 1960, 127 (1960).

[93]. Sukharev, V. M. and Chistyakov, N. M., Terapevt. Arkh.,
35, 38 (1963).

[94]. Shustov, V. Y., Vestsi Akad. Navuk Belarusk. S. S. R., Ser. Biyal. Navuk, 1960, 77 (1960).

[95]. Shustov, V. Y., Polskie Arch. Med. Wewnetrznej, 31, 211 (1961).

[96]. Lago, O. M., Sb. Nauchn. Tr. Ivanov. Gos. Med. Inst., 31, 85 (1965).

[97]. Kimura, K., Hara, R., and Iijima, N., J. Pharm. Soc. Japan, 72, 1249 (1952).

[98]. Sakovich-Lomako, L. T., Zdravookhr. Belorussii, 1962, 28 (1962).

[99]. Boiko, V. A., Dokl. Akad. Nauk Belorussk. S. S. R., 8, 332 (1964).

[100]. Silvestri, U., Boll. Soc. Ital. Biol. Sper., 36, 347 (1960).

[101]. Bertrand, G. and Macheboeuf, M., Compt. Rend., 182, 1504 (1926).

[102]. Bertrand, G. and Macheboeuf, M., Compt. Rend., 183, 257 (1926).

[103]. Bertrand, G. and Macheboeuf, M., Compt. Rend., 183, 5 (1926).

[104]. Bertrand, G. and Macheboeuf, M., Compt. Rend., 182, 1305 (1926).

[105]. Schwab, H., Compt. Rend., 207, 409 (1938).

[106]. Berenshtein, F. Y., Byull. Eksptl. Biol. Med., 12, 178 (1941).

[107]. Berenshtein, F. Y., Fiziol. Zhur. S. S. S. R., 33, 209 (1947).

[108]. Dixit, P. K. and Lazarow, A., Am. J. Physiol., 213, 849 (1967).

[109]. Hermann, H., Chatonnet, J., and Vial, J., Arch. Intern. Pharmacodynamie, 98, 129 (1954).

[110]. Berenshtein, F. Y., Sapozhkov, S. V., Korneiko, A. V.,
Sak, Z. M., and Kholod, V. M., Materialy 1-go (Peruogo)
S'ezda Belorussk. Fiziol. Obshchestva Sb., 1962, 40
(1960).

[111]. Szilágyi, T., Szatai, I., and Csaba, B., Acta Physiol.
Acad. Sci. Hung., 15, 75 (1959).

[112]. Sushko, E. P., Dokl. Akad. Nauk Belorussk. S. S. R.,
13, 952 (1969).

[113]. Chaix, P., Chauvet, J., and Jezequel, J., Biochim.
Biophys. Acta, 4, 471 (1950).

[114]. Mascherpa, P., Arch. Intern. Pharmacodynamie, 43, 371
(1932).

[115]. Dodds, E. C., Noble, R. L., Rinderknecht, H., and
Williams, P. C., Lancet, 1937, 309 (1937).

[116]. Noble, R. L., Rinderknecht, H., and Williams, P. C.,
J. Physiol., 96, 293 (1939).

[117]. Organon, N. V., Neth., 97, 112 (1961).

[118]. Sobel, H., Sideman, M., and Arce, R., Proc. Soc. Exptl.
Biol. Med., 104, 86 (1960).

[119]. Kikkawa, H., Ogita, Z., and Fujito, S., Science, 121,
43 (1955).

[120]. Kikkawa, H., Ogita, Z., and Fujito, S., Proc. Japan
Acad., 30, 30 (1954).

[121]. Doi, K. and Abe, K., Igaku to Seibutsugaku, 37, 197
(1955).

[122]. Kikkawa, H., Ogita, Z., and Fujito, S., Kagaku, 24,
528 (1954).

[123]. Yumikura, T. and Abe, K., Igaku to Seibutsugaku, 36,
71 (1956).

[124]. Abe, K., Med. J. Osaka Univ., 6, 605 (1955).

[125]. Abe, K., Igaku to Seibutsugaku, 37, 64 (1955).

[126]. Kikkawa, H., Ogita, Z., Abe, K., and Doi, K., Science, 128, 1431 (1958).

[127]. Kertéz, D., Nature, 168, 697 (1951).

[128]. Polonovski, M., Gonnard, P., and Svinareff, O., Congr. Intern. Biochim., Résumés Communs., 2e Congr., Paris, 1952, 282 (1952).

[129]. Khodorov, B. I. and Belyaev, V. I., Tsitologiya, 6, 680 (1964).

[130]. Khodorov, B. I. and Belyaev, V. I., Biofizika, 10, 625 (1965).

[131]. Blaustein, M. P. and Goldman, D. E., Science, 153, 429 (1966).

[132]. Mambrini, J. and Benoit, P. R., C. R. Soc. Biol., 163, 581 (1969).

[133]. Fischman, D. A. and Swan, R. C., J. Gen. Physiol., 50, 1709 (1967).

[134]. Imai, S. and Takeda, K., J. Physiol. (London), 190, 155 (1967).

[135]. Frank, G. B., J. Physiol. (London), 163, 254 (1962).

[136]. Donskikh, E. A., Tr. Inst. Norm. Patol. Fiziol. Akad. Med. Nauk S. S. S. R., 10, 48 (1967).

[137]. Babskii, E. B. and Donskikh, E. A., Dokl. Akad. Nauk S. S. S. R., 178, 248 (1968).

[138]. Khodorov, B. I., Biofizika, 8, 707 (1963).

[139]. Khodorov, B. I. and Belyaev, V. I., Biofizika, 11, 108 (1966).

[140]. Khodorov, B. I., Protoplasmich. Membrany Ikh Funkts. Rol, 1965, 46 (1965).

[141]. Kleinfeld, M., Stein, E., and Aguillardo, D., Am. J. Physiol., 211, 1438 (1966).

[142]. Lederer, E. and Lourau, M., Biochim. Biophys. Acta, 2, 278 (1948).

[143]. Lecoq, R., Chauchard, P., and Mazoué, H., Thérapie, 7, 345 (1952).

[144]. Lecoq, R., Chauchard, P., and Mazoué, H., Excerpta Med., Sect. II, 7, 93 (1954).

[145]. Nasel'skiǐ, N. B., Mikroelementy v Sel'sk. Khoz. i Med. Sb., 1956, 597 (1956).

[146]. Garvin, J. E., J. Cell Physiol., 72, 197 (1968).

[147]. Allison, F., Jr., Lancaster, M. G., and Crosthwaite, J. L., Am. J. Pathol., 43, 775 (1963).

[148]. Allison, F., Jr. and Lancaster, M. G., Ann. N. Y. Acad. Sci., 161, 936 (1964).

[149]. Reinhard, B. and Patscheke, H., Therapiewoche, 18, 2113 (1968).

[150]. Wacker, W. E. C. and Vallee, B. L., J. Biol. Chem., 234, 3257 (1959).

151]. Wacker, W. E. C., Gordon, M. P., and Huff, J. W., Biochemistry, 2, 716 (1963).

[152]. Lark, K. G. and Adams, M. H., Cold Spring Harbor Symposia Quant. Biol., 18, 171 (1953).

[153]. Fais, D., Biokhimiya, 28, 1018 (1963).

[154]. Eichhorn, G. L., Nature, 194, 474 (1962).

[155]. Kaindl, K. and Altmann, H., Oesterr. Studienges. Atomenergie SGAE-BL-1, 1964.

[156]. Altmann, H., Biophysik, 1, 329 (1964).

[157]. King, M. V., Nature, 201, 918 (1964).

[158]. Hellerman, L. and Perkins, M. E., J. Biol. Chem., 112, 175 (1935).

[159]. Hellerman, L. and Stock, C. C., J. Biol. Chem., 125, 771 (1938).

[160]. Stock, C. C., Perkins, M. E., and Hellerman, L., J. Biol. Chem., 125, 753 (1938).

[161]. Edlbacher, S. and Baur, H., Z. Physiol. Chem., 254,
        275 (1938).

[162]. Vincent, D., Aloy, R., and Govinet, R., Trav. Membres
        Soc. Chim. Biol., 23, 1463 (1941).

[163]. Frommel, E., Herschberg, A. D., and Piquet, J., Compt.
        Rend. Soc. Phys. Hist. Nat. Genève, 60, 97 (1943).

[164]. Miyaji, T. and Greenstein, J. P., Arch. Biochem.
        Biophys., 32, 414 (1951).

[165]. Langenbeck, W., Müller, K. A., and Lange, K., Z. Physiol.
        Chem., 314, 130 (1959).

[166]. Cennamo, C., Montecuccoli, G., and Bonaretti, G.,
        Boll. Soc. Ital. Biol. Sper., 42, 29 (1966).

[167]. Brown, J. H. and Bowles, M. E., Toxicon, 3, 205 (1966).

[168]. Webster, L. T., Jr., J. Biol. Chem., 240, 4164 (1965).

[169]. Sugai, K., J. Biochem. (Japan), 36, 91 (1944).

[170]. Lerner, A. B., Fitzpatrick, T. B., Calkins, E., and
        Summerson, W. H., J. Biol. Chem., 187, 793 (1950).

[171]. Speck, J. F., J. Biol. Chem., 178, 315 (1949).

[172]. Ray, W. J., Jr., J. Biol. Chem., 244, 3740 (1969).

[173]. Yamamoto, M., Kekkaku, 30, 473 (1955).

[174]. Egami, H., J. Chem. Soc. Japan, 60, 849 (1939).

[175]. Saito, T., J. Biochem. (Japan), 40, 265 (1953).

[176]. Guirard, B. M. and Snell, E. E., J. Am. Chem. Soc., 76,
        4745 (1954).

[177]. Courtois, J. E. and Manet, L., Congr. Intern. Biochim.,
        Résumés Communs., 2e Congr., Paris, 1952, 254 (1952).

[178]. Ellfolk, N., Acta Chem. Scand., 9, 771 (1955).

[179]. Kato, A., Yoshioka, Y., Watanabe, M., and Suda, M.,
        J. Biochem. (Japan), 42, 305 (1955).

[180]. Yoshioka, Y., Osaka Daigaku Igaku Zass., 7, 377 (1955).

[181]. Adams, J. B. and Poulos, A., Biochim. Biophys. Acta,
        146, 493 (1967).

[182]. Kratochvil, B., Boyer, S. L., and Hicks, G. P., Anal. Chem., 39, 45 (1967).

[183]. Gavard, R., Compt. Rend., 238, 1620 (1954).

[184]. Liu, W. I. and Wang, T. P., Sheng Wu Hua Hsueh Yu Shing Wu Wu Li Hsueh Pao, 3, 319 (1963).

[185]. Malmström, B. G., Arch. Biochem. Biophys., 58, 381 (1955).

[186]. VandeVelde, A. J. J., Koninkl. Vlaam Acad. Wetenschap, Belg. Klasse Wetenschap, 9, 12 (1947).

[187]. VandeVelde, A. J. J., Koninkl. Vlaam Acad. Wetenschap, 12, 3 (1950).

[188]. Frieden, E., Biochim. Biophys. Acta, 9, 696 (1952).

[189]. O'Sullivan, W. J. and Morrison, J. F., Biochim. Biophys. Acta, 77, 142 (1963).

[190]. Streffer, C., Biochim. Biophys. Acta, 92, 612 (1964).

[191]. Weitzel, G. and Schaeg, W., Z. Physiol. Chem., 316, 250 (1959).

[192]. Ichimura, M., Hirose, Y., and Katsuya, N., Nippon Nogei Kagaku Kaishi, 39, 291 (1965).

[193]. Imada, S., Japan J. Gastroenterol., 11, 88 (1939).

[194]. Schroeder, H. A., J. Nutr., 94, 475 (1968).

[195]. Whitehouse, M. W., Staple, E., and Kritchevsky, D., Arch. Biochem. Biophys., 87, 193 (1960).

[196]. Ishihara, M., Sato, K., Oyama, M., Shimokosu, A., Hase, Y., and Konno, S., Engei Shikenjo Hokoku, Ser. A., 1968, 29 (1968).

[197]. Ishihara, M., Hase, Y., Yokomizo, H., Konno, S., and Sato, K., Engei Shikenjo Hokoku Ser. A., 1968, 39 (1968).

[198]. Millikan, C. R., J. Australian Inst. Agr. Sci., 13, 180 (1947).

[199]. Hunter, J. G. and Vergnano, O., Ann. Appl. Biol., 40, 761 (1953).

[200]. Crooke, W. M., Hunter, J. G., and Vergnano, O., Ann.
        Appl. Biol., 41, 311 (1954).

[201]. Crooke, W. M., Ann. Appl. Biol., 43, 465 (1955).

[202]. Adiga, P. R., Sastry, K. S., Venkatasubramanyam, V.,
        and Sarma, P. S., Proc. Soc. Exptl. Biol. Med., 109,
        151 (1962).

[203]. Sastry, K. S., Adiga, P. R., Venkatasubramanyam, V.,
        and Sarma, P. S., Biochem. J., 85, 486 (1962).

[204]. Adiga, P. R., Sastry, K. S., and Sarma, P. S., Biochim.
        Biophys. Acta, 64, 546 (1962).

[205]. Rausch, C. G., Proc. Iowa Acad. Sci., 72, 477 (1965).

[206]. Valuiskii, P. P., Mikroelem. Zhivotnovod. Rastenievod.,
        Akad. Nauk Kirg. S. S. R., 1966, 38 (1966).

[207]. Sunderman, F. W., Donnelly, A. J., West, B., and
        Kincaid, J. F., A. M. A. Arch. Ind. Health, 20, 36
        (1959).

[208]. Sunderman, F. W., Range, C. L., Sunderman, F. W., Jr.,
        Donnelly, A. J., and Lucyszyn, G. W., Am J. Clin.
        Pathol., 36, 477 (1961).

[209]. Sunderman, F. W., Jr., Am. J. Clin. Pathol., 39, 549
        (1963).

[210]. Beach, D. J. and Sunderman, F. W., Jr., Proc. Soc.
        Exptl. Biol. Med., 131, 321 (1969).

[211]. Sunderman, F. W., Jr. and Esfahani, M., Cancer Res.,
        28, 2565 (1968).

[212]. Sunderman, F. W., Jr. and Selin, C. E., Toxicol. Appl.
        Pharmacol., 12, 207 (1968).

[213]. Sunderman, F. W., Jr., Cancer Res., 28, 465 (1968).

[214]. Kasprzak, K. I. and Sunderman, F. W., Jr., Toxicol.
        Appl. Pharmacol., 115, 295 (1969).

[215]. Hackett, R. L. and Sunderman, F. W., Jr., Arch. Environ.
        Health, 19, 337 (1969).

[216].   Sunderman, F. W., Jr., Res. Commun. Chem. Pathol.
         Pharmacol., 1, 161 (1970).

[217].   Beach, D. J. and Sunderman, F. W., Jr., Cancer Res.,
         30, 48 (1970).

[218].   Sunderman, F. W., Jr., Cancer Res., 27, 1595 (1967).

[219].   Sunderman, F. W., Jr., Dis. Chest., 54, 41 (1968).

[220].   Sunderman, F. W., Jr., Cancer Res., 27, 950 (1967).

[221].   Hueper, W. C., Am. J. Med., 8, 355 (1950).

[222].   Williams, W. J., Brit. J. Ind. Med., 15, 235 (1958).

[223].   Hueper, W. C., Texas Repts. Biol. Med., 10, 167 (1952).

[224].   Hueper, W. C., A. M. A. Arch. Pathol., 65, 600 (1958).

[225].   Raben, A. S. and Antonev, A. A., Vestn. Dermatol.
         Venerol., 40, 19 (1966).

[226].   Cormia, F. E., Can. Med. Assoc. J., 32, 270 (1935).

[227].   Phatak, S. S. and Patwardhan, V. N., J. Sci. Ind.
         Research (India), 9B, 70 (1950).

[228].   Phatak, S. S. and Patwardhan, V. N., J. Sci. Ind.
         Research (India), 11B, 173 (1952).

[229].   Weber, C. W. and Reid, B. L., J. Nutr., 95, 612 (1968).

[230].   Weber, C. W. and Reid, B. L., J. Anim. Sci., 28, 620
         (1969).

[231].   Sandell, E. B., Colorimetric Determination of Trace
         Metals. New York: Wiley (Interscience), 1959, p. 668.

[232].   Smith, J. C. and Schwarz, K., J. Nutr., 93, 182 (1967).

[233].   Nielsen, F. H. and Sauberlich, H. E., Proc. Soc. Exptl.
         Biol. Med., 134, 845 (1970).

[234].   Kikkawa, H., Ogita, Z., and Fujito, S., Kagaku, 25,
         139 (1955).

[235].   Goldenberg, H. and Sobel, V. E., Proc. Soc. Exptl.
         Biol. Med., 81, 695 (1952).

[236]. Silverstein, A. M. and Maltaner, F., New York State
        Dept. Health, Ann. Rept. Div. Labs. and Research, 1952,
        14 (1952).
[237]. Knight, A. H. and Crooke, W. M., Nature, 178, 220
        (1956).
[238]. Paschoud, J. M., Dermatologica, 112, 323 (1956).
[239]. Wellenreiter, R. H., Michigan State University,
        Personal Communication.

Chapter 12

NEWER ASPECTS OF COPPER AND ZINC METABOLISM

R. I. Henkin

Section on Neuroendocrinology
Experimental Therapeutics Branch
National Heart and Lung Instutite
Bethesda, Maryland

I. INTRODUCTION

The purpose of this paper is to describe some of the recent
advances made in the study of copper and zinc metabolism in
our laboratory over the past three years. These studies fall
into two general categories: one, methodological advances made
in the measurement of these metals in biological fluids and in
their binding to their carrying proteins, and two, application
of these methodological advances to the study of the manner in
which these metals are involved in several physiological
processes. These processes include (a) the normal physiological
variations which occur in copper and zinc concentrations in
various body fluids, (b) the interrelationships between copper
and zinc and steroidal hormones, (c) the interrelationships
between copper and zinc in maternal-fetal metabolism, and
(d) the interrelationships between metals and sensory processes,
particularly that of gustation.

II. METHODOLOGICAL ADVANCES IN MEASUREMENT OF COPPER AND ZINC

A. Simultaneous Estimation of Copper and Zinc in
Biological Fluids

It is generally agreed that atomic absorption spectrophotometry (AAS) has proven to be a useful technique for the
measurement of copper and zinc in biological fluids. However,
estimation of these metals in several biological fluids has
generally required extensive sample preparation in order to
concentrate these metals to obtain a satisfactory signal-to-noise
ratio. Sample preparation has included ashing of dried
fluids[1], precipitation of plasma proteins[2], extraction into
organic solvents[3], or various combinations of these techniques[4,5]. These steps lengthen the total procedure and can
introduce systematic errors[6]. Some methods using only sample

dilution[7] can produce clogging of the spectrophotometer
burner due to the low dilution of sample used. In addition,
previous methods required separate procedures prior to the
estimation of either copper or zinc.

We have developed a technique for the simultaneous
estimation of copper and zinc in biological fluids requiring
only sample dilution. This shortens the time required to
perform these determinations and decreases the volume of sample
needed. This technique has proved accurate, specific, reliable,
and reproducible.

The instrument used to perform the measurements was an
Instrumentation Laboratory atomic absorption spectrophotometer
Model 153[*/]. This instrument is manufactured with two optical
channels. In one channel (Channel A) a grating monochromator
is used, and in the other (Channel B) an interference filter is
used for wavelength selection. Zinc is determined in Channel A
at the 213.9-nm wavelength, copper in Channel B, using a
324.7-nm filter. The instrument is equipped with a three-slot
Boling burner. All instrumental adjustments are made according
to the manufacturer's manual of standard conditions.

The reagents used for the procedure were as follows.

(1) Diluent. Sixty ml of analytical grade n-butyl alcohol
were diluted to 1000 ml with deionized distilled water. The
blank reading of this solution did not differ from zero when
measured by AAS at the major copper and zinc absorption lines,
respectively.

(2) Sodium Choloride (NaCl) Solution. Analytical grade
NaCl was dissolved in deionized distilled water to make a final
concentration of 1.5 Eq/L.

---

* The instrument was manufactured by the Instrumentation
Laboratory, Inc., Lexington, Massachusetts.

(3) Standard Solutions. Copper reference standard
solution So-C-194 and zinc reference standard solution So-Z-13,
obtained from the Fisher Scientific Company, were used as
stock solutions. These solutions contain 1000 ppm copper and
zinc, respectively. Equal volumes of each of these solutions
were mixed, 10 ml NaCl solution were added, and the mixture
was diluted to 100 ml with deionized distilled water so that
standard solutions containing 10, 25, 50, 100, and 200 µg/100 ml
of both copper and zinc in 150 mEq/L NaCl were obtained.

(4) Working Standard Solutions. One part of each solution
was diluted with nine parts of diluent with a Fisher diluter,
Model 250. To accomplish this, 4.5 ml of diluent and 9.5 ml
of each standard solution were delivered into a plastic vial,
capped, and thoroughly mixed. These solutions were used to
calibrate the instrument.

(5) Unknown Solutions. 4.5 ml of diluent and 0.5 ml of
each sample of serum, urine, or CSF were mixed in the same
manner as were the working standard solution.

Plastic vials and caps*/ were used without pretreatment
for the diluted samples and working standards. The readings
of both deionized distilled water and 0.1 N HCl allowed to
stand in the capped vial for one week did not differ from zero
when measured by AAS at the major copper and zinc absorption
lines. All glassware was soaked for at least 18 hours in
6 N HCl, thoroughly rinsed in deionized distilled water, and
dried before use. Pipettes used in making standard solutions
were "aged" in aliquots of the particular solutions used.

For the estimation of copper and zinc, the digitial display
of the A and B Channels was set at zero with the autozero and
zero controls while the diluent was aspirated. Then the

---

* Purchased from Celluplastics, Inc., New York, New York.

combined copper and zinc working standard (100 µg/100 ml) was
aspirated and the digital displays set at 100. The other
concentrations of working standards were then aspirated to
verify the calibration accuracy and the linearity of instrument
performance. Following calibration, samples were aspirated
and the results on the digital displays were recorded manually.
Diluent was aspirated between samples and a working standard
(100 µg/100 ml) was aspirated after every ten samples. If there
were any deviations from 0 or 100 on either digital display,
the calibration controls were readjusted before further samples
were aspirated. The concentrations of copper and zinc in
aliquots of laboratory pools of human serum, urine, and CSF
were estimated with each set of samples.

Determination of copper and zinc was carried out in
laboratory pools of human serum, urine, and CSF each day for
30 days and on one day for ten consecutive determinations.
The results are summarized in Table I. In this study the
the within-day variation in CSF copper and zinc was larger than
the day-to-day variation over a 30 day period due to the lack
of precision of analyses at extremely low concentrations of
the metals.

The specificity and accuracy of the present method was
compared with that of a standard colorimetric procedure[8]
by comparative estimation of concentration of copper in serum
from patients with Wilson's disease who were either untreated
or treated with D-penicillamine. These samples were chosen
because they are significantly lower than normal, and reliable
sensitivity for low concentrations of copper is important due
to the low urinary excretion and CSF concentration of this
metal under normal physiological conditions. The results
obtained in 15 patients indicate no systematic differences
between the two methods (Table II).

TABLE I

Variations in Estimates of Copper and Zinc in Serum, Urine, and CSF

Sample		Mean of daily determinations over 30 days (µg/100 ml)	SD[a]	SEM[b]	CV[c] (percent)	Mean of 10 determinations on one day (µg/100 ml)	SD[a]	SEM[b]	CV[c] (percent)
Serum	Cu	221	2.2	0.41	1.0	221	0.99	0.31	0.4
	Zn	112	2.0	0.38	1.8	111	1.1	0.35	1.0
Urine	Cu	14	2.1	0.33	15.0	14	0.88	0.28	6.3
	Zn	131	2.2	0.36	1.7	132	1.7	0.55	1.3
CSF	Cu	16	1.2	0.27	7.5	16	1.6	0.5	10.0
	Zn	15	1.1	0.25	7.3	15	1.9	0.6	12.7

a/ SD, standard deviation.

b/ SEM, standard error of mean.

c/ CV, coefficient of variation.

TABLE II

Comparison of Estimates of Serum Copper Concentration by a Colorimetric[a]
and by Present Atomic Absorption Methods

| Sample number | Serum copper concentration (μg/100 ml) | | Difference | Percent difference |
	Colorimetric method	Atomic absorption method		
1	18	15	-3	+18
2	10	10	0	0
3	46	40	-6	-14
4	12	18	+6	+40
5	11	13	+2	+17
6	10	15	+5	+40
7	61	56	-5	- 8
8	45	41	-4	- 9
9	40	44	+4	+10
10	32	37	+5	+14
11	10	11	+1	+10
12	<10	6	0	0
13	<10	8	0	0
14	32	35	+3	+ 9
15	<10	8	0	0
Mean ± SD[b]	23 ± 17.8	24 ± 16.4		+ 8.5

a/ Dicyclohexanone oxalyl dihydrazone complex method[8].

b/ SD, standard deviation.

The specificity and accuracy of the present method was also compared with that of a standard colorimetric procedure for the estimation of zinc in serum and urine[9]. The comparison of results indicates that there is no systematic difference between the values obtained with the two methods at low, normal or high concentrations of the metal (Table III).

In the present method, samples were diluted with a solution of 6% n-butyl alcohol for several reasons. First, a relatively small amount of sample could be used since this concentration of n-butanol in the diluted sample enhanced the signal of the copper and zinc absorption by about 30%. Second, sample protein concentrations could be decreased, particularly in serum, to produce a less viscous fluid for aspiration into the flame[10]. Third, various possible interfering substances, such as Ca, P, and Mg could be diluted to relatively insignificant levels.

Standard solutions were prepared in 150 mEq/L NaCl because of a constant enhancement in copper absorption of about 50% at sodium concentrations between 125 and 500 mEq/L. Concentrations of NaCl lower than 125 mEq/L did not produce this effect. The sodium concentration used constituted physiological levels in serum and did not interfere with the estimation of copper in urine or CSF or with zinc in any of these fluids. Phosphorus at physiological concentrations and potassium at concentrations less than 200 mEq/L did not interfere with the determination of either metal in these fluids[11] by the present technique.

Using the present method, recoveries of copper and zinc added to laboratory pools of human serum, urine, and CSF are summarized in Tables IV and V. With the addition of solutions containing equal concentrations of copper and zinc ranging from 5 to 100 µg/100 ml to each pool, recovery of each metal did not vary by more than 1.1% (Table IV). With the addition of

TABLE III

Comparison of Estimates of Serum and Urinary Zinc by a Colorimetric[a] and by Present Atomic Absorption Methods

| Sample number | Zinc concentration (µg/100 ml) | | Difference | Percent difference |
	Colorimetric method	Atomic absorption method		
Serum				
1	84	84	0	0
2	131	130	-1	-0.8
3	94	96	+2	+2.1
4	72	70	-2	-2.1
5	76	76	0	0
6	92	90	-2	-2.2
7	68	70	+2	+2.9
8	69	70	+1	+1.4
9	112	111	-1	-0.9
10	68	66	-2	-3.0
Mean ± SD[b]	87 ± 21.2	86 ± 20.9		-0.3

a/ Diphenylthiocarbazone complex method[9].
b/ SD, standard deviation.

TABLE III (continued)

Comparison of Estimates of Serum and Urinary Zinc by a Colorimetric [a]

and by Present Atomic Absorption Methods

| Sample number | Zinc concentration (µg/100 ml) | | Difference | Percent difference |
	Colorimetric method	Atomic absorption method		
Urine				
A	88	84	-4	-4.7
B	7	8	+1	+13.3
C	17	16	-1	-6.1
D	14	9	-5	-43.5
E	29	22	-7	-27.5
F	44	41	-3	-7.1
G	41	38	-3	-7.6
H	17	19	+2	+11.1
I	36	38	+2	+5.4
J	12	10	-2	-18.2
Mean ± SD [b]	30 ± 24.0	29 ± 24.0		-8.5

a/ Diphenylthiocarbazone complex method[9].

b/ SD, standard deviation.

TABLE IV

Recovery of Copper and Zinc Added in Equal Quantities to
Pooled Serum, Urine, and CSF

Copper and zinc added	Average obtained		Expected		Percent recovered	
	Cu	Zn	Cu	Zn	Cu	Zn
	(µg/100 ml)		(µg/100 ml)			
Serum (4)[a/]						
0	133	83				
5.0	138	88	138	88	100	100
10.0	143	93	143	93	100	99.1
25.0	160	107	158	108	101.3	99.1
50.0	186	130	183	133	101.6	97.8
75.0	207	158	208	158	99.5	100
100.0	229	179	233	183	98.3	97.8
Mean ± SEM					101.1 ± 0.5	99.2 ± 0.4
Urine (5)[a/]						
0	21	144				
5.0	26	150	26	149	100	100.7
10.0	32	156	31	154	103.2	101.3
25.0	47	171	46	170	102.2	100.6
50.0	72	193	71	194	101.4	99.5
100.0	123	253	121	244	101.6	103.7
Mean ± SEM					101.7 ± 0.5	101.2 ± 0.7
CSF (6)[a/]						
0	16	15				
5.0	21	20	21	20	100	100
10.0	27	25	26	25	103.8	100
25.0	42	40	41	40	102.4	100
100.0	117	115	116	115	100.9	100
200.0	218	215	216	215	100.9	100
Mean ± SEM					101.6 ± 0.7	100 ± 0

[a/] Number in parentheses indicates number of samples tested in this manner.

increments of either metal in the presence of high concentrations
of the other metal, recovery of each metal did not vary by more
than 1% (Table V).

With the technique described, copper and zinc concentrations
were determined in the serum and urine of 82 normal subjects,
45 women and 37 men, ages 12 to 55 (mean, 25 years). All
blood samples were drawn before 9:00 A.M. from fasted subjects
and urines were collected over a 24 hour period during which

TABLE V

Recovery of Copper and Zinc Added Differentially to
Pooled Serum, Urine and CSF

Added Copper and Zinc (µg/100 ml)		Serum (µg/100 ml)		Urine (µg/100 ml)		CSF (µg/100 ml)	
		Copper	Zinc	Copper	Zinc	Copper	Zinc
0	/0	127	/ 87	13	/ 65	7	/ 13
10	/100	137	/187	23	/164	17	/114
25	/100	153	/187	38	/165	32	/113
50	/100	177	/187	63	/165	63	/113
100	/100	227	/187	113	/165	107	/114
200	/100	325	/186	212	/164	206	/113
0	/0	126	/ 87	12	/ 65	7	/ 13
100	/10	226	/ 97	112	/ 75	107	/ 24
100	/25	227	/113	112	/ 90	106	/ 39
100	/50	227	/137	113	/114	107	/ 64
100	/100	227	/187	113	/168	106	/113
100	/200	227	/286	113	/267	107	/214

they were refrigerated. The results are summarized in Table VI.
Estimation of these metals was also carried out in serum and
CSF of patients with neurological disorders who underwent
pneumoencephalography (Table VI). None of these patients had
any evidence of tumor and all were treated with anticonvulsant
medication at the time of sample collection.

The results obtained with the present method, compared
with those of other investigators for each biological fluid
studied (Table VII), indicated that there were no systematic
differences in the estimation of copper and zinc by any of these
methods. However, the data collected with the present method
resulted in a somewhat smaller range of variability for both
serum and urinary copper and zinc. In addition, these values
were obtained more quickly and simply than with other methods.

Previous measurements of copper and zinc concentrations
in CSF have been reported only with the cumbersome,
time-consuming technique of activation analysis or spectrophotometry[12,13]. With the present technique, copper and
zinc concentrations in CSF can be determined more quickly,
simply, and reproducibly and at least as accurately (Table III).

With the method described simultaneous copper and zinc
concentrations may be determined in 30 to 50 samples of biological
fluids per hour with a minimum of sample and glassware handling.

B. Estimation of Copper and Zinc Binding in Biological Fluids

Significant amounts of copper and zinc exist in most
biological fluids bound to protein. In serum copper exists
mainly bound in a fairly tight manner to the β globulin
ceruloplasmin. Various investigators have estimated that
85 to 95% of the copper in serum is bound to this protein. Zinc
also exists in serum mainly bound to protein. Estimates made

TABLE VI

Copper and Zinc Concentrations in Serum, Urine, and
CSF of Normal Subjects and in Patients with Seizures

Condition	Number	Sex	Serum (µg/100 ml)		Urine (µg/24 hour)		CSF (µg/100 ml)	
			Copper	Zinc	Copper	Zinc	Copper	Zinc
Normal subjects	82	M,F[a]	106 ± 2[b]	92 ± 2	36 ± 5	353 ± 23		
	45	F	107 ± 3	90 ± 3	38 ± 7	347 ± 48		
	Range		(82-147)	(63-122)	(10-114)	(141-779)		
	37	M	105 ± 2	94 ± 3	35 ± 7	360 ± 22		
	Range		(80-135)	(63-147)	(16-63)	(301-510)		
Patients with seizures	26		129 ± 7	85 ± 3			7.6 ± 1.7	6.6 ± 2.1
	Range		(80-190)	(60-117)			(1-28)	(1-35)

a/ M, Male; F, Female.

b/ Mean ± SEM.

in our laboratory suggested that 75 to 85% of zinc is normally
protein bound. Zinc, however, is bound to several proteins in
serum. Difficulties in identifying these proteins have arisen
since zinc is fairly loosely bound to its binding proteins in
serum. Nevertheless these proteins have been identified as an
α_2 macroglobulin[14], a π protein or transferrin itself[15],
and several other nonspecific protein moieties[16]. Urine
appears to be one of the major biological fluids in which there
is little or no binding of these metals to protein.

Our interest in this problem was to develop a technique
by which an estimate of copper-protein and zinc-protein binding
could be obtained quickly, easily, and reproducibly in biological fluids. The technique utilized for these determiniations
was that of ultrafiltration.

The instrument used for measurements was the Instrumentation
Laboratory atomic absorption spectrophotometer, Model 153,
assembled and operated as described above. The ultrafiltration
equipment used for measurements were Diaflo membranes, Type
XM 50*/. This membrane is made of an inert, nonionic polymer
in which there is no adsorption of strongly coordinated ionic
or inorganic solutes. This membrane was made into a cone shape
and called "Diaflo membrane, cone shape" (CF 50A)*/. Also
required was a Diaflo conical support (CS 1A)*/, and a Diaflo
test tube, plastic, 50 ml (CT 1)*/.

The ultrafiltration equipment was assembled by placement of
the cone shaped membrane into a nonporous, plastic conical
support with a small hole in the bottom. This system was, in
turn, placed into a graduated 50 ml plastic test tube. The
assembled parts were placed into an International Model 2
centrifuge.

---

*Manufactured by the Amicon Corp., Lexington, Massachusetts.

TABLE

Comparison of Results of Present Methods in

Reference	Subject Number	Sex	Technique	Mean conc. (μg/100 ml)	Copper Serum SD[a] or SEM[b]
Present method	82	M,F[c]	AAS	106	2[b]
	37	M		105	2[b]
	45	F		107	3[b]
	26	M,F%[d]		129	7[b]
Dawson[44]	24	M,F	AAS	108	
	12	M		95	
	12	F		122	
Sprague and Slavin[7]	4	M,F	AAS	105	2[b]
Berman[45]	60	M,F	AAS	133	
Parker[46]	28	M,F	AAS	105	15.9[b]
	18	M		106.5	15.9[b]
	10	F		102.6	16.4[a]
Butt[1]	37	M	AAS	87	
	45	F		105	
Sunderman[5]	58	M	AAS	119	19[a]
	21	M			

AAS- atomic absorption spectrophotometry

a/ SD, standard deviation.

b/ SEM, standard error of mean.

c/ F, female; M, male.

d/ %, patients with seizures.

VII-a

Normal Subjects with those of other Investigators

	Urine or [CSF]		
Range	Mean conc. (µg/24 hr.)	SD[a] or SEM[b]	Range
	36	5[b]	
(80-135)	35	7[b]	(16-63[c])
(82-147)	38	7[b]	(10-114)
(80-190)	[7.6	1.7[b]	(1-28)]
(70-165)	52		(26-64)
(78-111)			
(70-165)			
(80-170)			(20-50)
(70-165)			
	18.4	8.4[a]	(7.5-33.8)

TABLE

Comparison of Results of Present Methods in

Reference	Subject Number	Sex	Technique	Copper Serum Mean conc. (μg/100 ml)	SD[a] or SEM[b]
Ch'en[48]	10	M	S	105	
Canelas[49]	20	M,F s	S	108.1	9.7[a]
	50	M,F[c]		164.9	38.2[a]
Cartwright[50]	120	M	S	110	15.7[a]
	85	F		120	17.8[a]
Kjellin[12]	15	M,F c	AA		
	8	M			
	7	F			

S-spectroscopy

AA-activation analysis

s-patients with epilepsy

c-patients with psychonurosis

[a] SD, standard deviation.

[b] SEM, standard error of mean.

[c] F, female; M, male.

VII-a (continued)

Normal Subjects with those of other Investigators

Range	Urine or [CSF]		
	Mean conc. (μg/24 hr.)	SD[a] or SEM[b]	Range
(65-154)	18	14[a]	(0-70)
(90-125)	[42.6	5.7[a]	(30-50)]
(85-286)	[21.2	14.6[a]	(1-54)]
(68-161)			
(83-165)			
(100-200)	[16	4[a]	(7-23)]
	[15		(7-21)]
	[17		(14-23)]

TABLE

Comparison of Results of Present Methods in

| | | | | Zinc | |
| | | | | Serum | |
Reference	Subject Number	Sex	Technique	Mean conc. (μg/100 ml)	SD[a] or SEM[b]
Present method	82	M,F[c]	AAS	92	2[b]
	37	M		94	3[b]
	45	F		90	3[b]
	26	M,F%[d]		85	3[b]
Sprague and Slavin[7]	4	M,F	AAS	107	2.7[b]
Parker[46]	23			89.9	10.3[a]
Butt[1]	37	M	AAS	157	
	45	F		159	
Davies[47]	36	F	AAS	95	13[a]
Woodbury[13]	11		AAS	85	15[a]

AAS-atomic absorption spectrophotometry.

a/ SD, standard deviation.

b/ SEM, standard error of mean.

c/ F, female; M, male.

d/ %, patients with seizures.

VII-b

Normal Subjects with those of other Investigators

| | Urine or [CSF] | | |
Range	Mean conc. (μg/24 hr.)	SD[a] or SEM[b]	Range
	353	23[b]	
(63-147)	360	22[b]	(301-510)
(63-122)	347	38[b]	(141-779)
(60-117)	[6.6	2.1[b]	(1-35)]
	4.0	2.6[a]]	

The reagents used were as follows.

(1) Standard Solutions. One part of each standard solution (described above) was diluted with 9 parts of diluent (described above) with a Fisher diluter, Model 250. To accomplish this, 4.5 ml of diluent and 0.5 ml of each standard solution was delivered into a plastic vial, capped, and thoroughly mixed. These solutions were used as standards in each ultrafiltration run.

(2) Deionized Distilled Water. The blank reading of this solution did not differ from zero when measured by atomic absorption spectrophotometry at the major cooper and zinc absorption lines, respectively.

(3) Human Serum Albumin. The human serum albumin was from the Cohn Fraction V, Hyland Laboratories, Costa Mesa, California.

(4) Unknown Solutions. One to 2 ml of each sample of serum, urine, or CSF was delivered to each ultrafiltration assemblage and placed in the International Model 2 centrifuge.

The ultrafiltration technique involved an initial preparation of the membranes to establish that the system was free of contaminants of copper or zinc. To accomplish this 1 to 2 ml volumes of deionized, distilled water, with and without EDTA, albumin, and serum (from a laboratory pool of serum) were successively placed in the filter cone of the ultrafiltration assembly. These were centrifuged at 2000 rpm (1000 × g) for 30 minutes at 20°C. The ultrafiltrate was collected in the 50 ml plastic test tube, the retained material remaining behind in the filter cone. The copper and zinc concentration of the ultrafiltrate was determined in each ultrafiltration system by the AAS method described above. The reading of the filtrate from the final water sample did not differ from zero when measured by AAS at the major copper and

zinc absorption lines, respectively. Less than 50 mg/100 ml
protein was measured in the ultrafiltrate after centrifugation
of the pooled serum, the protein concentration determined on a
total solids (TS) meter. If more than 50 mg/100 ml protein
was found during the preparation the filter cone was discarded.

For each unknown determination, 1 to 2 ml of sample was
placed singly or in duplicate into the prepared ultrafiltration
assembly and centrifuged at 2000 rpm (1000 × g) for 30 minutes
at 20°C. In duplicate 1 to 2 ml of standard solution were also
placed into prepared ultrafiltration assemblies and centrifuged
along with the unknown solutions. Following centrifugation
copper and zinc concentrations were estimated in the diffusible
filtrate. For convenience we have called the ultrafilterable
copper and zinc "free" and have expressed this either as
µg/100 ml of serum or percent of total measureable copper and
zinc. By the refractometric technique of the total solid
meter less than 50 mg/100 ml protein was found in each sample.
If more protein was found, the sample and membrane were
discarded and the sample rerun in another membrane assembly.

Determination of "free" copper and zinc was carried out
in 12 aliquots of 2 volumes of a laboratory pool of human serum
in a single centrifugation run. The results are summarized in
Table VIII. Estimation of "free" zinc varied from 49 to 52
µg/100 ml with a mean and standard deviation (SD) of 50 ± 2;
estimation of "free" copper varied from 12 to 17 µg/100 ml with a
mean and SD of 13 ± 2. The total zinc and copper in these
samples, similarly determined were 98 ± 1 and 130 ± 1,
respectively (Table VIII).

The specificity and accuracy of the present method in
serum was compared with that of a standard procedure for the
estimation of ceruloplasmin in serum[17]. This was difficult

TABLE VIII

Determination of "Free" Copper and Zinc by Ultrafiltration in
Replicate Samples from a Laboratory Pool of Human Serum

Sample number	"Free" Cu^{2+} ($\mu g/100$ ml)	"Free" Zn^{2+} ($\mu g/100$ ml)
1	12	50
2	14	52
3	13	49
4	12	46
5	12	47
6	15	51
7	17	53
8	13	49
9	15	47
10	14	52
11	12	49
12	11	49
Mean ± 1 SD[a]	13 ± 2	50 ± 2
Total Mean ± 1 SD	130 ± 1	98 ± 1

[a] SD, standard deviation.

since quantitative values for copper or zinc binding in serum
or other biological fluids are not well established. Various
estimates have been made relating the amount of copper bound
in serum to that bound to ceruloplasmin. From these studies
approximately 95% of the protein bound copper in serum may be
presumed to be bound to ceruloplasmin; ceruloplasmin itself
has been estimated to contain 0.28% copper[18]. On the basis
of this value the amount of ceruloplasmin bound copper has
been estimated in the serum of 17 patients with various diseases

whose total serum copper concentrations ranged from 37 to 255
µg/100 ml (Table IX). These estimated values were compared
with estimates of bound copper obtained by the ultrafiltration
method described above. Comparison of these bound copper values
revealed a mean difference of 5% with the estimates by either
method not varying systematically from one other (Table IX).

Since little is known about zinc-binding proteins in serum,
comparison of the values presented in this paper with those
obtained with other methods is not practical.

Using the present method it was not possible to estimate
recovery of copper and zinc added to laboratory pools of serum
since large amounts of both metals are adsorbed to several
large and small molecular species in serum.

With the technique described free and bound copper and
zinc concentrations were determined in the serum and urine of
24 normal subjects, 14 women and 10 men, ages 18 to 40 (mean,
25 years). All blood samples were drawn before 9:00 A.M. in
the fasting state; urines were collected over a 24 hour period
during which they were refrigerated. Results, summarized in
Table X, indicate that approximately 10% of the total serum
copper is free, the remaining 90% is bound to protein, primarily
ceruloplasmin. Twice as much zinc in serum is free, that is,
20% of the total serum zinc, the remaining 80% is bound to
serum proteins.

Only free copper and zinc were found in each urine sample
analyzed. This correlates well with the observation that for
all practical purposes there was no protein in any of the urine
samples analyzed.

Although this method provides a useful procedure for
obtaining an estimate of free and bound copper and zinc in

TABLE IX

Comparison of Ceruloplasmin Bound and Protein Bound Copper
by the Copper Oxidase and Ultrafiltration Methods

Patient	Total copper (µg/100 ml)	Bound copper by ultrafiltration (µg/ml)	Bound copper by ultrafiltration (percent)	Ceruloplasmin (mg/100 ml)	Copper bound to ceruloplasmin (µg/100 ml)	Δ (percent)
EM	107	103	4	39	111	+ 8
JM	155	147	5	48	134	-13
ET	91	76	16	32	89	+13
ME	132	121	8	42	118	- 3
SS	130	110	15	46	129	+19
MB	102	92	10	38	106	+14
BC	133	114	14	49	137	+23
JG	96	83	14	35	98	+15
LD	117	112	4	43	120	+ 8
FC	120	96	20	44	123	+27
PZ	98	93	5	37	103	+10
BW	118	108	8	39	109	+ 1
SD	136	128	6	40	112	-16
AT	107	102	5	37	103	+ 1
RP	255	250	2	81	227	-23
JL	207	196	5	67	188	- 8
JH	37	34	8	15	42	+ 8
Mean	126	116	9	44	121	+ 5

TABLE X

"Free" and "Bound" Copper and Zinc in Serum Determined
by Ultrafiltration Method in 24 Normal Volunteers

	Cu(II) (μg/100 ml)	Zn(II) (μg/100 ml)
Free	11 ± 1	19 ± 2
Bound	94	77
Total	105 ± 4	96 ± 4

serum, it also has several unexplored limitations. The
specificity of this method has yet to be clearly established.
Although it is possible to determine marked differences in free
copper and zinc between normal, physiologically altered and
pathological conditions, the application of the method to small
changes in binding cannot be assumed. Similarly, the failure
to estimate recoveries by this technique limits the conclusions
that may be drawn from data collected by its application. An
inherent problem is that "binding" is assumed to occur only to
proteins of molecular weight 50,000 and above for both copper
and zinc due to the nature of the membrane chosen for ultrafiltration.

Nevertheless, the simplicity, reproducibility, and
consistency of this method and the ease and speed by which the
results can be obtained (that is, 10 to 30 samples may be
processed per hour) suggest that it can provide a useful approxi-
mation to the amount of copper and zinc that exists free and
bound in serum.

III.   COPPER AND ZINC METABOLISM IN BIOLOGICAL
       AND PATHOLOGICAL PROCESSES

A.   Circadian Variation of Copper and Zinc in Man

It is well known that there is in man a circadian variation
in the serum and urinary excretion of several electrolytes and
for sodium and potassium this has been related to the serum
concentration and/or urinary excretion of adrenal cortical
hormones and their metabolites[19,20]. We were interested in
determining whether or not a circadian pattern of variation
existed in serum and urine for copper and zinc. Also, since we
had previously shown that copper and zinc metabolism were
influenced by carbohydrate active steroid excretion[21], we were
also interested in determining whether or not any circadian
pattern of variation was affected by carbohydrate-active
steroid.

The subjects were 10 normal volunteers who remained confined
to a metabolic ward throughout the study. All subjects took
500 ml of a constant liquid diet which contained 105 μg Cu^{2+},
1350 μg Zn^{2+}, at 8:00 A.M., 4:00 P.M., and 12 midnight and
400 ml of distilled water at 12:00 noon, 8:00 P.M., and 4:00 A.M.
All studies began at 8:00 A.M. and lasted five days. Urine was
collected in 4 hour periods in plastic containers throughout
the study. Blood was taken in the middle of each 4 hour period
during the second and third days of the study. All urine and
blood were collected and handled as noted above. In two
subjects, after the first three days of the study, prednisolone,
2.5 mg was given orally every 6 hours beginning at 8:00 A.M. for
three days and blood and urine were collected as noted.

Total copper and zinc in blood and urine were determined
by the method described above. Ceruloplasmin was measured in

each serum sample[16] and expressed as mg/100 ml of serum.
Each urine sample was analyzed for creatinine[22]. All blood
and urine samples from each subject were analyzed at the same
time.

Presentation of the data was expressed as percent change
for the mean of all 10 subjects at each time period and plotted
as mean ± 1 standard error of mean (SEM) for clarity and to
correct for different baseline values. There were no systematic
differences in representing the data in this manner.

There is a circadian variation in serum copper concentration. It is higher than the mean from 10:00 A.M. to 2:00 P.M.,
equal to the mean from 6:00 P.M. to 10:00 P.M., and significantly
lower than the mean from 2:00 A.M. to 6:00 A.M. (Fig. 1). This
pattern persisted for up to 56 hours which was the longest study

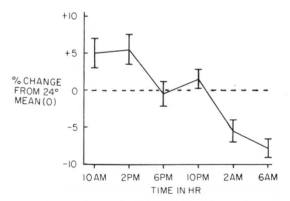

Fig. 1 Changes in total serum copper, expressed at each
time point over one 24 hour period as the mean percent change
from each subject's 24 hour mean (M) plus and minus one
standard error of the mean (SEM). Each point in this figure
and in Figs. 2-5 represents the M ± SEM of 10 subjects, under
constant conditions.

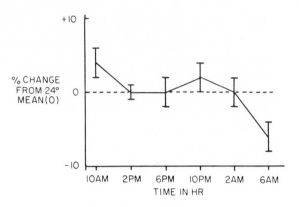

Fig. 2   Changes in serum ceruloplasmin, expressed at each
time point over one 24 hour period as the mean percent change
from each subject's 24 hour M + 1 SEM.

conducted. Serum concentrations of ceruloplasmin showed a
similar but less marked circadian pattern of variation (Fig. 2).

   There is a circadian variation in serum zinc concentration
which is similar to that for copper. It is higher than the mean
from 10:00 A.M. to 10:00 P.M. and significantly lower than the
mean between 2:00 A.M. and 6:00 A.M. (Fig. 3). This pattern
of variation also persisted for as long as 56 hours.

   Urinary excretion of copper showed no obvious circadian
pattern of variation by this method of calculation but excretion
tended to be lower from 8:00 P.M. to 4:00 A.M. than at other
times during the 24 hour period (Fig. 4). This was true whether
the data were expressed as micrograms excreted per 4 hour or
as micrograms per milligram creatinine per 4 hour. Recalcu-
lation of the data by fitting a 24 hour cosine to them resulted
in the detection of a significant circadian rhythm in urinary
copper excretion. Urinary zinc excretion showed no obvious
circadian pattern of variation but appeared to be higher in the
urine collected after eating (Fig. 5).

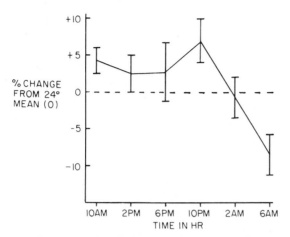

Fig. 3 Changes in total serum zinc, expressed at each time point for one 24 hour period as the mean percent change from each subject's 24 hour M ± 1 SEM.

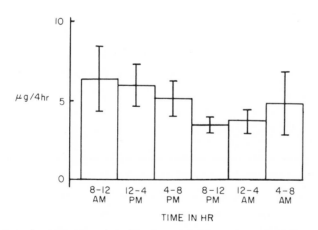

Fig. 4 Changes in urinary excretion of copper over one 24 hour period expressed as the M ± SEM of each 4 hour collection period.

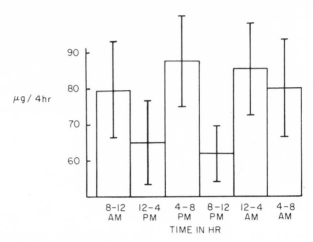

Fig. 5 Changes in urinary excretion of zinc over one
24 hour period expressed as the M ± 1 SEM of each 4 hour
collection period.

Administration of carbohydrate active steroids (CAS) did
not suppress the circadian variation for serum concentration of
copper or zinc although the normal pattern for serum zinc was
less apparent. The absolute levels of serum copper and zinc
were generally higher during prednisolone administration
(Fig. 6 and 7); no change in the level or pattern of serum
ceruloplasmin occurred. The pattern of excretion of urinary
copper and zinc did not change significantly following CAS
administration although the absolute levels were uniformly
higher (Fig. 8 and 9).

The circadian pattern of variation noted for serum copper
has been noted previously[23] but that for ceruloplasmin and
for zinc is herein noted for the first time. It is tempting
to speculate that the pattern for serum copper may be due to
changes in serum ceruloplasmin.

It is difficult to explain the absence of a circadian
pattern of variation for urinary zinc excretion in the face of

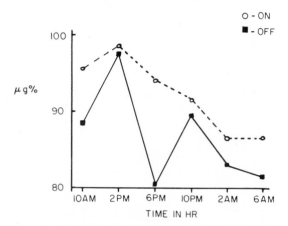

Fig. 6 Within-day changes in total serum copper in
two subjects receiving 2.5 mg prednisolone orally every
6 hours. Each point represents the mean of two absolute values
and indicates that on prednisolone serum copper is elevated.

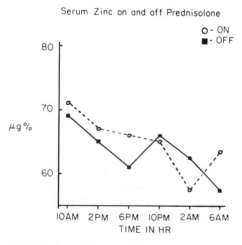

Fig. 7 Within-day changes in total serum zinc in two
subjects receiving 2.5 mg prednisolone orally every 6 hours.
On prednisolone four of six values are elevated.

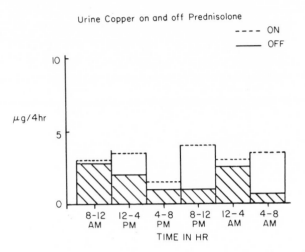

Fig. 8 Within-day changes in urinary excretion of copper in two subjects receiving prednisolone. Values expressed as excretion in μg/4 hour, indicate that on prednisolone more copper is excreted.

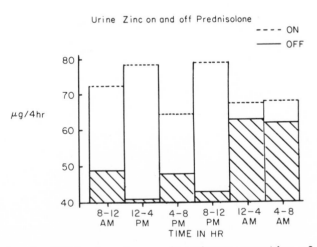

Fig. 9 Within-day changes in urinary excretion of zinc in two subjects receiving prednisolone. Values, expressed as excretion in μg/4 hour, indicate that on prednisolone more zinc is excreted.

an obvious serum pattern of variation and in contrast to previous
reports of the presence of such a pattern[24]. A circadian
pattern of variation for urinary copper excretion has been
previously observed[25].

Administration of prednisolone did not alter the pattern
of variation of serum or urinary copper or zinc. However, the
levels of these metals in both serum and urine were increased.
Whether this effect is due to the direct action of prednisolone
on altering protein binding of copper and zinc or to renal
mechanisms for handling these metals is being determined in our
laboratory at the present time. We have previously shown that
administration of CAS does increase urinary excretion of both
metals but also that administration of larger concentrations of
CAS decreases rather than increases serum concentrations of
of these metals[21]. How this hormone affects gastrointestinal
absorption and mobilization of these metals from tissues is also
being investigated.

B. Maternal-Fetal Metabolism of Copper and Zinc

Copper and zinc are particularly important metabolic
substances for both mother and fetus. We and other investigators[26,27] have noted wide differences between maternal and
fetal concentrations of these metals; for example, the fetal
serum concentrations of copper and zinc are one-tenth and twice,
respectively, the maternal concentrations and the fetal liver
copper concentrations are 4 to 5 times the amount found in
normal adult liver[28]. These differences prompted us to
investigate the maternal-fetal interrelationships of these metal
by demonstrating differences in maternal and fetal binding.

At the time of delivery venous blood was obtained from 15
normal mothers and from the umbilical cord of their 15 normal
babies. Each pregnancy and delivery was uncomplicated, single,
vaginal, and at term. Amniotic fluid was obtained from four of

these patients. Blood was obtained, total concentrations of
copper and zinc were measured simultaneously, and measurements
of ultrafilterable copper and zinc were determined by membrane
ultrafiltration as noted above.

The results of these studies, shown in Table XI, indicate
that mean total maternal serum copper concentration was 221
μg/100 ml and was approximately twice the normal nonpregnant
value. Mean total maternal serum zinc concentration was 48
μg/100 ml and was approximately one half the normal adult female
value. Mean maternal free serum copper was 8% of total maternal
value and was not significantly different from the nonpregnant
level. Mean maternal free zinc was 67% of total zinc and was
about 2.5 times the normal nonpregnant value.

Mean fetal total serum copper concentration was 29
μg/100 ml. The percentages of free copper and zinc in fetal
serum were 16% and 32%, respectively.

Mean total concentrations of copper and zinc in amniotic
fluid were 6 and 32 μg/100 ml, respectively. The percentages
of free copper and zinc were 83 and 92, respectively.

There are no significant differences in serum copper,
ceruloplasmin, or zinc in either maternal or fetal serum
relative to fetal sex (Table XII).

Copper and zinc are both critically important trace
elements involved in the growth and development of many organ
systems. Copper is essential to the normal development of the
nervous system and plays a significant role in the maintenance
of the myelin sheath[29,30]. Numerous copper-containing enzymes
and cofactors have been described and their importance to body
metabolism is well known[31-33]. Zinc is essential to the
growth of animal tissues[34,35] and is an integral part of

TABLE XI

Total and Free Copper and Zinc in Maternal and
Umbilical Cord Serum and in Amniotic Fluid

Subject	Maternal				Umbilical cord				Amniotic fluid			
	Total serum (μg/100 ml)		Free (percent)		Total serum (μg/100 ml)		Free (percent)		Total serum (μg/100 ml)		Free (percent)	
	Cu	Zn	Cu	Zn	Cu	Zn	Cu	Zn	Cu	Zn	Cu	Zn
1	149	55	16	77	17	100	10	26	10	10	100	100
2	217	60	10	93	25	88	21	21	13	29	31	100
3	145	55	8	31	19	88	11	22	2	25	100	96
4	198	65	7	51	50	102	4	29	1	65	100	72
5	187	31	13	90	22	80	38	31				
6	295	60	4	68	35	73	20	27				
7	253	43	10	100	18	79	11	53				
8	330	55	8	69	38	72	16	60				

TABLE XI (continued)

Total and Free Copper and Zinc in Maternal and
Umbilical Cord Serum and in Amniotic Fluid

Subject	Maternal				Umbilical cord				Amniotic fluid			
	Total serum (µg/100 ml)		Free (percent)		Total serum (µg/100 ml)		Free (percent)		Total serum (µg/100 ml)		Free (percent)	
	Cu	Zn	Cu	Zn	Cu	Zn	Cu	Zn	Cu	Zn	Cu	Zn
9	223	56	4	64	28	97	14	28				
10	170	38	4	30	25	70	12	27				
11	295	60			35	73						
12	258	37			42	83						
13	202	27			46	77						
14	187	31			22	80						
15	200	43			18	83						
Mean (± 1 SEM)[a]	221 (14)	48 (3)	8 (1)	67 (8)	29 (3)	83 (3)	16 (3)	32 (5)	6 (3)	32 (12)	83 (17)	92 (7)
Normal mean[b] (± 1 SEM)	107 (3)	90 (3)	12 (2)	28 (2)								

a/ SEM, standard error mean.

b/ 45 females, ages 18–42.

TABLE XII

Comparison of Maternal and Fetal Total Serum Concentrations
of Copper and Zinc and Ceruloplasmin with Respect to Fetal Sex

| | Male | | Female | |
	Maternal	Fetal	Maternal	Fetal
Total serum copper (μg/100 ml)	$236 \pm 29^{a/}$	28 ± 4	192 ± 6	36 ± 14
Ceruloplasmin (mg/100 ml)	90 ± 7	10 ± 2	88 ± 6	6 ± 6
Total serum zinc (μg/100 ml)	48 ± 5	83 ± 3	48 ± 17	91 ± 1

$\underline{a/}$ Mean $\pm$ 1 SEM.

several enzymes and other cofactors[36]. Because of these
diverse and important functions, these trace elements play an
essential role in maternal metabolism and fetal development.

At term the total serum concentration of copper in the
mother is approximately twice the normal nonpregnant value
(Tables XI and XIII). However, the percentage of free copper
is not significantly changed. This increase in total copper
is primarily due to an increase in the amount of copper bound
to ceruloplasmin, which is increased as a result of the
elevated levels of maternal estrogen.

Indeed, measurement of ceruloplasmin in the serum of
these mothers indicated that all the bound copper was complexed
with ceruloplasmin. Also the values of bound copper obtained
by ultrafiltration in the present work and by estimation of
ceruloplasmin copper in a previous study[26] are in general
agreement (Table XIV).

TABLE XIII

Comparison of Serum Copper and Zinc Concentrations
in Nonpregnant and Pregnant Women

	Nonpregnant	Pregnant
	(μg/100 ml)	
Serum copper		
Bound	94	203
Free	13 $\pm$ 2	18 $\pm$ 2
Total	107 $\pm$ 3[a]	222 $\pm$ 14[a]
Serum zinc		
Bound	65	16
Free	25 $\pm$ 2	32 $\pm$ 2
Total	90 $\pm$ 3	48 $\pm$ 3

[a] Mean $\pm$ SEM.

At term the maternal total serum concentration of zinc is
approximately one half that of normal nonpregnant values. This
is primarily due to a significant decrease in zinc binding
presumably due either to diminished quantities of zinc binding
proteins or alterations in binding affinities. This decrease
appears to be an example of one of the few instances wherein
binding may diminish during pregnancy. However, in spite of
this decrease in zinc binding, the absolute level of free
zinc in the pregnant woman at term remains unchanged from the
nonpregnant state (Tables XI and XIII).

In the fetus as in the mother, almost the entire bound
fraction of copper is carried by ceruloplasmin. Scheinberg
indicated that 22 μg of copper/100 ml of serum was bound to
ceruloplasmin in the fetus whereas 8.5 μg were free[26]. Our

TABLE XIV

Comparison of Mean Total, Bound and Free Serum Copper Concentrations by Techniques of Present Study (AAS and Ultrafiltration)
and by Colorimetric and Ceruloplasmin-Estimation Techniques[26]

Serum copper	Present techniques	Colorimetric techniques
	(µg/100 ml)	
Maternal		
Bound	203	189[c]
Free	18 ± 2	11[c]
Total	221 ± 14[a]	216 (118-302)[b]
Fetal		
Bound	24	22[c]
Free	5 ± 2	8.5[c]
Total	29 ± 3	36 (12-67)

[a] Mean ± SEM.

[b] Mean (range).

[c] Estimated from determination of ceruloplasmin and calculation
of ceruloplasmin copper as 0.34% of protein concentration.
Note that the sum of free and bound copper by colorimetric
techniques does not equal the total concentration.

results obtained by a different method are in close agreement
(Table XIV).   Widdowson and others have demonstrated a
significant elevation of copper concentration above normal
adult levels in several fetal tissues[27,28], which may be a
manifestation of tissue binding. This is of interest since
fetal serum binding of copper is quantitatively not different
from that of normal adults.

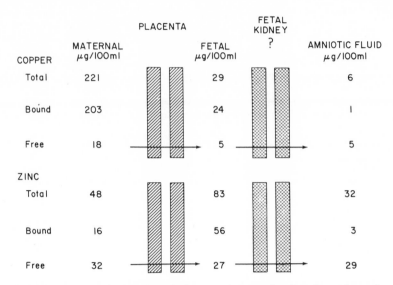

		PLACENTA		FETAL KIDNEY	
COPPER	MATERNAL μg/100ml		FETAL μg/100ml	?	AMNIOTIC FLUID μg/100ml
Total	221		29		6
Bound	203		24		1
Free	18		5		5
ZINC					
Total	48		83		32
Bound	16		56		3
Free	32		27		29

Fig. 10 Total bound and free copper and zinc in maternal
and fetal serum and amniotic fluid. Free metals appear to
move by passive transfer.

Mean fetal serum zinc concentrations, both bound and free,
are not significantly different from adult, nonpregnant levels.
Thus whatever effects the changes noted in the mother at term
does not appear to be active in the fetus.

The relationships between maternal and fetal serum copper
and zinc and between fetal serum and amniotic fluid copper
and zinc are shown in Fig. 10. Presumably, since only free
metals are available for transfer, there is a maternal-fetal
gradient of 13 µg/100 ml for copper and of 5 µg/100 ml for zinc.
Thus both copper and zinc appear to move across the placenta
by passive transfer. Likewise the concentrations present in
amniotic fluid are compatible with the passive transfer of
these trace elements into this fluid and with the predominant
origin of amniotic fluid as fetal urine[37].

C. The Role of Metals in Sensory Function

As previously noted it is well known that copper plays
an important role in the function and/or maintenance of
myelin[29,30]. In this general sense an important role for
some metals in neural function has already been described.
However, there may be a more specific role for some metals in
neural function, especially the role of the transition metals
in several aspects of sensory function, particularly in
gustation. Data collected in our laboratory over the past
3 years indicate that copper, zinc, and nickel play important
roles in maintaining normal gustatory function.

Decreased taste acuity (hypogeusia) for each of four
qualities of taste occurred in 32% of the patients without
Wilson's disease treated with D-penicillamine (β,β-dimethyl-
cysteine, D-pen)[38] (Fig. 11). These patients also had
abnormally low, or lowered, serum copper and ceruloplasmin
concentrations (Fig. 11). Since only 4% of patients with
Wilson's disease treated with D-penicillamine, exhibited
hypogeusia[38,39], we hypothesized that D-penicillamine produced
hypogeusia by lowering copper content. This hypothesis was
tested by administering cupric salts to patients with hypogeusia
while continuing D-penicillamine therapy. Taste sensitivity
returned to normal in each patient treated with copper after
the serum copper and ceruloplasmin concentrations returned
to normal.

These experiments in man were repeated in rats.
Administration of D-penicillamine produced hypogeusia as
indicated by elevated preference thresholds for salt and sugar.
Administration of copper with continued administration of the
drug returned taste acuity to control levels[40].

Ingestion of $NiAc_2$ lowered detection and recognition
thresholds to normal for four taste qualities proportionately

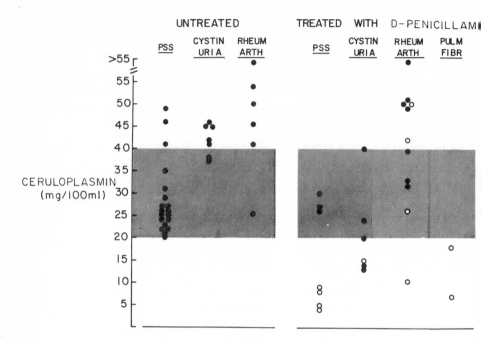

Fig. 11   Serum ceruloplasmin and taste acuity in patients
with various diseases before and after treatment with
D-penicillamine.   Closed circles indicate patients with normal
taste acuity, open circles indicate patients with hypogeusia.
PSS refers to patients with progressive systemic sclerosis or
scleroderma.   The hatched area represents the range of normal
serum ceruloplasmin concentrations.

in a patient with disease-induced hypogeusia[39].   The change
was similar to that previously produced by ingestion of $CuSO_4$
and $ZnCl_2$ in this patient[39].   In a patient with drug-induced
hypogeusia $ZnCl_2$ had this same effect[38], a change similar to
that previously produced by ingestion of $CuSO_4$[38].   All of
these changes were reversed soon after ingestion of the metals
was stopped[41].

With these concepts in mind we found a large group of
patients who had marked hypogeusia, dysgeusia (unpleasant
taste sensations), hyposmia (decreased olfactory acuity),
and dysosmia (unpleasant olfactory sensations) without any
obvious abnormality of either copper or zinc metabolism.
Because this symptom complex had not been previously described,
it was apparent that these patients represented a new syndrome
which we called "idiopathic hypogeusia" for lack of a better
term and to indicate our inability to define a specific
etiology for the development of this condition.

On the basis of our previous data and hypotheses which
related taste acuity to some undefined aspects of trace metal
metabolism we decided to treat several of these patients, in
a single blind study, with placebo and with $ZnSO_4$ orally. We
chose $ZnSO_4$ because it was the most easily tolerated of the
transition metals with which we had experience. By measurement
of detection and recognition thresholds for four taste
qualities[42] and through the use of forced scaling techniques[43], we were able to quantitate taste acuity prior to
and after treatment with either placebo or $ZnSO_4$ therapy.
Subjective responses of the patients with respect to intensity
of dysgeusia and changes in taste acuity were also closely
followed during treatment.

Initial results of the first 35 patients observed with
this disease indicated that they had both a severe hypogeusia,
noted upon threshold measurements (Table XV), and abnormalities
of taste response judgment, note upon measurement of forced
scaling responses (Fig. 12). Following treatment with placebo
there were no consistent, objective changes in taste acuity,
although patients not uncommonly reported some subjective
improvement; following treatment with $ZnSO_4$ there was improvement in taste acuity and in the ability to scale taste responses

TABLE XV

Median Detection and Recognition Thresholds for Four Taste

Qualities in 35 Patients with "Idiopathic Hypogeusia"

Taste quality	Patients		Normal subjects	
	MDT/MRT[a] (mM/L)	Range	MDT/MRT[a] (mM/L)	Range
NaCl	150/300	12–∞/30–∞[b]	12/30	6–60/6–60
Surcrose	90/150	12–∞/12–∞	12/30	6–60/6–60
HCl	30/60	3– >500/6– >500	3/6	15–6/8–6
Urea	800/800	300– >5000/300– >5000	120/150	90–150/90–150

a/ MDT, median detection threshold; MRT, median recognition threshold.

b/ ∞, inability to detect or recognize saturated solutions of NaCl or sucrose.

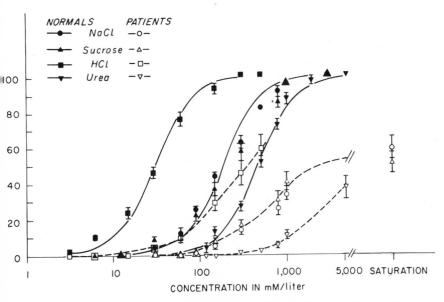

Fig. 12   Forced scaling responses for taste in 22 normal
subjects and in the 35 patients first observed with
idiopathic hypogeusia. Responses are reported as means
(± 1 SEM) for each group, normal or hypogeusic, with respect
to percent taste response (ordinate, 1 to 100) for a range of
concentrations (abscissa, 3 mM/L to 5 M/L) of drops of HCl
for sour, NaCl for salt, sucrose for sweet, and urea for bitter.
As noted in the figure not all concentrations were presented
for representatives of each taste quality. The patients with
hypogeusia did not scale the solutions presented as highly as
did the normal subjects and the mean response values for the
patients did not reach 100% for any concentration presented
even though the concentrations were as high as 0.5 N for HCl,
saturated solutions for NaCl and sucrose, and 5 M for urea.

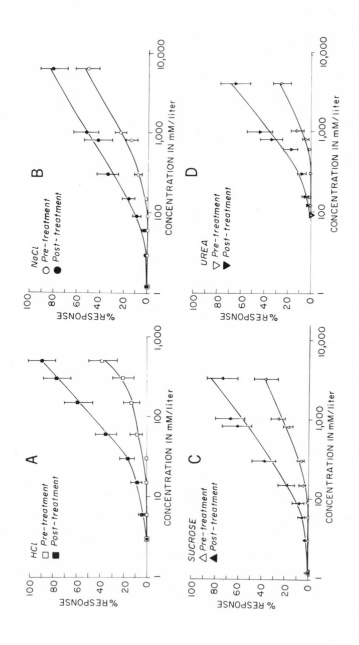

in more than 50% of the patients studied. The results of studies for the first 11 patients with this disease following treatment with $ZnSO_4$ in a single-blind study are shown for threshold changes and changes in serum and urinary zinc (Table XVI) and for forced scaling measurements (Fig. 13). In addition, each patient with dysgeusia or dysosmia reported that these unpleasant symptoms either lessened significantly or disappeared. During treatment serum concentrations of and urinary excretion of Zn^{2+} increased significantly (Table XVI).

Stopping the administration of $ZnSO_4$ after improvement in taste acuity had occurred and switching once again to placebo therapy without the patient's knowledge were followed by a gradual return of dysgeusia and hypogeusia in each patient in whom this regiment was carried out. The time period over which these changes occurred varied and appeared to be dependent primarily on the length of time during which $ZnSO_4$ was administered. Stopping the administration of $ZnSO_4$ also produced

◁ Fig. 13 Mean (± 1 SEM) forced scaling responses in the first 11 patients with idiopathic hypogeusia before and after treatment with $ZnSO_4$, 100 mg daily (as Zn^{2+}) given orally in divided doses. The abscissa indicates concentration of tastant put into the oral cavity, in mM/L; the ordinate indicates percent response of the patient to the drop of tastant over a range from 1 to 100% (that concentration of tastant judged as the saltiest, sourest, sweetest, or bitterest tastant ever appreciated. Mean responses before treatment (open symbols) were significatly lower than mean responses after treatment (closed symbols) indicating a significant improvement in the ability of the patients to obtain taste information from the drops of solutions placed in the oral cavity.

TABLE XVI-a

Median Detection and Recognition Thresholds for Four Taste Qualities and Total

Concentrations of Zinc in Serum and Urine of 11 Patients with

Idiopathic Hypogeusia Before and After Therapy with Zinc Sulfate

| Patient | Sex | Age | Preceding event | Pretreatment | | | | | |
				NaCl (mM/L)	Sucrose (mM/L)	HCl (mM/L)	Urea (mM/L)	Serum (μg/100 ml) Zn	Urine (μg/24°) Zn
ED	M	58	None	800/800[a]	300/300[a]	150/150[a]	5000/5000[a]	63	284
EM	F	51	URI[b]	90/90	30/30	15/500	800/800	87	270
AC	M	53	URI	800/S[d]	150/50	60/500	1000/1000	78	632
MB	M	51	URI	150/150	30/30	30/60	800/800	87	610
AS	M	55	URI	150/150	30/30	15/30	800/800	90	748
JP	M	64	None	300/1000	300/300	30/>500	800/5000	73	448
LD	M	46	None	150/150	150/150	30/60	800/1000	92	810
AM	M	59	URI	150/150	30/30	30/30	300/300	76	580

TABLE XVI-a (continued)

Median Detection and Recognition Thresholds for Four Taste Qualities and Total Concentrations of Zinc in Serum and Urine of 11 Patients with Idiopathic Hypogeusia Before and After Therapy with Zinc Sulfate

Patient	Sex	Age	Preceding event	Pretreatment					
				NaCl (mM/L)	Sucrose (mM/L)	HCl (mM/L)	Urea (mM/L)	Serum (µg/100 ml) Zn	Urine (µg/24°) Zn
JM	M	60	None	∞/∞^{c}	∞/∞	>500/>500	>5000/>5000	92	453
JL	M	68	None	∞/∞	∞/∞	>500/>500	>5000/>5000	76	752
LG	F	60	None	90/300	30/30	15/>500	500/500	91	483
Median				150/300	150/150	30/500	800/1000	82 ± 3	552 ± 55
Normal Values				12/30 6-60/6-60	12/30 6-60/6-60	3/6 0.5-6/0.8-6	120/150 90-150/90-150	92 ± 2	353 ± 23

$\underline{a}/$ Numerator of fraction, detection threshold; denominator of fraction, recognition threshold.

$\underline{b}/$ URI, upper respiratory infection.

$\underline{c}/$ ∞, inability to detect or recognize saturated solutions of NaCl or sucrose.

$\underline{d}/$ S, saturated solution of NaCl.

TABLE XVI-b

Median Detection and Recognition Thresholds for Four Taste Qualities and Total
Concentrations of Zinc in Serum and Urine of 11 Patients with
Idiopathic Hypogeusia Before and After Therapy with Zinc Sulfate

| Patient | Sex | Age | Preceding event | NaCl (mM/L) | Sucrose (mM/L) | HCl (mM/L) | Urea (mM/L) | Post treatment | | Duration in months |
								Serum Zn (μg/100 ml)	Urine Zn (μg/24°)	
ED	M	58	None	60/60[a]	12/12[a]	60/60[a]	500/500[a]	91	970	11
EM	F	51	URI[b]	30/30	30/30	3/3	150/300	173	1820	1
AC	M	53	URI	12/12	12/60	6/6	120/120	112	1056	4
MB	M	51	URI	60/60	12/12	0.8/6	120/120	168	1479	3
AS	M	55	URI	30/30	12/12	3/6	90/90	118	2144	1/2
JP	M	64	None	300/500	90/90	6/60	500/500	125	1444	2
LD	M	46	None	30/60	30/30	6/15	90/90	105	2646	1/2
AM	M	59	URI	30/30	12/12	3/3	90/90	72	1240	1/4

TABLE XVI-b (continued)

Median Detection and Recognition Thresholds for Four Taste Qualities and Total Concentrations of Zinc in Serum and Urine of 11 Patients with Idiopathic Hypogeusia Before and After Therapy with Zinc Sulfate

Patient	Sex	Age	Preceding event	Post treatment						
				NaCl (mM/L)	Sucrose (mM/L)	HCl (mM/L)	Urea (mM/L)	Serum (μg/100 ml) Zn	Urine (μg/24°) Zn	Duration in months
JM	M	60	None	5000/5000	150/150	60/60	2000/5000	165	1802	1
JL	M	68	None	S/∞ c,d/	300/300	150/>500	5000/5000	89	1540	2
LG	F	60	None	12/30	30/30	6/6	150/150	140	2541	1/2
Median				30/60	30/30	6/6	150/150			
Normal Values										

a/ Numerator of fraction, detection threshold; denominator of fraction, recognition threshold.

b/ URI, upper respiratory infection.

c/ ∞, inability to detect or recognize saturated solutions of NaCl or sucrose.

d/ S, saturated solution of NaCl.

a sudden fall in serum concentrations of Zn^{2+} with a more
prolonged, gradual decrease in urinary Zn^{2+} excretion which
generally mirrored the fall in taste acuity to abnormal levels
and the return of dysgeusia.

The mechanisms by which taste acuity is affected by Zn^{2+}
are not known. These questions are now being critically analyzed
and evaluated and a double-blind study of patients with this
disease is now being carried out.

IV. SUMMARY

Copper and zinc metabolism affects several physiological
systems. In order to identify these systems simpler and more
effective tools for the estimation of these metals in biological
fluids were required. For these reasons we developed a new
method for the simultaneous estimation of copper and zinc in
biological fluids which is faster and simpler to perform than
other available methods and which provides results that are as
accurate as methods that are more difficult or more time
consuming. In addition, a simple method for the estimation of
the binding of copper and zinc to their respective carrying
proteins in serum was developed.

Using these techniques copper and zinc metabolism was
investigated in several physiological conditions. These
included the study of the circadian pattern of variation of
these metals in blood and urine, the influence of carbohydrate
active steroids or their metabolites on these metals, the
maternal-fetal transport of these metals and the role that
these metals play in gustation.

REFERENCES

[1]. Butt, E. M., Nusbaum, R. E., Gilmour, T. C., Didio, S. L.,
      and Mariano, S., Arch. Env. Health, 8, 52 (1964).

[2]. Davies, I. J. T., Musa, M., and Dormandy, T. L., J.
      Clin. Path., 21, 359 (1968).

[3]. Willis, J. B., Anal. Chem., 34, 614 (1962).

[4]. Parker, M. M., Humoller, F. L., and Mahler, D. J.,
      Clin. Chem., 13, 40 (1967).

[5]. Sunderman, F. W. and Raszel, N. O., Am. J. Clin. Path.,
      48, 286 (1967).

[6]. Fuwa, K., Pulido, P., McKay, R., and Vallee, B. L.,
      Anal. Chem., 34, 614 (1962).

[7]. Sprague, S. and Slavin, W., Atomic Absorption Newsletter,
      228 (1965).

[8]. Morel, A. G., Windsor, J., Sternlieb, I., and
      Schienberg, I. H., Laboratory Diagnosis of Liver Disease
      (W. Sunderman, ed.) St. Louis, Missouri: W. H. Green,
      1968.

[9]. Kagi, J. H. R., and Vallee, B. L., Anal. Chem., 30,
      1951 (1958).

[10]. Reinhold, J. G., Pascoe, E., and Kfoury, G. A., Anal.
      Biochim., 25, 557 (1968).

[11]. Zettner, A., Advances in Clinical Chemistry (H. Sobotka,
      ed.) New York: Academic Press, 1965.

[12]. Kjellin, K., J. Neurochem., 10, 89 (1963).

[13]. Woodbury, J., Lyons, K., Carretta, R., Hahn, A., and
      Sullivan, J. F., Neurology, 18, 700 (1968).

[14]. Parisi, A. F. and Vallee, B. L., Biochem., 9, 2421-2426
      (1970).

[15]. Andran, R. and Steinbach, M., Protides of the Biological
      Fluids (H. Peeters, ed.) Amsterdam: Elsevier, 14,
      pp. 189-192, 1966.

[16]. Himmelhoch, S. R., Sober, H. A., Vallee, B. L.,
Peterson, E. A., and Fuwa, K., Biochem., 5, 2523-2530
(1966).

[17]. Holmberg, C. G. and Laurell, C. B., Scand. J. Clin.
Lab. Invest., 3, 103-107 (1951).

[18]. Morel, A. G., DenHamer, C. J. A., and Scheinberg, I. A.,
J. Biol. Chem., 244, 3494-3496 (1969).

[19]. Doe, R. P., Flink, E. B., and Goodsell, M. G.,
J. Clin. Endocrin., 19, 196-206 (1956).

[20]. Bartter, F. C. and Delea, C. S., Ann. N. Y. Acad. Sci.,
98, 969-983 (1962).

[21]. Henkin, R. I., Meret, S., and Jacobs, J. B., J. Clin.
Invest., 48, 38a (1969).

[22]. Chasson, A. L., Grady, H. J., and Stanley, M. A.,
Am. J. Clin. Path., 35, 83-88 (1961).

[23]. Munch-Petersen, S., Scand. J. Clin. Lab. Invest., 2,
48-52 (1950).

[24]. Drinker, K. R., Fehnel, J. W., and Marsh, M., J. Biol.
Chem., 72, 357-383 (1927).

[25]. Butler, E. J. and Newman, G. E., J. Clin. Path., 9,
157-161 (1956).

[26]. Scheinberg, I. H., Cook, C. D., and Murphy, J. A.,
J. Clin. Invest., 33, 963 (1954).

[27]. Ketcheson, M. R., Barron, G. P., and Cox, D. H.,
J. Nutr., 98, 303 (1969).

[28]. Widdowson, E., Proc. VIIIth Int. Congress of Nutri.,
Excerpta Med. Found, 1971.

[29]. Bennetts, H. W. and Beck, A. B., Commonw. Australia
CSIR Bull., 147, 1 (1942).

[30]. Innes, J. R. M., Vet. Rec., 48, 1539 (1936).

[31]. Morrison, M., Horie, S., and Mason, H. S., J. Biol.
Chem., 238, 2220 (1963).

[32].   Yamada, H. and Yasunobu, K. T., J. Biol. Chem., 237,
        3077 (1962).

[33].   Wintrobe, M. M., Cartwright, G. E., and Gubler, C. J.,
        J. Nutri., 503, 395 (1953).

[34].   Hurley, L. S., Am. J. Clin. Nutri., 22, 1332 (1969).

[35].   Prasad, A. S., Oberleass, D., Wolf, P., and
        Horwitz, J. P., J. Lab. Clin. Med., 73, 486 (1969).

[36].   Parisi, A. F. and Vallee, B. F., Am. J. Clin. Nutri.,
        22, 1222 (1969).

[37].   Eastman, N. J. and Hellman, L. M., Obstetrics (13th ed.)
        New York: Appleton-Century-Crofts, 1966 p. 213.

[38].   Henkin, R. I., Keiser, H. R., Jaffe, I. A., Sternlieb, I.,
        and Scheinberg, I. H., Lancet, 2, 1268-1271 (1967).

[39].   Henkin, R. I., Graziadei, P. P. G., and Bradley, D. F.,
        Ann. Intern. Med., 71, 791-821 (1969).

[40].   Kare, M. R. and Henkin, R. I., Proc. Soc. Exper. Biol.
        Med., 131, 559-569 (1969).

[41].   Henkin, R. I. and Bradley, D. F., Life Sciences, 9,
        701-709 (1970).

[42].   Henkin, R. I., Gill, Jr., J. R., and Bartter, F. C.,
        J. Clin. Invest., 42, 727-735 (1963).

[43].   Giroux, E. L. and Henkin, R. I., Life Sciences,
        (submitted for publication) (1970).

[44].   Dawson, J. B., Ellis, D. J., and Newton-John, H.,
        Clin. Chim. Acta, 21, 33 (1968).

[45].   Berman, E., Atomic Absorption Newsletter, 4, 296 (1965).

[46].   Parker, M. M., Humoller, F. L., and Mahler, D. J.,
        Clin. Chem., 13, 40 (1967).

[47].   Davies, T. J. T., Musa, M., and Dormandy, T. L.,
        J. Clin. Path., 21, 359 (1968).

[48].   Ch'en, P. E., Chinese Med. J., 75, 917 (1957).

[49]. Canelas, H. M., Assis, L. M., de Jorge, F. B.,
       Tolosa, A. P. M., and Cintra, A. B. U., Acta Neurol.
       Scan., 40, 97 (1964).

[50]. Cartwright, G. E. and Wintrobe, M. M., Am. J. Clin.
       Nutr., 14, 224 (1964).

Chapter 13

TIN AS AN ESSENTIAL GROWTH FACTOR FOR RATS[*]/

K. Schwarz

Laboratory of Experimental Metabolic Diseases
Medical Research Programs
Veterans Administration Hospital
Long Beach, California
and
Department of Biological Chemistry
School of Medicine
University of California
Los Angeles, California

Having discovered the essential physiological roles of selenium[1] and chromium[2], the latter in close collaboration with Walter Mertz and with the staunch assistance of Edward Roginski, I am glad to be able to contribute this chapter on tin. We recently added tin to the list of elements essential for growth and well-being of a mammalian species, the rat[3]. This finding resulted from the development of a systematic, novel approach to the production of new trace element deficiency diseases and to the detection of hitherto unidentified essential elements initiated in our laboratory almost 10 years ago.

* Supported by USPHS Grant AM-08669.

I. RESEARCH TECHNIQUES

Following the discoveries of selenium and chromium, we
decided after several exploratory studies to combine ultraclean-room and modern isolator techniques with highly purified,
chemically defined diets containing amino acids in lieu of
protein. We constructed a trace-element-"sterile" isolator
system that is based on the use of plastics for all components.
There is no metal, glass, or rubber used anywhere in the system.
The isolator was originally a modification of the Trexler
isolator for germ-free research[4]. An earlier version of the
system has been described[5]. A greatly improved model has
been in operation in our laboratory since 1968[6]. It is shown
in Fig. 1. The isolator has six working sleeves; a vinyl
zipper extends over the entire top to facilitate cleaning and
setting-up operations. The isolator holds a rack with 32
animals in individual cages. An air lock facilitates passage
of articles in and out of the trace-element-sterile area. A
major operational improvement is the introduction of calcium
chloride hexahydrate $(CaCl_2 \cdot 6H_2O)$ in the plastic refuse trays
under the cages which not only keeps the humidity in the
isolator at a relatively constant level but also prevents
microbial deterioration and completely eliminates undesirable
odors.

The isolator system works so well as a single barrier to
trace element contamination that we found it unnecessary to
apply the more elaborate ultraclean-room techniques originally
planned. However, it is advantageous to use a laminar-flow
air filter in the clean animal room housing the isolators.
The filter removes dust from the air down to a particle size
of 0.35 μ. Each isolator, in addition, is equipped with two
individual air filter units which remove not only dust but

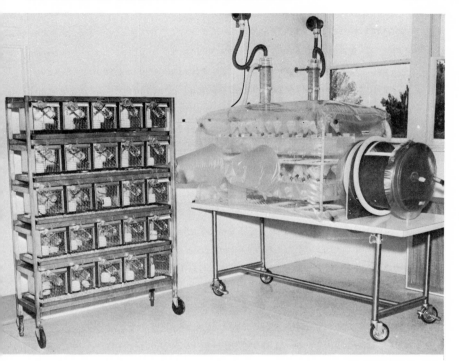

Fig. 1   Trace-element-controlled isolator and conventional caging.

also bacteria, yeasts, and molds from the air. The experiments are not carried out under germ-free conditions.

The system lends itself to definitive experiments on any known element provided analytical methods are available that are sensitive enough and diets can be developed that are free of the element under study. The diet is the main source of trace element contaminants. The rations contain an optimal mixture of L-amino acids and all other chemically known nutritional factors in adequate and balanced amounts, including the nine trace elements identified previously as being required by the rat. In our experience salts are the main source of

undersirable impurities in such diets. Extensive use has been
made of emission spectrography which is applied to each batch
of each dietary ingredient. It permits the semiquantitative
screening for 28 different elements. Batches of amino acids,
salts, and other dietary constituents of high purity are
selected after emission spectrographic analysis and other
analytical screening procedures. The exact composition of the
basal diet is described elsewhere[5].

Weanling rats maintained on the basal amino acid diet
inside the trace-element-controlled isolator system show signs
of deficiency within 1 to 2 weeks after initiation of the
experiment (Fig. 2). They grow poorly, lose hair, develop a
seborrhealike condition, and are lacking in energy and tonicity.
The condition is nutritional in origin since rats maintained on
laboratory chow in the isolator are perfectly normal. The
symptoms observed in the trace-element-sterile environment are
caused primarily by lack of hitherto unrecognized trace elements
because supplements of 1% ash from yeast largely, but not
entirely, prevent their occurrence. Chemical fractionation
of yeast ash has provided evidence for the involvement of more
than one element in the prevention of the deficiency symptoms[7].

If we classify the elements of the periodic system with
respect to their biological or potential physiological function
in the mammalian organism (Fig. 3), we find that the 11 elements
which constitute the bulk of living matter are all very small
in atomic size. They are among the lowest 20 elements. All
elements presently known to be essential have slightly higher
atomic numbers. At the present state of knowledge there is
no overlap between the essential trace elements and those that
make up the bulk of living tissue. An additional noteworthy
observation is that not one of the 39 elements with higher
numbers (not including the artificial transuranium elements)

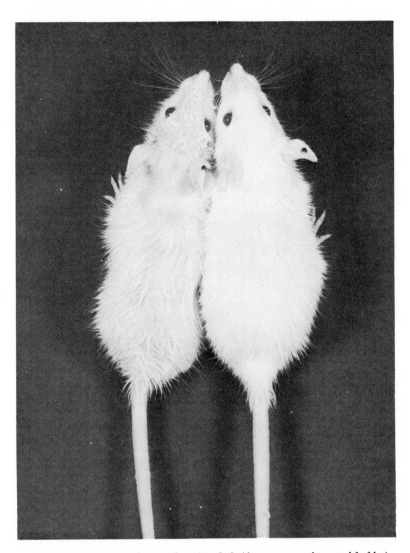

Fig. 2 Comparison of rats fed the same amino acid diet
in conventional and controlled environments. Left: animal
fed basal diet after 2 weeks in the control environment.
Right: control animal fed basal diet kept outside in metal
cage with glass water bottle and food cup.

TRACE ELEMENTS FOR THE MAMMALIAN ORGANISM

| ☐ established | ═ possible |
| ≡ under special consideration | ╱ unlikely |

Ia	IIa	IIIb	IVb	Vb	VIb	VIIb	VIII	VIII	VIII	Ib	IIb	IIIa	IVa	Va	VIa	VIIa	O
H																	He
Li	Be											B	C	N	O	F	Ne
Na	Mg											Al	Si	P	S	Cl	Ar
K	Ca	Sc	Ti	V	Cr	Mn	Fe	Co	Ni	Cu	Zn	Ga	Ge	As	Se	Br	Kr
Rb	Sr	Y	Zr	Nb	Mo	Tc	Ru	Rh	Pd	Ag	Cd	In	Sn	Sb	Te	I	Xe
Cs	Ba	La	Hf	Ta	W	Re	Os	Ir	Pt	Au	Hg	Tl	Pb	Bi	Po	At	Rn
Fr	Ra	Ac	Th	Pa	U												

14 Rare Earth Elements

Ce	Pr	Nd	Pm	Sm	Eu	Gd	Tb	Dy	Ho	Er	Tm	Yb	Lu

Fig. 3   Established, possible, and potential trace elements for the mammalian organism. (Modified after Schwarz, 1968).

has been shown to have any physiological significance for animals. If we omit those elements for which physiological functions are most unlikely--namely, the inert gases, the artificial elements (technetium and promethium), and those elements that are highly radioactive--we are left with 56 elements that could be potential pretenders for trace element function. In Fig. 3, 24 elements are designated as "under special consideration" since they fulfill at least in part some of the postulates that may characterize essentiality (presence in the newborn or in milk, presence in the organism, in tissues, and in nutrients, existence of homeostatic mechanisms for maintenance of constant levels in the blood and tissues, and so on). Two of these, vanadium and nickel, are treated elsewhere in this monograph[8,9].

II. GROWTH EFFECTS OF TIN

We have identified tin as an element essential for growth of rats maintained under trace-element-sterile conditions in the isolator system.[*/] Table I demonstrates growth effects obtained with various tin compounds at dose levels supplying 1 ppm of the element to the diet. The first two experiments show effects of two organic tin compounds, trimethyl tin hydroxide, $(CH_3)_3SnOH$, and dibutyl tin maleate, $(C_4H_9)Sn(OOCCH^{2-})_2$. The experiment was carried out in 1968. Positive responses are clearly evident. The results demonstrate that experimentation with tin at that time was approximately at the stage at which the experiments with vanadium[8] and nickel[9] are today.

From 1968 to 1969 we made a series of step-by-step improvements in the basal diet, with the effect that it is now much more deficient in tin than the basal diet A of Table I. This diet produces much less growth of animals in the control groups. The addition of tin at 100 µg levels in the form of either inorganic salts or organic tin derivatives produces constant growth effects amounting to 30 to 50% of the initial growth rate. Organotin compounds, however, show chemical

---

[*] More recently, the same results have been obtained in all plastic cages outside the isolator.

TABLE I

Growth Effects of Various Tin Compounds in Rats in Trace-Element-Controlled Environment

(Duration of Experiments 26 to 29 days)

Compounds	Dose level (μg Sn/100 g)	Number of animals	Average daily weight gain (grams)	Increase (percent)	P value
Basal A[a]					
Control		5	1.89 ± 0.06[b]		
Trimethyl tin hydroxide, $(CH_3)_3SnOH$	100	4	2.22 ± 0.09	18	0.02
Dibutyl tin maleate, $(C_4H_9)_2Sn(OOCCH^{2-})_2$	100	5	2.16 ± 0.14	14	0.1
Basal B[a]					
Control		7	1.27 ± 0.11		
Stannic sulfate, $Sn(SO_4)_2 \cdot 2H_2O$	100	7	1.67 ± 0.07	31	0.01
Potassium stannate, $K_2SnO_3 \cdot 3H_2O$[c]	100	8	1.55 ± 0.10	22	0.1
Basal C					
Control		8	0.84 ± 0.07		
Stannic sulfate, $Sn(SO_4)_2 \cdot 2H_2O$	100	7	1.16 ± 0.06	38.2	0.02
Stannous tartrate, $SnC_4H_4O_6$	100	8	1.12 ± 0.09	33.4	0.05

a/ Reprinted from Ref. [3] by courtesy of Academic Press.

b/ Mean ± standard error.

c/ Better formulated as $K_2[Sn(OH)_6]$.

specificity with respect to their potency. A dose response
curve obtained with various levels of tin as stannic sulfate,
$Sn(SO_4)_2 \cdot 2H_2O$, is shown in Table II. One ppm of tin produces
a near-optimum result.

The identification of tin as an element essential for the
growth of rats comes as an unexpected surprise to those
familiar with the literature. To our knowledge tin has never
before been shown to exert any physiological role in animals
or man. Even references to effects of tin in plants are found
only sporadically in the literature.

Tin belongs with carbon, silicon, germanium, and lead to
the fourth main group of elements. It has many chemical and
physical properties in common with the other members of this
group. Its atomic number is 50; its atomic weight is 118.7.
It is noteworthy that aside from the paramount role of carbon
in living matter of our planet and the role of silicon as a
structural building material in plants, none of the other
elements of this group have been implicated in biological
functions until today.

In its chemical properties tin is similar to carbon in
its tendency to form truly covalent linkages. A great number
of organotin compounds have been synthesized. Many of them
are of industrial or practical usefulness as catalysts.
Others, especially the triethyl and tripropyl tin derivatives,
are used as bacteriostatic and fungistatic agents.[*/] Even
stannic chloride is largely covalent in its chemical nature.
It has little ionic character. Other tin salts, however,
are ionic by nature. In addition to its capacity to form

---

[*] These compounds were found much less active than stannic
sulfate in the promotion of growth of rats in the
trace-element-controlled environment system.

TABLE II

Growth Effect of Tin, as Stannic Sulfate, in Rats in Trace-Element-Controlled Environment[a]

(Duration of Experiment 28 days)

Compound	Dose level (μg Sn/100 g)	Number of animals	Average daily weight gain (grams)	Increase (percent)	P value
Control		5[b]	1.10 $\pm$ 0.05[c]		
Stannic sulfate, Sn(SO$_4$)$_2$·2H$_2$O	50	8	1.37 $\pm$ 0.10	24	0.02
Stannic sulfate	100	8	1.68 $\pm$ 0.10	53	<0.001
Stannic sulfate	200	8	1.75 $\pm$ 0.10	59	<0.001

[a] Reprinted from Ref. [3] by courtesy of Academic Press.

[b] Two control animals died in the course of the experiment. One animal was eliminated because it was outside of the normal error.

[c] Mean $\pm$ standard error.

covalent organic compounds, trivalent tin has a strong tendency
to form coordination complexes with 4, 5, 6, and 8 ligands.
Thus it could well contribute to the tertiary structure of
proteins or other biologically important macromolecules such
as nucleic acids. It could also function as the active site
of metalloenzymes. The oxidation-reduction potential of
$Sn^{2+} \rightleftharpoons Sn^{4+}$ is at -0.13 V. This is well within the range of
physiological oxidation-reduction reactions. As a matter of
fact it is very close to the potential of the flavin enzymes.

Trace amounts of tin occur widely distributed in tissues
and nutrients (Table III) but the element has been considered
an "environmental contaminant" instead of an essential dietary
trace factor. A relatively recent review of tin in man and
foods, for instance, treated tin as an abnormal trace metal
and concluded that "the evidence is convincing that measurable
tin is not necessary for life or health"[10]. This conclusion
was based mainly on the fact that with the prevailing
inadequate methods of analysis, "zero" levels of tin were found
in the newborn and in organs of natives of some foreign
countries. The analytical methods applied to tin in tissues
involved drying of specimens at 110°C and subsequent ashing
at 450°C. It is possible that under these conditions losses
of tin could occur, especially if the element was present in
the form of organotin compounds. Even stannic chloride has a
boiling point of 114°C. Stannous acetate boils at 240°C, and
the great majority of organotin derivatives evaporates below
200°C. It is obvious, therefore, that values reported in the
literature for tin are highly questionable if they were obtained
with the ashing methods described. We have investigated the
behavior of some organotin compounds under these conditions
and have found recoveries of 0%. The chemical nature of the
tin compounds found in biological specimens is unknown. It
may be expected that the findings related here open up a new,
and hopefully fruitful, field of bioinorganic chemistry.

TABLE III
Tin in Foods[a]

	(μg/g)	(μg/100 cal)
Foods of Animal Origin		
Beef, ground, lean	2.76	153
Beef and fat, ground	3.44	90
Pork, lean chop	0.84	26
Lamb chop	1.36	72
Chicken breast, frozen	1.73	92
Halibut steak	1.21	121
Codfish steak, 1	3.67	459
Greysole, fillet	3.21	382
Lobster, claw meat	0.60	50
Oysters, frozen	1.38	276
Beaver heart	7.28	
Ruffed grouse liver	0.50	
Eggs, chicken	0.91	57
Milk, from udder into polyethylene	0.19	29
Milk, dry skim, packaged	0.96	29
Cheese, tinfoil wrapped	0.32	8

[a] Reprinted from Ref. [10] by courtesy of Pergamon Press.

TABLE III (continued)
Tin in Foods[a]

	(µg/g)	(µg/100 cal)
Foods of Plant Origin		
Peas, split, dried, packaged	8.50	281
Peas, fresh	1.06	166
Beans, navy, dried	5.80	191
Beans, string, fresh	0.28	187
Potato, raw	0.97	111
Spinach	1.23	473
Spinach, fresh, packaged	6.47	2488
Kale	0.86	430
Asparagus, fresh	9.07	5039
Mushrooms, fresh	1.08	1543
Rye, winter	1.9	57
Rye flour from seed	0.0[b]	
Barley	0.65	18
Corn meal	0.11	3
Wheat flour (Japan)	0.47	14
Wheat flour (U.S.)	0.0[b]	
Wheat bread	2.48	100
Oats, seed	2.28	
Rice, packaged	0.28	8
Tea, packaged, bags	2.28	

[a] Reprinted from Ref. [10] by courtesy of Pergamon Press.

[b] "0" equals less than 0.05 µg Sn/g fresh weight.

ACKNOWLEDGMENT

Dr. J. Cecil Smith, Jr., and Dr. Mercedes Petersen
collaborated in the earlier phase of this work, and Dr. David
B. Milne and Betty Vinyard collaborated in the recent
developments concerning tin. The efficient technical assistance
of David Evans, Maureen Conley, and George El-Bogdadi is
gratefully acknowledged.

REFERENCES

[1]. Schwarz, K., and Foltz, C. M., J. Am. Chem. Soc., 79,
3292 (1957).

[2]. Schwarz, K., and Mertz, W., Biochem. Biophys., 85,
292 (1959).

[3]. Schwarz, K., Milne, D. B., and Vinyard, E., Biochem.
Biophys., 40, 22 (1970).

[4]. Trexler, P. C., Ann. N. Y. Acad. Sci., 78, 29 (1959).

[5]. Smith, J. C. and Schwarz, K., J. Nutr., 93, 182 (1967).

[6]. Schwarz, K., Trace Element Metabolism in Animals
(C. F. Mills, ed.) Livingstone, Edinburgh, 1970,
pp. 25-38.

[7]. Schwarz, K., unpublished results.

[8]. Hopkins, L. L., Jr. and Mohr, H. E., The Newer Trace
Elements in Nutrition (W. Mertz and W. E. Cornatzer, eds.)
New York: Marcel Dekker, in press.

[9]. Nielsen, F. H., The Newer Trace Elements in Nutrition
(W. Mertz and W. E. Cornatzer, eds.) New York: Marcel
Dekker, in press.

[10]. Schroeder, H. A., Balassa, J. J., and Tipton, I. H.,
J. Chron. Dis., 17, 483 (1964).

Chapter 14

DECREASED INCORPORATION OF L-CYSTINE-^{35}S
INTO SKIN PROTEIN OF ZINC-DEFICIENT RATS

J. M. Hsu

Biochemistry Research Laboratory
Veterans Administration Hospital
The Johns Hopkins University
and the Department of Biochemistry
Baltimore, Maryland

I. ABSTRACT

Studies were carried out in young rats to determine the effect of zinc deficiency on the distribution of ^{35}sulfur and incorporation of L-cystine-^{35}S into skin protein. Results indicate that urinary excretion of ^{35}sulfur in zinc-deficient rats was about three times more than in zinc-supplemented rats. Conversely the uptake of ^{35}sulfur in the skin and hair of zinc-deficient rats was only 30% of normal value. Zinc deficiency also drastically reduced the amount of cystine-^{35}S incorporation into skin protein at 4, 8, 16, and 24 hour postinjection. This defect was not due to food intake and can be restored on zinc repletion. An additional experiment reveals that zinc-deficient rats had a reduced capacity to utilize L-proline-^{14}C for the formation of skin protein as compared to zinc-supplemented rats. These observations as a whole strongly suggest that zinc is essential in the synthesis of skin keratin and collagen.

II. INTRODUCTION

Initial studies on cystine metabolism revealed that a 30% reduction was observed in the incorporation of cystine-1-^{14}C into the liver and kidney proteins of zinc-deficient rats[1]. These findings were interpreted as evidence of an impairment in protein synthesis during zinc deficiency. Later investigation[2], however, indicated that after cystine-^{35}S injection, 24 hour urinary excretion of total ^{35}sulfur from zinc-deficient rats was two to three times higher than that of zinc-supplemented controls. The great loss of radiosulfur in the urine cannot be explained on the basis of a relatively small decrease of protein formation in the two tissues examined. Since one of the pronounced and universally recognized symptoms induced by dietary deprivation of zinc is skin lesions and since it is known that epidermis has a high cystine content, it is desirable to study the effect of zinc deficiency on skin function. The purpose of this investigation was to determine whether the rate of incorporation of L-cystine-^{35}S into skin protein is altered by the lack of zinc ion. For comparison other tissue proteins including pancreas, liver, testes, and muscle were also examined.

III. MATERIALS AND METHODS

A. Animals and Diet

Young male albino rats of the Sprague-Dawley strain weighing 40 to 50 g and obtained from a commercial laboratory[*] were used in all experiments. The animals were randomly separated into two groups unless otherwise stated. One group was fed on a zinc-deficient diet composed of 65.97% sucrose, 15.0% dried egg albumin, 3.0% salt-free casein hydrolysate, 10.0% corn oil, 5.74% salt mixture[**] and 0.29 vitamin supplement.[†] The zinc content of the diet was 2 ppm as

---

[*] Sprague-Dawley rats purchased from Zivic Miller Laboratories, Inc., 3848 Hieber Road, Allison Park, Pennsylvania 15101.

[**] Furnished per 100 g of diet; (in grams) $CaHPO_4$, 2.716; $CaCO_3$, 0.957; $NaHPO_4$, 0.670; NaCl, 0.383; KCl, 0.670; $MgSO_4$, 0.287; $FeC_6H_5O_7 \cdot 5H_2O$, 0.019; $MnSO_4$, 0.021; KIO_3, 0.001; and $CuSO_4 \cdot 5H_2O$, 0.001.

[†] Furnished per 100 g of diet (in milligrams) thiamine HCl, 0.24; riboflavin, 0.60; pyridoxine·HCl, 0.30; Ca-pantothenate, 2.00; niacin, 4.00; inositol, 10.00; biotin, 0.60; folic acid, 0.20; vitamin B_{12}, 0.002; choline, chloride, 100.00; 2-methyl-1-4-napthoquinone, 1.00; and α-tocopherol, 6.00; (IU) vitamin A, 2500; and vitamin D_3, 300.

determined by a direct-reading spectrphotometer.[*/] The second
group, used as controls, received the same diet supplemented
with 65 ppm of zinc as zinc carbonate. All rats were housed
individually in stainless steel cages. Feed and deionized
distilled water were offered ad libitum in all experiments,
except to the pair-fed control group of rats.

B. Injection of Labeled Compounds

After 16 hour fasting, each rat was weighed and injected
intramuscularly (2 to 5 μC/100 g body weight) with the labeled
compounds.[**/] In some experiments in which urine and feces were
collected rats were transferred to individual stainless steel
metabolism cages after isotope administration. They were fed
as usual during the collection period.

C. Measurement of Radioactivity

All measurements of radioactivity were made in a Tricarb
liquid scintillation spectrometer. The diotol composed of
4.6 g 2,5-diphenyloxazole (PPO), 0.091 g 1,4-bis-(methyl-5
phenyloxazol-2-yl) benzene, 73 g napthalene, 210 ml methanol,
350 ml dioxane, and 350 ml toluene was used as scintillator
solution. The distribution of radioactivity in various tissues
was expressed as percentage of the injected dose. All values
for tissue protein radioactivity were expressed as
disintegrations per minute per milligram protein (DPM/mg protein).

---

*   Jarrell-Ash atomic absorption spectrophotometer,
Jarrell-Ash Company, Waltham, Massachusetts.

**   The following radiochemicals were obtained from New England
Nuclear Corporation, Boston, Massachusetts: L-Cystine-^{35}S
(39.5 mCi/mmole), and L-proline-UL-^{14}C (254.4 mCi/mmole).

D. Preparation of Various Tissue and Excreta for Measurement of Radioactivity

The liver, kidney, gastrointestinal tract (GI tract), and testes were homogenized with ice-cold distilled water to make a 5% homogenate(w/v). One half milliliter of tissue homogenate in duplicate was added to a counting vial containing an equal amount hyamine hydroxide. The mixture was heated at 55-60°C for 30 minutes or more until the tissue homogenate was completely digested, then 15 ml scintillation fluid was added and the radioactivity measured. Each carcass composed of bones and muscles and the skin-hair of each animal were separately dissolved in about 200 ml of 20% KOH in 50% ethanol, heated at 70-75°C for 4 hours and diluted to 600 ml with water. Portions were suspended in scintillation solution and their radioactivity determined. Urine was diluted to constant volume, filtered, and an aliquot was added to scintillation solution and counted. Feces were homogenized with 50% ethanol, made to volume, and shaken for 30 minutes at room temperature. An aliquot was centrifuged and the supernatant fluid was counted.

E. Measurement of Incorporation of Labeled Amino Acid into Tissue Protein

Immediately after decapitation, the liver, pancreas, kidney, and testes were excised and weighed and portions of each tissue were homogenized in a Porter-Elvehjem glass homogenizer. To 1 ml homogenate was added 2 ml ice-cold 10% trichloroacetic acid (TCA) and the TCA suspensions were kept at 4°C overnight. Protein was prepared for measurement of radioactivity as follows: The TCA suspension was centrifuged and the sediment was washed three times successively with 8 ml of 6% TCA containing 4.74 mg of unlabeled L-cystine. The

residue was then dissolved in 3 ml of 88% formic acid and
0.6 ml of 30% hydrogen perioxide and the mixture was allowed
to stand 30 minutes at room temperature. To the formic acid
treated solution, 5 ml of 10% TCA was added and the resulting
precipitate was separated by centrifugation. To remove the
residual TCA as well as some of the lipid, the precipitate was
extracted with 5 ml of a 95% ethanol saturated with sodium
acetate. Further lipid extraction was completed with 5 ml of
a 3:1 ethanol ethyl ether mixture and 5 ml of anhydrous
ethyl ether. The extra ether was evaporated by drying the
precipitate in air at room temperature for 5-10 minutes. While
the protein precipitate was still slightly wet, 4.0 ml of a
0.4 N KOH solution was added and the mixtures were incubated
for 30 minutes at 40°C. The resulting KOH hydrolyzate was
used for the determinations of protein radioactivity and
protein content.

Tissue protein concentrations were estimated by the method
of Lowry, Rosebrough, Farr, and Randall[3] with bovine serum
albumin as standard. Radioactive protein was determined by
adding 0.5 ml of hyamine hydroxide solution to an equal amount
of KOH hydrolyzate and the sample was shaken until clear.
To the hyamine solution 15 ml of scintillator fluid was added,
and the sample was counted. All samples were corrected for
quenching by the internal standard techniques of Herberg[4].

In some experiments protein from gastrocnemius muscle was
also prepared for measurement of radioactivity by the
procedures similar to those described for liver with the
exception of using 0.4 N NaOH instead of distilled water to
make a 5% homogenate.

To study skin protein a portion of dorsal skin was
immediately removed and then shaved, cleaned, weighed, minced,
and homogenized for 10 minutes with water in "Virtis" 45
homogenizer. The skin suspension was further ground to make

a final 5% homogenate. Their radioactive proteins were measured
by the method described above.

F. Measurements of Skin Trace Elements and Minerals

A piece of dorsal skin was shaved, carefully cleaned with
distilled and deionized water, chopped into several pieces,
and weighed. The hairless skin was kept at 95°C for 18 hours
in a constant-temperature oven. The dried skin was used to
determine various trace elements by Jarrell-Ash atomic
absorption method[5].

IV. RESULTS

Table I presents the results of radioactive distribution
after cystine-^{35}S injection. The increased urinary excretion
of ^{35}sulfur indicates that the zinc-deficient rats oxidized
cystine at a faster rate than the zinc-supplemented controls.
The liver, kidney, and testes of rats fed a zinc-deficient diet
contained more radioactivity from cystine-^{35}S than did those of
the zinc-supplemented rats and more ^{35}sulfur was also retained
in the gastrointestinal tract and carcass of the deficient
rats. However, the most interesting discovery is that the
amount of radioactivity found in the skin and hair of
zinc-supplemented rats was four times greater than that of
zinc-deficient animals. In pair-fed zinc-supplemented controls
the skin and hair also contained significantly higher
radioactivity as compared to zinc-deficient rats.

The incorporation of cystine-^{35}S into skin protein was
studied at time intervals from 4 to 24 hour postinjection.
The results in Table II indicate that at 4 hours the specific
activity present in the skin of zinc-deficient rats was
one-seventh of that of zinc-supplemented rats, ad libitum
fed rats, and one-fifth of that of pair-fed controls. Although
more cystine-^{35}S was incorporated into skin protein of

TABLE I

Distribution of ^{35}S at 24 Hours after L-Cystine-^{35}S Injection

	Percent of injected ^{35} sulfur		
	Zn-supplemented ad lib	Zn-supplemented pair-fed	Zn-deficient
Urine	11.35 ± 0.99 [a,b]	10.60 ± 2.18 [c]	32.82 ± 5.06
Feces	Trace	Trace	Trace
Liver	1.27 ± 0.15 [c]	1.52 ± 0.35	2.73 ± 0.95
Kidney	0.53 ± 0.07 [c]	0.63 ± 0.13	0.94 ± 0.20
Testes	0.25 ± 0.03	0.29 ± 0.07	0.45 ± 0.15
Gastrointestinal Tract	2.29 ± 0.04 [b]	4.97 ± 0.14	6.24 ± 0.21
Skin and Hair	77.71 ± 2.13 [b,e]	58.82 ± 4.11 [d]	20.61 ± 2.34
Carcass	8.72 ± 0.85 [e]	25.24 ± 1.34 [d]	34.58 ± 2.18

a/ Mean ± SD. Six rats in each group and they were on experimental diet for 18 days.

b/ Difference between Zn-supplemented ad lib and Zn-deficient rats is statistically significant (P<0.01).

c/ Difference between Zn-supplemented ad lib and Zn-deficient rats is statistically significant (P<0.05).

d/ Difference between Zn-supplemented pair-fed and Zn-deficient rats is statistically significant (P<0.01).

e/ Difference between Zn-supplemented ad lib and Zn-supplemented pair-fed rats is statistically significant (P<0.01).

TABLE II

Incorporation of L-Cystine-^{35}S into Skin Protein

Type of diet	Days of feeding	Number of rats	Hours after injection	Specific activity (DPM/mg protein)
Zinc-supplemented ad lib	14	7	4	1302 $\pm$ 585[a,b]
Zinc-supplemented pair-fed	14	5	4	881 $\pm$ 319[c]
Zinc-deficient	14	6	4	174 $\pm$ 66
Zinc-supplemented ad lib	16	5	8	1444 $\pm$ 136[b]
Zinc-supplemented pair-fed	16	6	8	1337 $\pm$ 108[c]
Zinc-deficient	16	5	8	506 $\pm$ 118

TABLE II (continued)

Incorporation of L-Cystine-^{35}S into Skin Protein

Type of diet	Days of feeding	Number of rats	Hours after injection	Specific activity (DPM/mg protein)
Zinc-supplemented ad lib	16	6	16	1080 ± 227[b]
Zinc-deficient	16	6	16	352 ± 83
Zinc-supplemented ad lib	15	5	24	1267 ± 112[b]
Zinc-supplemented pair-fed	15	5	24	1117 ± 295[c]
Zinc-deficient	15	5	24	306 ± 115

[a] Mean ± SD.

[b] Difference between Zn-supplemented ad lib and Zn-deficient rats is statistically significant (P<0.01).

[c] Difference between Zn-supplemented pair-fed and Zn-deficient rats is statistically significant (P<0.01).

zinc-deficient rats at 8 hours than that at 4 hours after
isotope injection, the amounts were still only 35% of the
normal value. Similar trends were found between zinc-supplemented and zinc-deficient rats at the end of 16 and 24 hours
of cystine-^{35}S incorporation into skin protein.

Results of the effect of zinc deficiency on the incorporation of cystine-^{35}S into other tissue proteins are given in
Table III. No significant differences were observed in the
protein-^{35}S activity of the liver, kidney, testes, and muscle.
However, more cystine-^{35}S was incorporated into the pancreas
protein of rats fed diets low in zinc than in rats fed the
diet containing an adequate level of zinc.

The effect of zinc repletion of cystine-^{35}S incorporation
into skin protein was determined by daily intraperitoneal
injections of 400 µg of zinc as zinc chloride on the last
three days of the experiment. Results summarized in Table IV
indicate that skin protein in zinc-repleted rats had
radioactivity similar to that in zinc-supplemented rats. In
the pancreas similar findings were noted between the two groups.
Thus the defects in incorporation observed in zinc-deficient
rats seemed to be reversible.

Results given in Table V reveal that the concentrations
of zinc, copper, manganese, sodium, and potassium found in the
skin were about the same in zinc-deficient rats and
zinc-supplemented rats.

V. DISCUSSION

Recently several investigators have attempted to relate
zinc to protein synthesis. Macapinlac, Pearson, Barney and
Darby[6] failed to show any difference in the rate of incorporation of leucine-U-^{14}C in the testes protein between
zinc-supplemented and zinc-deficient rats. Likewise O'Neal,

TABLE III

24 Hours Incorporation of Cystine-^{35}S into other Tissue Protein

Type of diet	(DPM/mg protein)				
	Pancreas	Liver	Kidney	Testes	Muscle
Zinc-supplemented ad lib	341 ± 35[a,b]	213 ± 39	397 ± 48	301 ± 38	120 ± 32
Zinc-supplemented pair-fed	458 ± 82[b]	216 ± 28	382 ± 9	304 ± 24	129 ± 44[a]
Zinc-deficient	587 ± 64	201 ± 46	382 ± 61	257 ± 61	84 ± 28

[a] Mean ± SD. Six rats in each group and they were on experimental diet for 15 days.

[b] Difference between Zn-supplemented ad lib or pair-fed and Zn-deficient rats statistically significant (P<0.05).

TABLE IV

Effect of Zinc-Repletion on Incorporation of Cystine-^{35}S into Tissue Proteins

Type of diet	Body weight before repletion (grams)	Body weight three days after repletion (grams)	Specific activities (DPM/mg protein)		
			Skin	Pancreas	Liver
Zinc-supplemented pair-fed	105 ± 4[a,c]	110 ± 5	343 ± 53	155 ± 35	99 ± 6
Zn-deficient and repleted[b]	83 ± 12	92 ± 14	309 ± 86	180 ± 32	107 ± 9

a/ Mean ± SD. Six rats in each groups were killed 24 hours after L-cystine injection (2 μCi/100 g body weight).

b/ Each rat received an intraperitoneal injection of 400 μg zinc daily on last three days of 18-day experiment.

c/ Difference between Zn-supplemented pair-fed and Zn-repleted rats is statistically significant (P<0.05).

TABLE V

Effect of Zinc Deficiency on the Content of Skin

(Zinc, Copper, Manganese, Sodium, and Potassium)

Type of diet	Zinc (μg/g dry weight)	Copper (μg/g dry weight)	Manganese	Sodium (mg/g dry weight)	Potassium (mg/g dry weight)
Zinc-supplemented ad lib	41.28 + 3.25[a]/	7.76 + 1.34	7.19 + 2.36	2.89 + 0.61	3.48 + 0.77
Zinc-supplemented pair-fed	36.21 + 9.02	7.83 + 3.39	7.74 + 1.81	3.01 + 0.77	3.85 + 1.04
Zinc-deficient	28.13 + 5.11	12.52 + 6.71	10.17 + 3.18	3.33 + 1.32	2.95 + 0.66

[a]/ Mean + SD. Six rats in each group and they were on experimental diet for 15 days.

Pla, Spivey Fox, Gibson, and Fry[7] were unable to find any
significant changes in the relative specific activities of the
brain protein isolated from the zinc-deficient and pair-fed
zinc-supplemented rats. On the other hand previous work from
this laboratory[1] indicated that rats fed a zinc-deficient diet
incorporated significantly less ^{14}C-labeled methionine into
liver and kidney proteins.

It occurred to us that studies of protein metabolism in
zinc deficiency might be carried out most profitably in the
skin of the rat since an inadequate intake of zinc causes
abnormalities of the dermal system in all the mammalian species
that have been examined. Data in the present investigation
clearly demonstrate that zinc-deficient rats show markedly
diminished capacity to incorporate injected cystine-^{35}S in
skin protein. To our knowledge this is the first biochemical
evidence in regard to the functional impairment of skin induced
by zinc deficiency. Since the major portion of the epidermal
layer of skin is made up of albuminoid proteins, keratins,
which have a high content of cystine[8], it would be of interest
to determine the relationship between zinc deficiency and the
biosynthesis of keratins.

To elucidate whether zinc deficiency affects the synthesis
of skin protein other than keratin, L-prolineUL-^{14}C (Sp. Act.
254.4 mCi/mmole) was employed. Results indicate that the skin
of zinc-deficient rats had a reduced capacity to utilize
proline for protein synthesis (242 $\pm$ 45 and 92 $\pm$ 64 DPM/mg
protein for the average of six pair-fed zinc-supplemented
and six zinc-deficient rats, respectively). Since proline
and hydroxyproline are major components of collagens, it
appears that zinc deficiency also impairs the formation of
skin collagens. This observation, if confirmed, supports the
finding that tensile strength of healing surgical incisions
was reduced in the integument of zinc-deficient rats[9].

The mechanism by which these changes in the rate of protein synthesis occurs is uncertain. The zinc level in the skin of zinc-deficient rats was lower than that of zinc-supplemented rats, but the difference was not statistically significant. The other possibility is an alteration in nucleic acid metabolism. The impairment of DNA synthesis in rat liver has been observed where zinc depletion was induced in partially hepatectomized rats by ethylenediaminetetraacetate perfusion[10]. Dietary zinc deficiency also decreases the rate of DNA synthesis from ^{3}H-label thymidine in liver of young rats without hepatectomy[11]. Thus the decreased incorporation of L-methionine-^{14}C into liver and kidney proteins[12] resulting from zinc deficiency may be caused by a basic defect in the synthesis of DNA. Whether this relationship exists in the skin remains to be elucidated.

REFERENCES

[1]. Hsu, J. M., Anthony, W. L., and Buchanan, P. J., Proceedings of the First International Symposium on Trace Element Metabolism in Animals (C. F. Mills, ed.) 1970, p. 151.

[2]. Hsu, J. M. and Anthony, W. L., J. Nutr., 1970, in press.

[3]. Lowry, O. H., Rosebrough, N. J., Farr, A. L., and Randall, R. J., J. Biol. Chem., 193, 265 (1951).

[4]. Herberg, R. J., Anal. Chem., 35, 786 (1963).

[5]. Hsu, J. M., Anthony, W. L., and Buchanan, P. J., J. Nutr., 97 279 (1969).

[6]. Macapinlac, M. P., Pearson, W. N., Barney, G. H., and Darby, W. J., J. Nutr., 95, 569 (1968).

[7]. O'Neal, R. M., Pla, G. W., Spivey Fox, M. R., Gibson, F. S., and Fry, B. E., Jr., J. Nutr., 100, 491 (1970).

[8]. Carruthers, C., <u>Biochemistry of Skin in Health and</u>
     <u>Disease</u>, Springfield, Illinois: C. C. Thomas, 1962,
     p. 27.

[9]. Sandstead, H. H. and Shepard, G. H., <u>Proc. Soc. Exp.</u>
     <u>Biol. Med.</u>, <u>128</u>, 687 (1968).

[10]. Fujioka, M and Lieberman, I., <u>J. Biol. Chem.</u>, <u>239</u>,
      1164 (1964).

[11]. Buchanan, P. J. and Hsu, J. M., <u>Fed. Proc.</u>, <u>27</u>, 1495
      (1968).

[12]. Hsu, J. M., Anthony, W. L., and Buchanan, P. J.,
      <u>J. Nutr.</u>, <u>99</u>, 425 (1969).

Chapter 15

RECENT ADVANCES IN EMISSION SPECTROSCOPY AND THE DETERMINATION
OF TRACE ELEMENTS IN BIOLOGICAL MATERIALS

W. A. Gordon

National Aeronautics and Space Administration
Lewis Research Center
Cleveland, Ohio

I. INTRODUCTION

In discussing the emission spectrometric approach in
connection with determination of trace metals in biological

345

materials, one is inevitably drawn to the problem of inadequate
detection limits. Certainly my association with
Dr. M. K. Hambidge in the determination of trace metals in blood
serum has made it apparent that this is the foremost problem.
Therefore advances in the spectrometric method in the area of
detection limits are of primary interest and will be emphasized
here.

The requirement for adequate detection limits, of course,
is not the only important requirement for the biological
materials. Other aspects of analytical procedures such as
accuracy, precision, and economy, for example, can be critically
important in the usefulness of a given technique. However, we
must first have a signal that we can measure above background
noise, and this is too often not the case when measuring trace
elements in biological materials.

For purposes of orientation we will briefly review the
methodology of emission spectroscopy. Figure 1 illustrates the
principles of operation. First, the sample must be vaporized
under conditions that break chemical bonds resulting in a
concentration of free atoms in a gaseous environment. This is
most conveniently accomplished in a high-temperature environment. In such an environment the atoms will absorb kinetic
energy and "leak" energy in the form of light. In practice the
spectroscopist has used just about anything that glows for this
purpose including arcs, sparks, hollow cathodes, plasma jets,
flames, microwave discharges, and lasers.

The light emitted in the excitation source is dispersed in
the spectrometer which images atomic "lines" of the elements on
the focal curve. (These intensities appear as lines only
because that is the geometry of the entrance slit.)
Photomultiplier detectors, or alternatively photographic
emulsions, are located to intercept the elemental lines. The

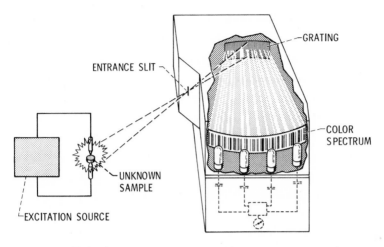

ENTRANCE SLIT

GRATING

COLOR
SPECTRUM

UNKNOWN
SAMPLE

EXCITATION SOURCE

Fig. 1 Emission spectroscopy; principle of operation.

currents produced by the detectors are proportional to specific elements in the sample. These currents are digitized and ultimately converted to concentrations by means of comparison standards. In principle any number of parallel detector channels can be included in this arrangement. In the instrument at the Lewis Research Center there are 22 parallel channels which allow the simultaneous determination of as many elements.

The critical steps in the emission procedure depicted in Fig. 1 are the sample vaporization and excitation of spectra. The conditions under which these processes are carried out will almost exclusively determine the precision and detection limits of the analytical procedure. It may be important to have reliable multichannel spectrometers and automatic data processing for the most effective utilization of the spectral information, but no amount of instrumentation, regardless of cost or sophistication, can in itself lower detection limits. The heart of the emission process is in the excitation and it is there that improvements in detection limits can best be approached.

The emission spectrometric procedures that are in use today
for the determination of trace metals vary greatly in experimental
detail. Sample sizes vary from a few micrograms to a gram or
so and the sample may be in liquid or solid form. Sample treatment often entails additions of powdered materials such as
lithium carbonate, graphite, and silver choloride, for example.
When arcs are used to excite the spectra, currents may vary
from a few amperes up to about 60 amperes, and the atmosphere
may be air or other gas mixtures under either static or flowing
conditions. Almost an infinite variety of combinations of these
and other conditions have been used in trace analysis. This
work on practical emission procedures has been done by empirically
testing various parameters, which have been identified through
practice of the art, to give the most favorable results for a
specific analysis problem. Conditions established for trace
analysis of nonbiological materials are not necessarily the best,
nor even useful, for biological materials. Therefore detailed
descriptions of specific emission procedures are usually not
very instructive and will be avoided in this paper.

Very little work has been done on the optimization of the
total emission process for trace analysis, and for good reason;
a theory for the complex emission processes is not available.
In recent years increasing attention has been given to developing
a theory for spectrochemical excitation. The first comprehensive
book on the subject appeared in 1966[1]. This theory was applied
to quantitative analysis using a direct-current arc in air[2].
Since the development of this theory is an important advance in
spectrochemical analysis, a brief description of it as it relates
to the problem of achieving low detection limits will be presented. By using this theory, even where it is not rigorously
applicable, it is possible to discern a continuous thread linking
the characteristics of many excitation sources now in use as
well as those under development. In this way the rationale for

the practical ways to excite atomic spectra, some of which will be discussed, comes into a little better focus. We can then better appreciate the important parameters for obtaining low detection limits and project the potential of future research.

II. THEORETICAL CONSIDERATIONS RELATED TO DETECTION LIMITS

The theory describes the behavior of particles in high-temperature plasmas under conditions in which the electrons, ions, and atoms are at thermodynamic equilibrium in the volume under observation. This condition prevails when random collisions of particles caused by thermal agitation are the only important means for transferring energy among the particles. Although it is rare when this model is rigorously applicable, it is roughly applicable to metal atoms in arcs, microwave discharges, lasers, and flames.

The relations for the atomic emission intensity from a neutral atom in a high-temperature environment are shown in Eq. (1).

$$I \approx (1- \alpha) \; N_0 Ag\nu \; \exp \, [- \; \Delta E/kT]$$

where

I = emission intensity

N_0 = atom number density

$Ag\nu$ = atomic constants descriptive of given element and transition

ΔE = energy of transition

k = Boltzmann N constant

T = plasma temperature

α = fraction of atoms ionized

From this relation we see that maximum line intensities that are necessary for low detection limits are achieved when (a) the maximum number of neutral atoms is supplied to the excitation zone, and (b) when the plasma temperature is optimum.

Surprisingly, the first condition is the most difficult to
achieve experimentally. Unfortunately the simple expedient of
vaporizing more sample is not usually the answer. Introducing
large densities of atoms into a high-temperature environment is
a fundmental problem in achieving low detection limits.

   We mentioned that the temperature must be an optimum one.
The emission intensity increases with temperature; but if the
temperature is too high, the neutral atoms will be depleted by
ionization resulting in loss of emission from the neutral states.
Figure 2 shows a graphical form of this equation for various
ionization potentials and excitation potentials as a function
of plasma temperature. It can be seen from the figure that for
a given spectral line, characterized by the ionization potential
of the element and the excitation potential for the spectral
line, there is an optimum temperature for maximum line emission.

   As an aid in orientation with respect to the temperature
scale of Fig. 2, it should be noted that flame temperatures lie

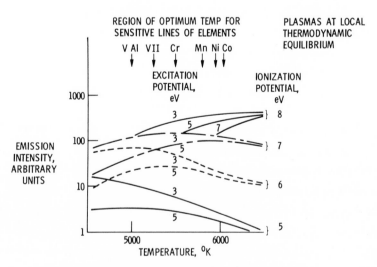

Fig. 2 Effect of excitation temperatures.

below 5000°K, whereas arcs, lasers, and microwave discharges produce temperatures from 5000°K to over 10,000°K. As is indicated on the figure, the newer trace elements such as Ni, V, Cr, and Sn are optimally excited in the temperature range between 5000°K and 7000°K. The optimum temperature for Se, however, is much higher than temperatures reached in most discharges in common use.

There is an aspect of this model that must now be considered because it can be of vital importance with biological materials. The temperature of the plasma is determined by the atomic composition of that plasma. So it is not simply a matter of introducing large numbers of sample atoms into a plasma at a fixed temperature. By doing so we may drastically alter the temperature. However, it is possible to adjust the composition of the sample so that an optimum temperature results. The modifying effect of sample atoms on the excitation temperature explains much of the problem of matrix effect and also explains why spectrographers are fond of mixing compounds known as "buffers" with their samples. Bearing in mind that many biological materials are rich in alkali metals and that easily ionized elements effect a greater change on excitation temperatures, we can see that this is an important consideration in obtaining low detection limits for transition elements in biological materials. Unless the sample composition is ideal, the resulting plasma temperature will not be the optimum one.

Having briefly considered the effect of line intensity on detection limits, let us now consider another equally important aspect, namely, the important parameters for obtaining minimum background intensities. The detection power of the excitation source can be express in terms of a ratio between the line intensity to the background intensity at the same spectral wavelength. (More precisely, the ration should be with respect to the variability of the line and background. For practical

purposes, however, we assume that for a given excitation source
the lower the background, the lower the variability in background
in direct proportion.)

The background from most high-temperature plasmas is due
to two basic causes: (a) radiation emitted by an electron losing
energy as it is deflected by a positive ion (bremsstrahlung) and
(b) energy emitted as a result of recombination of an ion and an
electron. In this discussion we do not consider light emitted
from incandescent electrodes nor do we consider band spectra.
These sources of background are not inherent in the plasma and
can be controlled experimentally.

One expression for the continuum emitted as a result of
electron-atom interactions in an arc is given in Ref.[1] and
shown in Eq. (2):

$$I_b = n_e n_i (kT)^{1/2} \exp [- (\nu_1 - \nu)/kT]$$

where

I_b = intensity of background

n_e = electron number density

n_i = ion number density

k = Boltzmann constant

T = plasma temperature

$(\nu_1 - \nu)$ = frequency dependent parameter

Although this relation agrees with experiment only qualitatively,
it is of interest to consider the parameters that might be
manipulated to obtain minimum background. From Eq. (2) we
conclude that as long as electrons and ions are present in the
plasma we will have to contend with background. However, we do
notice a difference in the dependency of line and background
intensities on particle density. Whereas the line intensity was
directly proportional to particle density [Eq. (1)], the
background is proportional to the square of particle density
[Eq. (2)]. The latter follows because at electrical neutrality

$n_e = n_i$, or $n_e n_i = n_e^2 = n_i^2$. As we reduce particle density, therefore, the background goes down faster than the line intensity. This suggests that thermal sources operated at lower particle densities are more advantageous for obtaining low detection limits than sources operated at higher particle densities. Although it is feasible to manipulate particle densities independently of plasma temperature, this is not easy to do without adversely affecting the maximum rate of sample introduction, thus resulting in loss of line intensity. The search for the optimum excitation conditions yielding the lowest detection limits is where theory ends and experimental work begins.

In summary, the three most important aspects of any emission spectrometric procedure designed to detect the smallest amounts of elements are (a) high rates of sample introduction into the excitation zone, (b) optimum excitation temperature, and (c) minimum background emission. The emission techniques with the lowest detection limits are compromises of the best combination of these three properties. A systematic development of excitation techniques with vastly improved detection limits must await further developments in excitation theory. In the meantime slow but positive progress is being made by empirical experimental evaluations. Now let us consider some new excitation sources that are illustrative of this progress.

III. RECENT INNOVATIONS IN PRACTICAL EXCITATION TECHNIQUES

Three practical approaches for exciting atomic spectra will be described. The first procedure was developed at the Lewis Research Center and involves the excitation of samples in an argon atmosphere in the presence of relatively large amounts of silver chloride vapor. This technique is hereafter referred to as the "argon-silver-arc." This procedure has been used routinely

at the Lewis Laboratory[3], and is incorporated into an automated
spectrometric facility. It has also been used by Hambidge[4]
for the determination of chromium in ashed blood serum and hair.

Two newer techniques that have recently been reported will
also be described. These are both based on microwave excitation
under conditions that have resulted in uncommonly low detection
limits.

A. Argon-Silver-Arc Technique

In this procedure samples are put into solution and a 10 µl
aliquot of the solution is deposited on a carbon rod and dried
to form a residue. In addition to containing the sample residue,
the carbon rods contain a few milligrams of silver chloride.
The carbon rod serves as the anode in a direct-current arc
operated in a static argon atmosphere. The sample residue is
evaporated along with the silver chloride under conditions that
allow detection of nanogram amounts of many metal elements.
The method is therefore applicable to microanalysis (very small
samples) as well as to trace analysis (low concentrations). The
advantages of this arcing procedure result from the enhancement
by silver chloride on line intensities, elimination of band
spectra, induced stability of the arc discharge by a special
cathode design, and a special anode design.

This arcing procedure has been integrated with an automated
spectrometer to provide rapid and automatic analyses of 10 samples
in the arc chamber. Figure 3 summarizes the procedural steps of
the automated procedure. As applied to biological materials
the material is ashed in a low-temperature asher and dissolved
in dilute hydrochloric acid. The concentration of ashed blood
serum is 1.3 mg/10 µl in 6 N HCl. A 10 µl aliquot of this
solution is added to the carbon electrode containing 4 mg AgCl,
and dried for a few seconds at 90°C. The silver chloride is

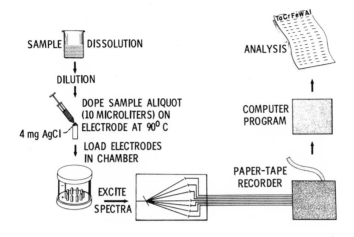

Fig. 3   Schematic procedure for analysis.

added to batches of carbon electrodes by first doping with 10 µl
of silver nitrate solution followed by addition of 10 µl of
hydrochloric acid solution. The solution concentrations are
such that 4 mg of silver chloride are precipitated in the carbon
matrix. After drying the sample solution, an intimate mixture
is formed between the sample residue and the silver chloride.
In addition to modifying the excitation conditions in the argon
arc, the silver chloride also serves to provide a high halide
activity during sample vaporization to prevent carbide formation
which can otherwise cause serious analytical errors. The pointed
anode was designed to introduce relatively high rates of solids
without disturbing the arc stability. The excitation temperature
of this arc has not been measured but temperatures of similar
arcs are about 6000°K.

A batch of 11 electrodes prepared in this way is loaded
into a gas-tight arc chamber and arced in a completely automated
sequence. The intensities from as many as 22 elements are
simultaneously recorded on punched-paper tape and converted to
absolute micrograms of elements by means of calibration curves

stored in the computer memory. With this procedure about
16 elements including, sodium, potassium, iron, phosphorous,
silicon, strontium, calcium, magnesium, copper, zinc, chromium,
molybdenum, nickel, manganese, aluminum, and vanadium can be
detected in 1.3 mg of ashed blood serum. Cobalt is not detected.
However, the elements molybdenum, nickel, and vanadium are
marginally detected and probably could not be measured precisely
without further improvements in detection limits. Since these
arcing conditions were established for metallurgical work,
additional development work aimed at optimizing conditions for
biological materials is indicated.

B. Low-Power Inductively Coupled
Microwave Discharge Technique

        This discharge technique has been of interest to spectro-
scopists as an excitation source for a number of years. Recently
the discharge was operated using conditions that resulted in
some very good detection limits[5]. The excitation assembly
without the power supply is shown in Fig. 4. In operation the
glow capillary is inserted into the excitation cavity. The
samples are introduced by drying a few microliters of solution
on a platinum wire filament. The sample is then vaporized by
applying current to the filament. A flow of argon sweeps the
sample vapor into the excitation zone where compounds are
dissociated and the atomic spectra are excited. The power supply
for this technique is similar to the familiar diathermy unit
which operates at 2450 MHz. The excitation temperature of the
plasma formed inside the capillary is in excess of 5000°K and
has been reported as high as 10,000°K. Limits of detection as
low as 10^{-11} to 10^{-12}g were reported with this source in Ref. [5].
The superior detection limits presumably result from the efficient
introduction of sample atoms into the high-temperature plasma.
Some aspects of this method for trace and microanalysis will be
summarized later.

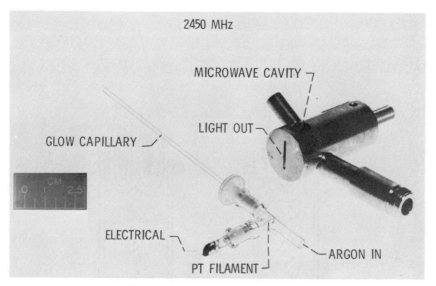

2450 MHz

MICROWAVE CAVITY ⌐

LIGHT OUT ⌐

GLOW CAPILLARY ╱

ELECTRICAL ⌐

ARGON IN

PT FILAMENT ⌐

Fig. 4 Microwave excitation assembly.

C. High-Power Inductively-Coupled Microwave Discharge (Plasma Torch) Technique

This excitation source can be thought of as a scaled-up version of the source just described. It operates at a power level of a few thousand watts, or about 50 times the power of the diathermy source, and at a frequency of 30 MHz. It also operates in flowing argon and produces excitation temperatures in the region of 10,000°K. This source has been under evaluation as an emission source for the past few years. Recently a more efficient way was discovered of introducing liquid samples which resulted in vastly improved detection limits[6]. Figure 5 shows how increased sample introduction was achieved. The torch is operated under conditions that open a hole in the center of the plasma and this allows the liquid sample to be introduced at a higher rate than was previously possible. In addition the authors used a rather elaborate arrangement to sonically nebulize and desolvate the liquid droplets prior to entry into

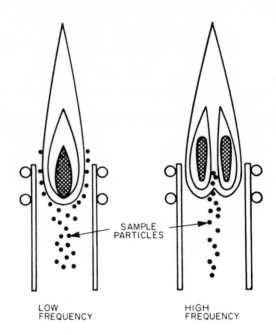

LOW   HIGH
FREQUENCY   FREQUENCY

Fig. 5   Aerosol entry into uniform versus toroidally shaped plasma.

the plasma. Apparently the single most important factor that previously limited the detectability of this source was the rate of sample introduction. The further development of this excitation source will be of interest to those interested in trace metals in biological materials.

IV. CONCLUDING REMARKS

Table I provides a summary comparison of detection limits for the techniques we have discussed and also some detection limits by flame spectroscopy and laser excitation. Estimates have been made from the literature which can be considered typical for the newer trace elements such as Cr, Ni, V, and Mo.

TABLE I

Comparison of Typical Powers of Detection of Some Emission Spectrometic Sources[a]

	Low-Power Microwave Plasma[b]	High-Power Microwave Plasma[c]	Laser[d]	Argon-Silver-Arc[e]	Flame
Absolute limit (g)	10^{-11}	10^{-9}	10^{-9}	10^{-9}	10^{-8}[f]
Limit in liquids (ng/ml)	---	3	---	---	5-1000
Limit in solids (ppm)	1-10	---	1-10	0.2	---
Reagent blank	Low	High	Low	Low	High
Quantity of sample at) Solid	μg	---	μg	μg	μg
detection limit) Liquid	μl	1	μl	μl	ml

a/ Author estimates.

b/ Runnels and Gibson.

c/ Dickinson and Fassel.

d/ Brech.

e/ Gordon.

f/ 10^{-10} in graphite furnace.

These estimates are only within about a factor of ten because
of variable definitions of detection limits. For the flame
and high-powered microwave discharge, detection limits are
determined using the best experimental conditions for each
element and are, therefore, not necessarily applicable to
simultaneous element determinations. For the other sources the
experimental conditions were the same for all elements.

The absolute detection limits given in Table I are a
measure of the detection power for microanalysis. These absolute
detection limits are not necessarily directly convertible to
trace detection limits because of the effect of other elements
also present in the samples. Therefore to estimate the detection power for trace analysis in liquid or solid samples, we
must know the effect of matrix elements on the spectral intensities. For those techniques in which this information is
known we can give an estimate of trace detection limits, otherwise no estimate is given. The use of a dashed line in Table I
indicates that a numerical estimate would not be meaningful
but does not necessarily mean that the technique is inapplicable
to the particular sample form, that is, solid or liquid. Also
listed in Table I are the sample amounts required for analysis
and the reagent blank. The reagent blanks are classified on
the basis of volume of reagent used. Although reagent blanks
can be corrected to some extent, they are limiting at progressively lower concentration.

The detection limit data in Table I illustrate the progress
that has been made in emission spectroscopy in detecting
smaller quantities of metals and metals at lower concentrations.
In evaluating these and other techniques for the determination
of trace metals in biological materials, other characteristics
of the techniques listed in Table I should also be taken into
consideration.

Further progress in lowering detection limits will continue to be concerned with optimization of excitation conditions. The rate of progress in this work is hindered by lack of a quantitative theory of the emission processes. Although quantitative description of the emission processes is the foremost unsolved problem in emission spectroscopy, progress in this direction will greatly benefit the development of practical analytical procedures with lower limits of detection.

REFERENCES

[1]. Boumans, P. W. J. M., Theory of Spectrochemical Excitation. New York: Plenum Press, 1966.

[2]. De Galen, L., Anal. Chim. Acta, 34, 2 (1966).

[3]. Gordon, W. A. and Chapman, G. B., Spectrochim. Acta, 25B, 123 (1970).

[4]. Hambidge, K., Rogerson, D. O., and O'Brien, D., Proceeding of the VIIIth International Congress on Nutrition, Prague, Sept. 1969.

[5]. Runnels, J. H. and Gibson, J. H., Anal. Chem., 39, 1398 (1967).

[6]. Dickinson, G. W. and Fassel, V. A., Anal. Chem., 41, 1021 (1969).

Chapter 16

GAS LIQUID CHROMATOGRAPHY OF TRACE ELEMENTS

M. L. Taylor, USAF, BSC

6570 Aerospace Medical Research Laboratory
Toxic Hazards Division (MRTC)
Wright-Patterson Air Force Base
Dayton, Ohio

I. INTRODUCTION

Certain elements have been shown to be required for the
proper nutrition of man. Others found within man have a

suspected nutritive function. Still other elements have been
implicated to be toxic when given in sufficient quantity and
appropriate form, yet their physiologic activity when present
in trace quantities may be entirely different. Whatever the
case may be, as more sensitive analytical techniques become
available to workers in the biological sciences, studies aimed
at determining the significance of elements present in trace
quantities in man, animals, and plants can be conceived and
carried through. Certainly if analytical methodology is
lacking for detecting trace and ultratrace quantities of metals
in plant and animal specimens, research to determine the
biological significance of these elements cannot be accomplished. In this presentation we want to outline the progress
made to date in the analysis of certain elements using a
relatively new approach--gas chromatography--and then to
enumerate a few cases in which this new method is being
employed to detect and quantitate metals in biological specimens.
The gas chromatographic approach is revolutionary in that it
has been used to perform ultratrace analysis of metals with an
accuracy and ease heretofore unheard of. On the general
subject of gas chromatography of elements, an excellent review
is the book by Moshier and Sievers, Gas Chromatography of
Metal Chelates[1]. Recent reviews by Sievers[2] and Ross and
Sievers[3] provide excellent coverage of newer developments
in the field.

At the outset it may seem incongruous that metals can be
analyzed by gas chromatography, a technique that, as the name
implies, is concerned with the analysis of materials in the
vapor state. Whereas certain of the metals have appreciable
vapor pressure at less than 500°C, most do not and since the
state of the art of gas chromatography requires that analysis
be performed within the ranges of -70° to 400°C, metals cannot

ordinarily be chromatographed as such but must be converted to derivatives that can be vaporized and are thermally and solvolytically stable within the temperature range indicated. Certain metal halides, for example, titanium tetrachloride, are reasonably easily volatilized and have been analyzed by gas chromatography[4,5]. As we might suspect the number of metal halides that are sufficiently volatile and thermally stable to permit their gas chromatographic analysis is rather limited. An alternative approach is to convert the metal to an organically bound form and obtain a suitable derivative. Indeed certain organic compounds have been discovered that can react with a wide variety of elements to form chelates which can be vaporized and chromatographed. Most of these compounds are β-diketones, the first of which to be examined was acetylacetone or 2,4-pentanedione.

$$
\begin{array}{c}
\text{O}\quad\text{O} \\
\text{"}\ \text{H}\ \text{"} \\
\text{H}_3\text{C–C–C–C–CH}_3 \\
\text{H}
\end{array}
$$

Acetylacetone

This compound was reported in 1958[6] to form chelates with certain metals which could then be chromatographed; more thorough studies soon followed in 1960[7,8]. The molecular structure of this type of metal chelate is exemplied in Fig. 1.

Since that time, a number of β-diketones have been examined. A significant improvement in the chromatographic behavior was achieved when halogen atoms were included in the molecular structure[8a]. These have subsequently proven to be far superior to the unfluorinated metal acetylacetonates. Thus trifluoroacetylacetone and hexafluoroacetylacetone,

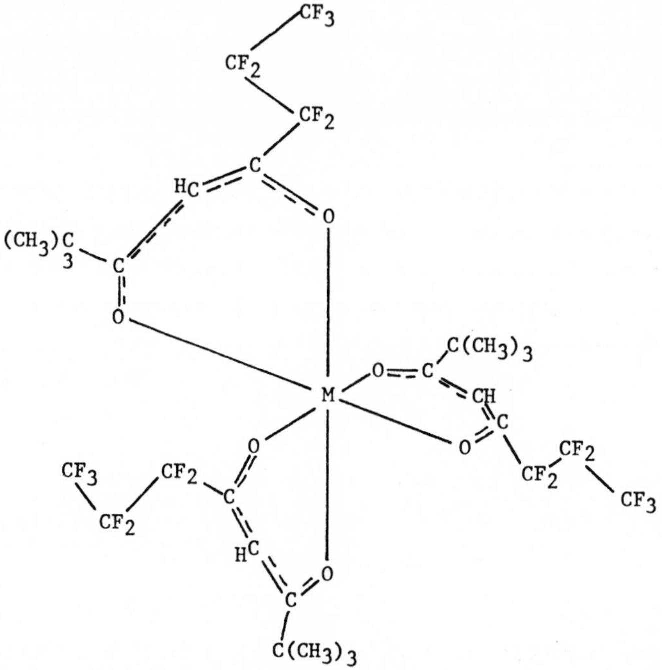

Cis metal(fod)$_3$

Fig. 1(a) Molecular structures of metal β-diketonates.

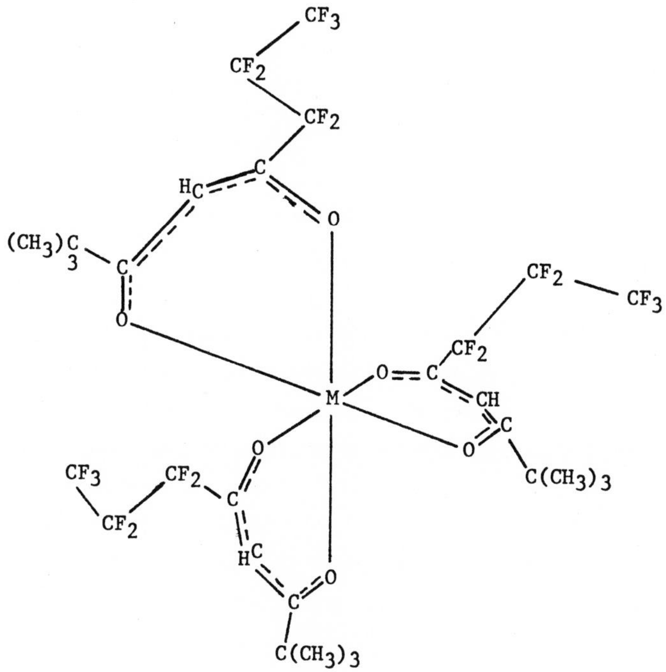

Trans metal(fod)₃

Fig. 1(b)   Molecular structures of metal β-diketonates.

$$F_3C-\overset{\overset{\displaystyle O}{\|}}{C}-CH_2-\overset{\overset{\displaystyle O}{\|}}{C}-CH_3$$

Trifluoroacetyl-
acetone H(tfa)

$$F_3C-\overset{\overset{\displaystyle O}{\|}}{C}-CH_2-\overset{\overset{\displaystyle O}{\|}}{C}-CF_3$$

Hexafluoroacetyl-
acetone H(hfe)

$$CH_3-\overset{\overset{\displaystyle CH_3}{|}}{\underset{\underset{\displaystyle CH_3}{|}}{C}}-\overset{\overset{\displaystyle O}{\|}}{C}-CH_2-\overset{\overset{\displaystyle O}{\|}}{C}-CF_2-CF_2-CF_3$$

Heptafluorodimethyloctanedione
H(fod)

as well as the fluorinated octane-dione have been found to be
extremely well suited to form volatile and stable derivatives
of a great number of members of the periodic table. In Fig. 2
the elements that have been converted to various β-diketonates
known to be volatile are depicted. Those accompanied by an
asterisk are ones that have actually been chromatographed in
the gas phase. It should be noted that not all of the β-diketones
employed are fluorinated; however, as will be seen in the
following discussion for purposes of trace analysis the
halogenated materials are much more promising. The fluorinated
chelates react with a great number of the metals to form highly
stable and volatile compounds, that is, compounds that are ideal
for gas chromatographic analysis.

     In an oversimplified way a gas chromatograph can be
considered as merely consisting of a column of inert material
for effecting a separation and a detector for detecting the
moment when each of the separated materials elutes from the
column and for responding proportionally to the amounts of

these materials present in the inert gas mobile phase. Fluorinated metal chelates not only behave well during separation
but also in detection. The most sensitive detector routinely
employed today in gas chromatography is the electron-capture
detector. The electron-capture detector requires that
electronegative atoms (fluorine, chlorine, bromine, iodine,
and oxygen) be present in the molecules of materials being
analyzed. In the case of highly fluorinated ligands such as
H(fod) or H(hfa) it is clear that a metal chelate formed from
either of these compounds would possess a large number of
electronegative atoms. The remarkable sensitivity of the
electron-capture detector for metal chelates is illustrated
in Table I.

The fluorinated β-diketones are quite remarkable from
another point of view. These compounds have been found by
Sievers, Connolly, and Ross[9] to react directly with a variety
of metals and metallic compounds. It is possible to dissolve
iron ore or steel directly in fluorinated β-diketones. It is
not necessary to convert the metal present in the sample to an
ionic form and therefore laborious digestion procedures using
acids or alkalies are in many cases not required. Often the
sample can simply be placed in a sealed tube and reacted
directly with the fluorinated ligand. The highly reactive
nature of this class of compounds has permitted remarkably
simple analytical procedures to be formulated. For example,
the chromium content in steel can be determined by direct
reaction[10]; likewise iron in iron ore can be determined
without preparatory steps[9]. Indeed even such strongly bound
compounds as beryllium oxide can be completely dissolved by a
fluorinated ligand according to the following equation.

$$BeO + 2H(tfa) \longrightarrow Be(tfa)_2 + H_2O$$

Li thd* fod hfa	**Be** fod* tfa* hfa* acac*											
Na thd fod hfa	**Mg** thd* dfhd* tfa*											**Al** fod* tfa* hfa* acac*
K thd hfa	**Ca** thd* dfhd*	**Sc** fod* tfa* thd* acac*	**Ti(IV)** hfa*	**V(IV)** tfa	**Cr(III)** fod* tfa* dfhd* acac*	**Mn(III)** tfa*	**Fe(III)** fod* tfa* hfa* dfhd*	**Co(III)** tfa* fod* thd*	**Ni(II)** fod* hfa* thd*	**Cu(II)** fod* tfa* hfa* acac*	**Zn** tfa* hfa* thd*	**Ga** tfa* hfa*
Rb hfa	**Sr** thd* dfhd*	**Y** fod* thd*	**Zr** tfa* thd* dfhd* hfa*	**Nb** hfa*	**Mo**	**Tc**	**Ru(III)** tfa* hfa*	**Rh(III)** tfa* hfa*	**Pd** fod* thd*	**Ag**	**Cd** hfa*	**In** tfa*
Cs hfa	**Ba** thd* dfhd*	57-71	**Hf** tfa* thd* dfhd* hfa*	**Ta** hfa*	**W**	**Re**	**Os**	**Ir**	**Pt**	**Au**	**Hg**	**Tl**
Fr	**Ra**	89-103 Th-tfa Th-thd* Am-thd										

Yb fod* thd*	**Lu** fod* thd*

La	Ce	Pr	Nd	Pm	Sm	Eu	Gd	Tb	Dy	Ho	Er	Tm
fod*	thd*	fod*	fod*		fod*	fod*	fod*	fod*	fod*	fod*	fod*	fod*
thd*		thd*	thd*		thd*	thd*	thd*	thd*	thd*	thd*	thd*	thd*

H(thd) = 2,2,6,6-Tetramethyl-3,5-heptanedione
H(fod) = 1,1,1,2,2,3,3-Heptafluoro-7,7-dimethyl-4,6-octanedione
H(hfa) = 1,1,1,5,5,5-Hexafluoro-2,4-pentanedione
H(dfhd) = 1,1,1,2,2,3,3,7,7,7-Decafluoro-4,6-heptanedione
H(tfa) = 1,1,1-Trifluoro-2,4-pentanedione
H(acac) = 2,4-Pentanedione

Fig. 2. Volatile β-diketonates of the elements.

TABLE I

Comparison of Absolute Detection Limits in Grams[a]

Metal	Gas Chromatograph[b]	Atomic Absorption	Neutron Activation	Emission Spectrography	Spark Source Mass Spectroscopy
Be	6×10^{-14}[c]	1×10^{-8}		2×10^{-10}	8×10^{-12}
Cr	2×10^{-14}	2×10^{-9}	1×10^{-6}	1×10^{-9}	5×10^{-11}
Rh	2×10^{-12}	2×10^{-8}	5×10^{-11}	2×10^{-6}	9×10^{-11}
Al	7×10^{-11}	1×10^{-6}	1×10^{-9}	3×10^{-9}	2×10^{-11}
Co	1×10^{-11}	2×10^{-9}	5×10^{-10}	1×10^{-6}	5×10^{-11}
Pd	1×10^{-10}	3×10^{-8}	5×10^{-11}	2×10^{-6}	3×10^{-10}
Ni	1×10^{-11}	2×10^{-9}	5×10^{-9}	8×10^{-8}	7×10^{-11}

a/ Data from Trace Analysis-Physical Methods, Morrison, Table 2, Wiley (Interscience) New York, 1965.

b/ Originial data.

c/ K. J. Eisentraut and D. G. Johnson, unpublished data.

As could be expected the potential of the chelation-gas chromatographic technique for trace and ultratrace analysis was quickly recognized by workers in many fields including those engaged in medical and biological research. Gas chromatographic methods for detection and quantitation of less than one trillionth of a gram of certain of .the elements have been recently developed. Let us now turn to some of the elements that are of biological interest and see what has been accomplished.

II. BERYLLIUM

The extreme toxicity of this element in certain instances has been known since the 1940s. Meehan and Smythe[11] have shown the element to be present in a great number of substances including human lung (nonpathological), liver, and smoking tobacco. The mechanism of beryllium toxicity is not currently well understood, yet owing to its potentially lethal effects in rather low concentrations, ultrasensitive methods for its detection are required. Currently used analytical methods for beryllium such as emission spectrography and morin spectrophotofluorimetry suffer from various deficiencies; extensive preparative steps are required, large sample sizes are required, precision and accuracy are only marginal. With the advent of gas chromatographic methods for analyzing metals we set about to develop a simple, yet rapid and ultrasensitive method for quantitating beryllium in biological specimens using the gas chromatographic approach.

Our initial efforts were directed toward detecting and quantitating beryllium that was added to various biological materials in vitro. Thus human urine as well as primate (monkey) blood, liver (monkey) homogenate, and plant (chicory) homogenate were doped with beryllium sulfate solutions. These doped samples were then analyzed by first chelating the

TABLE II

Average Recovery of Beryllium from Prepared Biological Samples

Sample	Be^{2+} conc prepared (g/ml)	Be^{2+} conc determined (g/ml)	Percent recovery
Urine	5.90×10^{-5}	4.76×10^{-5}	83.4
Plant extract	5.90×10^{-5}	5.40×10^{-5}	91.5
Tissue homogenate	5.90×10^{-5}	5.63×10^{-5}	95.4
Blood	5.90×10^{-5}	5.54×10^{-5}	93.5
Tissue homogenate	5.90×10^{-6}	5.72×10^{-6}	96.9
Blood	5.90×10^{-6}	5.61×10^{-6}	95.1

beryllium using trifluoroacelylacetone [H(tfa)] using a
sealed-tube reaction, then treating the reaction mixture to
remove unreacted ligand, and finally injecting aliquots of
the reaction mixture directly into the gas chromatograph.
Details of this procedure and the results have been
published[12]. An example of the results is given in
Table II.

The details of the analytical procedure for determining
beryllium in biological materials are as follows:

(1) Place 0.05 ml blood or urine, or 0.1 ml of a 25%
tissue homogenate in a glass ampule.*/

(2) Add 0.5 ml of a benzene solution containing
1 to 4 µl of trifluoroacetylacetone.**/

(3) Flame-seal ampule, allow to cool, shake vigorously,
and heat at 100 ± 5°C for 15 minutes (ampules on their sides
on metal grid in oven).

---

*   disPO$^{(R)}$ pipets were used to fabricate the ampules.

** Pierce Chemical Company, Rockford, Illinois.

(4) Allow ampule to cool to room temperature and open,
add 20 to 100 µl of 28% ammonium hydroxide and agitate for
10 to 15 seconds.

(5) Stopper ampule and centrifuge at 5000 rpm for
10 minutes.

(6) Chromatograph 0.5 to 1 µl samples of the benzene
layer on 6-ft glass column packed with 10% SE52 silicone gum
on Gas Chrom Z.

Temperature: column, 110°C; injector, 140°C; detector, 180°C.

Nitrogen flow: 100 cc/min electron-capture detection.

Varian Aerograph Model 2100 Gas Chromatograph was employed.

Certain features of the procedure deserve special comment.
It should be noted that only 50 µl of blood or 25 mg of tissue
are employed in the analysis. In addition no preliminary
preparative steps such as chemical digestion, ashing, or
extraction are required. The method is remarkably simple and
straight forward. Up to six ampules can be analyzed
simultaneously and the average time required to perform a
single analysis is 15 minutes.

Since publication of our early work we have moved ahead
to apply the method to blood and tissue samples obtained from
experimental animals administered aqueous beryllium solutions
intraveneously. In so doing we have also greatly extended
the lower limits of sensitivity of the technique. In studies
to be published elsewhere we have analyzed blood, liver, and
spleen samples obtained from rats treated with beryllium
sulfate solutions containing tracer levels of [7]Be[12a]. Gas
chromatographic findings were compared with radiochemical
analytical results. An example of these results is listed in
Table III.

TABLE III

Beryllium Levels in Blood and Liver (μg Be/g)

	Blood			Liver			
Rat Number	R[a/]	G[b/]	Percent[c/]	Rat Number	R	G	Percent
1	1.33	1.40	105	4	1.73	1.84	106
2	0.059	0.051	86	5	3.04	2.76	91
3	1.03	0.95	92	6	0.33	0.36	109

[a/] R, radiochemical.

[b/] G, gas chromatographic results. Individual results are averages of 3 to 6 replicate analyses.

[c/] Percentages shown are based on the radiochemical determination arbitrarily assumed to be the true value. In actuality the differences from 100% may reflect small errors in the radiochemical measurement as well as the gas chromatographic method. Independent measurements on accurately weighed-out samples of pure beryllium metal dissolved in acid, serially diluted, and subsequently analyzed indicate that the accuracy of the chromatographic method is not greatly different and one can confidently expect the actual relative error to be of the magnitude indicated.

The precision obtained in these analyses is indicated in Table IV together with a comparison against the radiochemical method.

Thus our results indicate that it is quite possible using metal chelation coupled with gas chromatography to achieve accurate and precise analyses of biological specimens containing beryllium at the subparts per million level (less than 1 μg/g).

TABLE IV

Replicate Analyses of Blood from Rat Number (1 µg/g)

Found (radiochemical)	Found (gas chromatographic)	Mean	Mean recovery (Percent)	Relative error (Percent)
1.33	1.44	1.40	105	5.3
	1.32			
	1.30			
	1.48			

Indeed recent findings in our laboratory indicate the lower limit of detectability for beryllium in blood using gas chromatography to be approximately 0.01 µg beryllium/g (actual biological sample size required is only 50 mg).

III. CHROMIUM

The biological importance of chromium has come to light only in recent years, and the physiologic role of this metal is still being explored. As the biological role of chromium is being elucidated workers in the field have determined the levels of chromium most often encountered in human blood to be extremely low--0.02 to 0.05 µg/ml. These ultratrace levels again call for an analytical technique that requires a reasonably small sample size yet is capable of detecting submicrogram amounts with suitable accuracy and precision. Savory, Musak, Roszel, and Sunderman, Jr.[13] recognized the potential of the gas chromatographic approach and have reported a procedure based on this method of analysis. Their method indeed illustrates that minute amounts of a metal contained in a biological matrix can be quantitated using gas chromatography. However, their procedure does require rather extensive sample preparation.

It is obvious that the procedure that will give the desired
results with the least effort is preferable, and thus the very
recent work of Hansen, Scribner, Gilbert, and Sievers[14] offers
the most attractive approach to ultratrace analysis of chromium.
The work of Taylor, Arnold, and Sievers[12] with beryllium
illustrated that a metal contained in a biological specimen
could be determined by direct reaction in a sealed tube followed
by gas chromatographic analysis. Hansen and coworkers have
somewhat modified the procedure and have applied it to the
analysis of chromium _in vivo_ and _in vitro_. Hansen's procedure
is to be published in detail elsewhere and it is suggested
that the reader refer to this forthcoming article for details
concerning the development of the method and the proof of its
efficacy using radiochromium. Here we will outline the
method proposed by Hansen for detection of chromium and then
summarize experiments performed using ^{51}Cr treated rats.

A. Rapid Method for Ultratrace Analysis of Chromium

(1) Add 0.05 ml of blood or plasma to ampule (4 in.
long x 3/16 in. i.d.) followed by 0.5 ml hexane containing
0.005 ml of trifluoroacetylacetone.

(2) Immerse ampules in ice bath, allow contents to cool,
then flame seal.

(3) Shake sealed ampule 15 seconds, wrap in aluminum
foil, place ampule on its side in an oven at 175°C for 30 minutes.

(4) Allow to cool 5 minutes, centrifuge 5 minutes, then
withdraw 0.4 ml of the hexane phase and place in a 2-dram vial
containing 0.5 ml of 1.0 N NaOH. Seal vial with polyeth-
ylene-lined cap. Shake 5 minutes then centrifuge vial 5 minutes.

(5) Immediately aspirate off the organic layer and
place in a clean 1-dram vial and tightly seal. Inject five

1.0 µl injections into the chromatograph (see conditions below) alternately with five 1.0 µl injections of the appropriate $Cr(tfa)_3$ standard solution. Use the average trans-$Cr(tfa)_3$ peak height obtained from the standard injections to calculate concentration of chromium in the unknown. Average time per sample (when samples are run in groups of four) is less than 1 hour.

B. Instrument Conditions

Chromatography was effected using a Hewlett-Packard Model 402 gas chromatograph equipped with a pulsed electron-capture detector (Tritium) and a 2 ft x 3/16 in. i.d. pyrex column packed with 5% Dow-Corning LSX-3-0295 silicone gum on 60 to 80 mesh Gas Chrom. P.

Temperature: column, 132°; detector, 190°.

Carrier gas: helium at 20 cc/min.

Purge gas: 5% methane - 95% argon at 100 cc/min.

Pulse mode interval setting: 150.

It is important to remember that both cis and trans isomers are formed in the reaction of chromium with H(tfa). These isomers are formed in approximately a 1:4 ratio (cis to trans) in the standards as well as the unknowns when conditions reported by Hansen, Scribner, Gilber, and Sievers[14] are employed. Therefore the height of the trans-$Cr(tfa)_3$ peak obtained from the unknown is directly comparable to the same peak in the standards. Care should be taken to use the specified reaction conditions in preparation of standards and analysis of unknowns so that the ratio of cis- to trans-$Cr(tfa)_3$ is not altered, thereby leading to erroneous results. The procedure is also quite remarkable in that in less than 1 hour, without any ashing or preconcentration, one can detect

and quantitate as little as 0.05 µg Cr/ml of blood or plasma.
It appears that quantitation of 0.005 µg Cr/ml will be feasible
without substantial modification of the method.

In vivo studies using ^{51}Cr were conducted in much the
same way as the ^{7}Be studies mentioned previously. Chromium
solutions containing tracer levels of ^{51}Cr were injected into
rats (0.5 ml Na$_2$ CrO$_4$ containing 100 µc of ^{51}Cr and 15 µg of
chromium intravenous, tail vein), the animals were bled at
intervals post injection (eye method) and the chromium present
in blood and plasma was determined by radiochemical means. These
blood and plasma samples were then reacted as in the recommended
procedure up through the point of extraction. Table V shows
the extraction efficiencies. These data indicate that the
normal metabolic processes occurring in the rat do not convert
chromium to a form that cannot be chelated and extracted.

Clearly this method has great promise as shown by the
in vivo results. Indeed Hansen, Scribner, Gilbert, and
Sievers[14] suggest that in addition to finding utility as a
method for determining chromium in biological fluids in various
nutrition studies, the gas chromatographic procedure should
be considered for use in determining circulating red blood cell
volumes and plasma volumes. It is suggested that the procedures
of Sterling and Gray[15] and Frank and Gray[16] could be
modified and instead of detecting injected ^{51}Cr by radiochemical
means, one could inject nonradioactive chromium and analyze the
respective blood fractions by means of gas chromatography.
This procedure would be most attractive in cases where injection
of radioactive material is contraindicated. Of course, the
required levels of chromium must be shown to be acceptable from
a clinical point of view.

TABLE V

Results of Chromium Extractions for In Vivo Rat Experiments[14]

Rat number	Hours in vivo	Extraction efficiency (Percent)	
		Blood	Plasma
1	1		94.3
2	1	85.0	
3	1	81.8	104.2
4	1	88.8	94.4
5	1	70.6	97.6
1	3		96.4
2	3	70.3	97.5
3	3	77.8	92.3
4	3	87.7	101.6
5	3	83.7	101.0
6	3	89.9	96.4
Mean		81.7	97.6

IV. COBALT

The presence of cobalt in vitamin B_{12} and the importance of this vitamin in the process of erythropoiesis are well recognized. The fact that vitamin B_{12} is an essential nutrient for all cells of the body is also recognized. A fantastically low level of this substance is required on a daily basis: 1 µg will maintain normal red cell maturation[17]. Yet it is also true that excess cobalt in the diet causes the opposite of anemia-polycythemia; and consequently here again we see a

rather delicate balance between salutary and detrimental
levels. Methods presently available for the detection of
cobalt in biological materials include emission spectrographic
procedures and colorimetric methods. Both of these procedures
require elaborate preparation, large samples (20 to 30 g tissues,
100 ml urine) and again accuracy and precision are not good[18].
Vitamin B_{12} is assayed by biological means employing microbes
but this method tends sometimes to be nonspecific. In view of
these facts Ross, Scribner, and Sievers[19] have recently
developed a new analytical procedure for the quantitative
determination of ionic cobalt and cobalt occurring as vitamin B_{12}
which utilizes gas chromatography and eliminates time-consuming
preparative steps.

Ross, Scribner, and Sievers[19] found that cobalt(II)
could undergo direct reaction with H(tfa) to form the corresponding chelate. Similarly, these workers found that H(fod)
could also react to form chelates with cobalt, but in this
case, depending on the reaction conditions, either
$Co(fod)_2 \cdot 2H_2O$ or $Co(fod)_3$ was formed. Whereas $Co(tfa)_3$ proved
to be superior where electron-capture detection was employed
[greater response obtained per milligram of $Co(tfa)_3$], it was
also found that concentrations less than 10^{-5} g/ml of $Co(tfa)_3$
are unstable. It was determined that the hydrated complex
formed from Co(II) and H(fod) is not satisfactory for gas
chromatographic analysis. Fortunately $Co(fod)_3$ proved
thermally and chemically stable and thus the following
analytical procedure is reported by Ross[19] which permits
detection of as little as 4×10^{-11} g of cobalt in the form of
$Co(fod)_3$.

A. Ultratrace Analysis of Cobalt

(1) An aliquot (1 ml) of the aqueous sample is transferred
to a 10 ml Pyrex culture tube fitted with a screw cap. A

small Teflon-coated stirring bar is placed in the culture tube
which is positioned over a stirring hot plate. The stirring
mechanism is turned on before the addition of any of the
reagents.

(2) A 0.1 ml aliquot of 0.5 N NaOH is added, followed
by 1.0 ml of 0.1 M H(fod) in benzene (Nanograd - Mallinckrodt)
and 0.2 ml of 35% hydrogen peroxide.

(3) A small piece of Teflon tape is placed over the mouth
of the culture tube and a cap is screwed on tightly to ensure
no leakage of vapors during the reaction.

(4) The reagents are placed in a water bath heated to
75°C and allowed to react for 30 minutes with continuous
stirring.

(5) The reagents in the culture tube are permitted to
separate into two layers and the organic layer is decanted
and put in a screw top vial.

(6) A 1 ml aliquot of 0.1 N NaOH is added to the organic
layer for backwashing. A thick, white precipitate forms
immediately. This precipitate is the sodium salt of H(fod)
which is not sufficiently soluble to be entirely dissolved in
this volume of aqueous layer. To this 4 ml of distilled water
are added and the contents shaken vigorously. The precipitate
usually disappears; however, if some remains, another washing
with distilled water will remove it. The organic layer is
again decanted and gas chromatographic analysis can now be made.

B. Instrument Conditions

Instrument, Hewlett Packard Model 402 Gas Chromatograph;
Column, 2 ft x 1/4 in. O.D. Pyrex tube packed with 5%
Dow-Corning LSX-3-0295 on 60 to 80 mesh Gas Chrom. P.

Temperatures: column, 135°C; injection port, 135°;
detector, 180°C.

Carrier gas: helium at 60 cc/min.

Auxiliary gas: 95% argon and 5% methane at 100 ml/min.

The sensitivity of the method can be increased several
fold if at the end of the procedure the cap is removed from
the tube, benzene is allowed to evaporate, and the organic
residue is redissolved in as little as 10 µl fresh benzene.
This is done at the end of the procedure while the organic and
aqueous layers are in contact.

The presence of hydrogen peroxide ensures conversion of
all cobalt present to Co(III) and thus the stable, gas
chromatographically suitable, Co(tfa)$_3$ is formed. The method
has been used to quantitate cobalt in aqueous solutions made
from cobalt(II) chloride, and significantly the procedure has
also been applied to the analysis of aqueous solutions of
vitamin B$_{12}$ (cyanocobalamin). The data in Table VI illustrates
results obtained on samples with weighed known amounts of
cyanocobalamin. Here it should be realized that no ashing or
preparative steps were required. These findings point to the
fact that ultratrace analysis of a compound of vital physiologic
importance can be readily accomplished. These workers are
now attempting to apply the technique to the analysis of cobalt
in liver tissue, serum and urine.

V. SELENIUM

This is the fourth element of biological significance that
has been shown to be amenable to detection by gas chromatography
at ultratrace levels. Unlike the three metals discussed
previously this element is not chelated by reaction with an
organic β-diketone but is treated with a chlorinated aromatic
amine to form a piaselenol as illustrated in the following
reaction[20].

TABLE VI

Analysis for Cobalt in Solutions Containing

Cyanocobalamin by Gas Chromatography

Cobalt (in cyanocobalamin) present (grams)	Cobalt (in cyanocobalamin) found by G. C., (grams)	Mean found (grams)	Mean recovery (percent)	Mean error	Relative error (percent)
4.35×10^{-10}	3.54×10^{-10}	3.67×10^{-10}	84.4	0.68×10^{-10}	15.6
	3.56×10^{-10}				
	4.11×10^{-10}				
	3.54×10^{-10}				
	3.60×10^{-10}				

$$\text{Cl}\underset{}{\overset{}{\bigcirc}}\overset{-\text{NH}_2}{\underset{-\text{NH}_2}{}} \quad \text{H}_2\text{SeO}_3 \quad \longrightarrow \quad \text{Cl} \overset{4\quad 3}{\underset{7\quad 1}{\bigcirc}} \overset{N}{\underset{N}{}} \text{Se} \; 2 \; + \; 3\text{H}_2\text{O}$$

Taking advantage of the fact that 4-chlorophenylenediamine
reacts quantitatively with selenous acid to form
5-chloropiaselenol and that this derivative is soluble in
toluene, Nakashima and Toei[21] have shown that selenium can be
quantitated using electron-capture gas chromatography. Thus
these workers prepared aqueous solutions of selenous acid,
adjusted the pH to less than 1, added a 0.5% solution of
4-chlorophenylenediamine, and extracted the derivative formed
into toluene.

Aliquots of the organic layer were injected into a gas
chromatograph equipped with an electron-capture detector. Using
this procedure amounts as low as 0.04 µg of selenium could be
determined. Work is now underway to see if this method is
amenable to the analysis of selenium in biological materials.
Other metals such as arsenic can possibly also be analyzed in
this fashion.

VI. SUMMARY

The preceding discussion points to the fact that gas
chromatography of metals is of considerable importance to those
engaged in quantitative analysis of submicrogram amounts of
elements. We have shown that workers in biomedical research
have successfully applied gas chromatographic methods in
conjunction with simple sealed tube reaction techniques to
perform trace analyses with ease and accuracy using remarkably
small sample size. Certainly new vistas are now open to all
researchers concerned with measuring ultratrace amounts of

elements in biological specimens. In general the methods
described here can be performed in any laboratory equipped
with the usual complement of instrumentation and thus are
attractive from the economic viewpoint. Gas chromatography
is an inherently simple technique and instrumentation is
inexpensive relative to other equipment used for trace analysis.

As indicated early in this discussion, many of the elements
of the periodic chart have been shown to react with a variety of
organic reagents to form volatile chelates. Thus the
possibility for analyzing many metals of biological importance
by the procedures described here is very real. Moreover we
strongly feel that in many instances the biological role of an
element can only be defined in detail after appropriate analytical
methodology is available. In our laboratory we are examining a
wide range of elements and plan to develop techniques for their
detection in biological materials in anticipation of future
biomedical investigations in connection with either environmental pollution or sophisticated physiological investigations
of the metabolism of man.

ACKNOWLEDGMENTS

Portions of the research reported in this paper were
conducted by personnel of the Aerospace Medical Research
Laboratory, Aerospace Medical Division, Air Force Systems
Command, Wright-Patterson Air Force Base, Dayton, Ohio. This
paper has been identified by Aerospace Medical Research
Laboratory as AMRL-TR-70-101. Further reproduction is authorized
to satisfy needs of the U. S. Government.

The experiments reported here were conducted according to
the Guide for Laboratory Animal Facilities and Care, 1965
prepared by the Committee on the Guide for Laboratory Animal

Resources, National Academy of Sciences, National Research
Council; the regulations and standards prepared by the Depart-
ment of Agriculture; and Public Law 89-544, Laboratory Animal
Welfare Act, August 24, 1967.

REFERENCES

[1]. Moshier, R. W. and Sievers, R. E., Gas Chromatography
      of Metal Chelates, Oxford: Pergamon Press, 1965.

[2]. Sievers, R. E., Coordination Chemistry (S. Kirschner,
      ed.) New York: Plenum Press, 1969, p. 270-288.

[3]. Ross, W. D. and Sievers, R. E., Developments in Applied
      Spectroscopy, Vol. 8, 1970, in press.

[4]. Juvet, R. S., Jr. and Wachi, F. M., Anal. Chem., 32,
      290 (1960).

[5]. Sievers, R. E., Wheeler, G., Jr., and Ross, W. D.,
      Anal. Chem., 38, 306-309 (1966).

[6]. Duswalt, A. A., Jr., Doctoral Dissertation, Lafayette,
      Indiana: Purdue University, 1958.

[7]. Brandt, W. W., Gas Chromatography 1960 (R. P. W. Scott,
      ed.) Washington: Butterworths, 1960, p. 305.

[8]. Biermann, W. J. and Gesser, H., Anal. Chem., 32, 1525
      (1960).

[8a]. Sievers, R. E., Ponder, B. W., Morris, M. L., and
      Moshier, R. W., Inorg. Chem., 2, 693 (1963).

[9]. Sievers, R. E., Connolly, J. W., and Ross, W. D.,
      Gas Chromatography, 5, 241 (1967).

[10]. Ross, W. D. and Sievers, R. E., 156 Am. Chem. Soc. Mtg.,
      Atlantic City, New Jersey, September 1968.

[11]. Meehan, W. R. and Smythe, L. E., Environ. Sci. Technol.,
      1, 839 (1967).

[12]. Taylor, M. L., Arnold, E. L., and Sievers, R. E., Anal.
      Lett., 1, 735 (1968).

[12a]. Taylor, M. L. and Arnold, E. L., unpublished data.

[13]. Savory, J., Musak, P., Roszel, N. O., and
Sunderman, F. W., Jr., Fed. Proc., 27, 3154, 177 (1968).

[14]. Hansen, L. C., Scribner, W. G., Gilbert, T. W., and
Sievers, R. E., to be published.

[15]. Sterling, K. and Gray, S. J., J. Clin. Invest., 29,
1614 (1950).

[16]. Frank, H. and Gray, S. J., J. Clin. Invest., 32, 991
(1953).

[17]. Guyton, A. C., Textbook of Medical Physiology (2nd ed.),
Philadelphia: W. Saunders, 1961, p. 150.

[18]. Jacobs, M. B., The Analytical Toxicology of Industrial
Inorganic Poisons (P. J. Elving and I. M. Kolthoff, eds.)
New York: Wiley (Interscience), 1967, p. 814-816.

[19]. Ross, W. D., Scribner, W. G., and Sievers, R. E.,
Proc. of 8th Intl. Symposium on Gas Chromatography
(R. Stock, ed.) Dublin, Ireland, September, 1970, to
be published.

[20]. Goto, M. and Toei, K., Talanta, 12, 124 (1965).

[21]. Nakashima, S. and Toei, K., Tananta, 15, 1475 (1968).

Chapter 17

DETERMINATION OF TRACE ELEMENTS IN BIOLOGICAL MATERIALS
BY SPARK-SOURCE MASS SPECTROMETRY

W. W. Harrison, M. A. Ryan, L. D. Copper, and G. G. Clemena

Department of Chemistry
University of Virginia
Charlottesville, Virginia

I. INTRODUCTION

Mass spectrometry can hardly be considered a new technique.
Early experiments by Aston date back more that 50 years and the
Nier-type instrument which is more recognizable with respect
to today's mass spectrometers goes back 30 years. The
significant advances in instrumentation in the 1940s and 1950s
allowed for rapid developments in mass spectrometry and a greater
realization and utilization of its unique capabilities. Organic
chemists were able to elucidate complicated chemical structures.
Analytical chemists found the technique extremely useful for
both qualitative and quantitative analysis. By use of the
proper inlet system, gases, liquids, and solids could be
successfully analyzed. The only limitation was that the sample
should be capable of producing a reasonable vapor pressure in
the order of 10 to 20 μ (0.01 to 0.02 Torr) at the conditions
employed so that the conventional electron-bombardment source
could ionize the molecular species for subsequent separation
according to mass and charge in a magnetic field. The fact
that the source compartments of mass spectrometers operate
at 10^{-5} to 10^{-6} Torr aids in the production of a vapor
population from liquid samples, and the ability to heat an
insertion probe to 150 to 350°C allows many solids to be
sufficiently vaporized for mass spectrometric analysis. However,
even a brief consideration of the vapor pressures of various
materials suggests that the mass spectrometric analysis of solids
using conventional ion sources would be generally restricted
to organics and to a relatively few inorganics. Furthermore
the mass spectra produced by the low energy source would be in
the form of molecular fragments rather than elemental
constituents.

Thus until recent years mass spectrometry has been considered
an extremely valuable tool, mainly for organic materials.

This, of course, leaves out a broad range of inorganics, such as metals, with volatilities too low to be amenable to ion formation with conventional sources. Elemental analysis in nonvolatile matrices was also not feasible. However, if the mild electron-bombardment source could be replaced with a more powerful unit capable of volatilizing and ionizing even high-melting solids, an entirely new field of capabilities would be opened. Fortunately such a source was already available and in use for emission spectroscopy. The high-voltage spark discharge was adapted to mass spectrometry with the result that even such materials as stainless steel could be analyzed. The highly energetic spark produced basically elemental spectra with great sensitivity so that trace element analysis now became possible, and spark-source mass spectrometry became very important in analyzing for trace impurities in metals and semiconductors.

Figure 1 shows a schematic layout of a spark-source mass spectrometer. The ions produced by the 500 kH$_z$ spark across the two electrodes are accelerated by a 20 kV potential into the electrostatic analyzer which acts as an energy filter to produce a more monoenergetic ion beam. The monitor collector samples a fixed portion of this beam and produces a current used to determine the total exposure charge. The portion of the ion beam that is allowed to pass the monitor enters the magnetic analyzer, is separated according to mass-to-charge ratio, and is recorded with respect to ion position and net intensity by an ion-sensitive photographic plate. Exposures are normally run from 10^{-13} to 10^{-7} C. Spark-source mass spectrometry (SSMS) has several advantages over other trace element survey techniques, such as spectrographic emission.

(1) Extreme Sensitivity. Detection limits for all elements are in the parts per billion (ppb) range, specific values depending on exposure times. By use of a wide range of exposures,

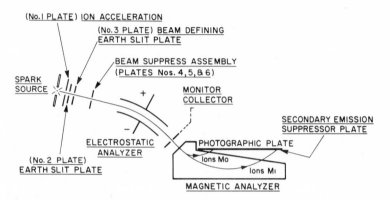

Fig. 1   Schematic of MS-702 Spark-Source Mass Spectrometer.

elements present at greatly variant concentrations may be
analyzed. For example, sodium and potassium at 5000 ppm may
be evaluated on a short exposure, with lead at 0.10 ppm read
on a long exposure.

(2) Response to Metals and Nonmetals. As opposed to
emission spectroscopy or atomic absorption, all metals and
nonmetals may be determined by SSMS. This allows data
collection from the halides, sulfur, phosphorus, boron, and so on.

(3) Uniform Sensitivity. The high-voltage spark produces
very efficient ionization of all elements to essentially the
same magnitude, providing the highly desirable situation in
which all elements have approximately the same sensitivity, in
sharp contrast to other analytical techniques.

(4) Minimal Matrix Effect. Again, the high-energy source
produces a leveling effect to yield no great change in
elemental sensitivity from one matrix to another.

It is thus obvious that SSMS has many critical advantages
that should make it a powerful technique in the area of trace
analysis. Limitations at present would include the considerable
expense of the SSMS facilities and also the precision and accuracy

of the method which are usually no better than $\pm$ 20%. The new electrical detection systems, which include precise electrode-control functions, are reported to provide significant improvements in precision and accuracy, however.

The application of SSMS to biological samples has been minimal. Most of the instruments are located at industrial laboratories which have other interests. Sasaki and Watanabe[1] indicated the usefulness of SSMS to biological materials, while Wolstenholme[2] had examined dried blood tissue using this technique. Evans and Morrison[3] showed quantitative data for a number of tissues. A previous report from this laboratory[4] discussed the analysis of human hair by SSMS.

II. EXPERIMENTAL

A. Apparatus

Table I shows a summary of the equipment and experimental conditions used in the spark-source mass spectrometric analysis.

B. Reagents

Extreme purity is required for all reagents. Blanks should be shot to determine total reagent contribution in any case. Ultra Superior Purity graphite (Ultra Carbon Corporation, Bay City, Michigan) was used as the matrix with which the sample was mixed for electrode preparation. A spectrographically pure standard yttrum oxide[*] was added as an internal standard. High-purity acids[**] were used for sample wet ashing.

---

* Johson, Matthey, and co. Inc., London, England.

** G. F. Smith Chemical Co., Columbus, Ohio and Suprapur, E M Reagents Division, Brinkman Instruments Co., Westbury, New York.

TABLE I

Equipment and Experimental Conditions

Analysis instrument	A. E. I. MS 702 Spark-Source Mass Spectrometer
Other equipment	Jarrell-Ash Model 23-100 Recording Microphotometer, Bristol Model 570 Dynamaster Recorder, Disc Chart Integrator Model 235A, Jarrell-Ash Model 3410 Processing Unit
Vacuum.	Magnetic analyzer, 10^{-8} Electrostatic analyzer, 10^{-8} Source, 5×10^{-6} (when sparking)
Spectrometer parameters . .	Spark voltage, 30 kV Repetition rate, 300 pulses/second Spark pulse length, 100 μsecond Electrostatic analyzer, 2 kV Accelerating voltage, 20 kV Primary slit, 0.002 mm Exposure range, 1×10^{-13} C to 1×10^{-7} C.
Microphotometer parameters. .	Slit, 3 μ Occulter, 1.2 mm Scanning speed, 1.0 mm/second
Recorder parameters	Response time (full scale), 0.4 second range, -0.05 to +1.05 mV Chart speed, 2.5 in./minute
Ion-beam chopper.	Chopping frequency, 200 to 20,000 Hz Pulse length, 5 μsecond
Detector.	2 x 10 in. Ilford Q-2 thin glass photographic plate
Developing conditions . . .	Developing, Eastman Kodak D-19 (1:1 ratio) at 20.0°C for 2-1/2 minutes under Wratten Series 1A safelight
Stop bath	14% Acetic acid solution for 30 second
Fixing.	Eastman Kodak Rapid Fixer with hardener for 3 minutes
Washing.	Running water for 15 minutes, distilled-deionized water for 1 minute
Drying.	Forced air for 15 minutes

C. Sample Preparation

No single specific preparation procedure can be described because of the several different types of biological samples investigated, including human hair, fingernails, blood serum, and tissue.

Vacuum drying of the samples at 100°C is done using a "drying pistol." Samples have been ashed by both low- and high-temperature dry ashing and also by wet ashing techniques using nitric and perchloric acids. Quartz apparatus is used for the ashing and subsequent preparation steps. The ash residue is mixed thoroughly with high-purity graphite, transferred to a plastic vial containing a ball pestle, and shaken for 15 minutes on a Wig-L-Bug[*]/ to achieve a homogeneous mixture.

D. Electrode Formation

A stainless steel moulding die[**]/ was used to prepare electrodes from the homogeneous sample-matrix mixture. A small polyethylene slug is drilled to provide two shafts into which the mixture is added by means of special loading funnels. In the case of quite small samples only the tips of the electrodes contained the sample, with pure graphite used for the remainder. The polyethylene slug is then pressed in the die at 10 tons pressure to form 10 mm × 1 mm electrodes.

E.   Internal Standard

Yttrium was used as an internal standard because of its availability in a highly pure form, the considered improbability of its normal occurrence in the sample, and its monoisotopic nature. Standard yttrium solutions were prepared that were

---

*   Crescent Dental Manufacturing Co., Chicago, Illinois.

** Associated Electrical Industries, Ltd., Manchester, England.

then used to dope the matrix to 100 ppmw yttrium by formation
of a homogeneous slurry, drying, and Wig-L-Bugging to produce
a stock quantity for mixing with the sample ash. Blanks were
run on the matrices and standard.

F. Data Treatment

Density measurement were taken as percent transmission
areas with a ball and disc integrator. A computer program
developed for the Burroughs B-5500 at the University of
Virginia corrected equivalent peak areas of the standard and
each unknown to exposure ratios which were used in a conventional
expression to calculate final concentration,

$$C_x = C_s \frac{E_s}{E_x} \frac{A_x}{A_s} \frac{I_s}{I_x} \frac{M_x^{1/2}}{M_s^{1/2}}$$

where x and s refer to the unknown and standard, respectively,
C is concentration in parts per million by weight, E is
exposure at equal peak areas, A refers to atomic weight
(correction from parts per million atomic to parts per million
weight), I is isotopic abundance of the specific isotopes used,
and M is isotopic mass, used to correct for photoplate
response[5]. Relative sensitivity factors, which were used
for most of the analyses, were computed from Jarrell-Ash SQ
Powder Standards, the graphite series at 1, 10, and 100 ppm.

III. RESULTS AND DISCUSSION

A. Matrix Requirements

The electrical nature of the spark-source requires that
the sample electrodes be electrically conducting in order for
the discharge and subsequent ionization to occur. Biological

compounds such as hair, nails, and tissue must be treated in
such a way that they can be made to conduct, or, rather, be
placed in a conducting sample matrix. Even if hair or nails
could be made to spark directly in their natural state, serious
problems would still result which would require sample
pretreatment. The organic constituents in the biological
samples produce an exceedingly complex spectrum which would
make identification and quantitation of the inorganic constituents virtually impossible. Therefore they must be removed
by one of the ashing procedures.

In principle the ashed samples may be mixed with any good
conductor. However, there are certain practical considerations
that dictate matrix properties.

(1) Purity. The matrix should be of the purest grade
possible. Since the bulk of the electrode will be made from
this material; purity requirements are stringent. Grades
known as "spectrographically pure" are often not satisfactory.
High-purity silver and gold are often used, but their trace
element concentration may be unacceptable, depending on the
manufacturer. A special grade of graphites is now available
which seems to be very low in impurities and consistent from
batch to batch.

(2) Physical Nature. Only a small amount of each
electrode, perhaps 1 mg, is consumed during the analysis. This
puts severe homogeneity requirements on the sample ash-matrix
mixture. Many metal powders are too course to allow the
proper intimate mixing of the ash and matrix. Again, the
graphite is much better in this respect because the Ultra
Superior Purity grade is extremely finely divided and provides
an excellent homogenization character.

(3) Chemical Nature. An ideal matrix might be monoisotopic, low atomic weight, with no tendency to form polyatomic

species or molecular units with sample elements. A
monoisotopic matrix removes fewer mass lines from analytical
use, the low atomic weight reduces interference from multiply
charged matrix ions, and the tendency to maintain the atomic
ionic state also reduces interferences. No matrix meets all
these requirements, of course. Graphite interferences are not
usually severe and are centered around the polycarbon lines
which must generally be avoided. Selection of proper spark
conditions can reduce molecular species.

B. Sensitivity Factors

Spark-source mass spectrometry is unusual in that the
standard against which calculations are made is not the analysis
element, that is, calcium standard for a calcium unknown, but
rather an internal standard--an element not normally present
in the sample which is added in a known amount. This one
standard then serves to define the concentrations of all the
analysis elements, which may be as many as 30 to 40. This
rather unorthodox approach is made possible in SSMS by the
relatively constant sensitivity that all elements have in the
spark and made necessary by the incompletely controllable
spark conditions which make the use of an external standard
somewhat hazardous. It is also true that reliable standards
containing 30 to 40 elements are not readily available.

The assumptions that the sensitivities of all elements
are equal is not true, and for best results "sensitivity
factors" are calculated from various standards. These
correction terms are then used routinely to adjust analysis
data to compensate for the different elemental sensitivities.
However, work in our laboratories has recently[6] pointed out
that external standards can indeed be useful if proper control
of electrode and spark parameters is maintained.

C. Biological Sample Problems

Whereas spark-source mass spectrometry is ideally suited for trace element studies in metal samples, biological samples pose a number of problems of which the analytical chemist must constantly be aware. The previously mentioned organic content that must be ashed is much more critical than in the case of other analytical techniques. A slight amount of residual organic will ordinarily have little effect on atomic absorption or spectrographic emission, but in SSMS this shows up as background lines at almost every nominal mass number. Therefore wet or dry ashing must be carried out with utmost care. Residual acid should also be removed in wet ashing.

The pretreatment necessary for biological samples greatly enhances the danger of contamination. The extraordinary sensitivity of SSMS requires "clean-room" conditions throughout merely to hold background contamination to a minimum. In the case of biological samples the acquisition step is often critical. Personnel who are charged with sample procurement and initial preparation such as rinsing may not be aware of the proper handling techniques to eliminate trace element contamination.

Standards are also a critical problem for biological samples. NBS standard and others, such as Johnson, Matthey, and Company, are available for metals to test SSMS techniques, at least in the parts per million levels. No such counterpart is at hand for parts per million and parts per billion trace element levels in biological samples. We have prepared our own standards, taking great precaution to assure homogeneous mixing. However, it would be much more desirable to check our technique against standards that had previously been monitored by several other laboratories.

D. Biological Analyses

Our interest in biological samples arose from a joint program with researchers in the Medical School of the University of Virginia during which atomic absorption was used to monitor several trace elements[7-9]. The results were sufficiently interesting to suggest a broader program. Atomic absorption is quite accurate and simple but is rather limiting in that normally only one element may be determined at a time, many elements in biological samples are below its working limits, and it is applicable only to metals. Furthermore the nature of the spectral source in atomic absorption dictates that the analyst must know which elements he wishes to analyze. SSMS thus became very attractive to our research interest as a broad survey technique that would give us qualitative and quantitative information for 20 to 40 elements simultaneously even from small amounts of sample. By this means we could monitor elements of prime interest and also check for any unusual patterns in other elements, metal and nonmetals, down to the parts per billion level. The following then is a brief summary of some of the sample types that we have studied over the past two years.

Analysis of Human Hair. Much of our work with human hair has been previously reported[4,9]. Hair analyses have been done in the past by spectrophotometry[10], atomic absorption[11], spectrographic emission[12], and neutron-activation analysis[13]. This sample is of both medical and forensic interest due to its capability of storing certain elements, particularly those that may be in excess in the body. Arsensic and lead have received notice in this regard, but other elements less well documented may behave in a similar manner.

Written instructions were given to each participant with regard to sample procurement. These samples were washed in a nonionic detergent (see Reference [9] for a more detailed description of the procedure), washed, and dried. Small samples led to the use of a wet ashing procedure wherein the residue could be conveniently handled in solution.

Figure 2 shows typical spectra resulting from SSMS analysis. The lower plate represents the blank or background which must be checked for contribution from the glassware, reagents, handling, and so on. The upper plate shows the mass lines for a hair ash sample in a graphite matrix. It is obvious that the polycarbon lines must be avoided for analytical purposes, but this is usually no problem as elements at these masses also have other isotopes that may be used. Elements present in high concentration in many biological samples, such as sodium, potassium, calcium, and phosphorous, may create interfering secondary emission which will darken the photoplate around the nominal mass and reduce the signal-to-background ratio.

Table II shows analysis results for two different hair samples analyzed by both SSMS and atomic absorption. The greater accuracy and precision of atomic absorption makes it an excellent complementary technique by which to check out SSMS, at least for those elements for which atomic absorption has sufficient sensitivity. Table III shows the precision attainable within a triplicate analysis of 10 mg samples taken from a common hair sample. There is possibly some inhomogeneity even within the stock sample since elemental concentrations have been shown to vary along the hair filament, but the inherent precision limitations are also quite certainly reflected in the data. Usually 25 to 30 elements are analyzed with confidence with another 5 or 6 elements often not reported due to possible interferences. We have monitored concentrations at 2 to 4 week intervals in several "normal" individuals to

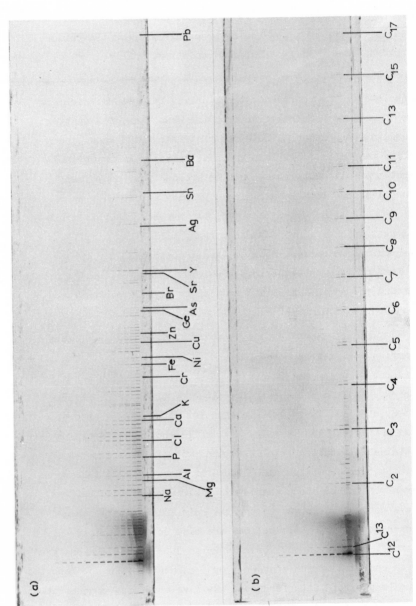

Fig. 2 Typical plates from the spark–source mass spectrometric analysis

TABLE II

Comparative Analysis of Two Different Hair Samples by Mass
Spectrographic and Atomic Absorption Methods
(Values given in µg/g, dry weight)

Element	Hair sample 1 (µg/g)		Hair sample 2 (µg/g)	
	SSMS	AA	SSMS	AA
Na	1205.0		516.4	
Mg	16.4	21.8	14.5	7.3 to 11.5[a]
Al	4.6		3.7	
Si	10.9		27.9	
P	120.2		208.9	
S	448.0		841.1	
K	72.6		225.7	
Ca	135.0	210.0	158.0	
Ti	3.9		24.0	
Cr	0.65		5.9	
Mn	1.7		1.8	
Fe	2.72	8.72	12.0	7.7 to 10.5[a]
Ni	0.45		3.4	
Co	0.24		0.34	
Cu	16.2	17.7	8.7	11.8 to 14.9[a]
Zn	246.0	236.0	181.0	122 to 172[a]
As	0.06		0.31	
Br	0.17		1.1	
Rb	0.2		0.23	
Sr	1.1		0.75	
Mo	0.13		0.28	
Ag	0.4		2.0	
Cd	0.34		0.96	
Sn	0.4		0.39	
I	0.03		0.14	
Ba	0.6		0.46	
Pb	14.5		21.8	

[a] Normal ranges for this subject from a previous atomic
absorption study.

TABLE III

Triplicate Analysis of 10 mg. Samples of a Common Hair Sample

(Values in μg/g, dry weight)

Element	Sample 1	Sample 2	Sample 3
Pb	52	47	45
La	0.83	0.49	N.D.[a/]
Ba	5.0	5.6	5.0
Sn	1.5	1.5	1.6
Cd	1.5	0.48	1.8
Ag	1.9	2.6	1.4
Mo	2.2	2.6	3.1
Zr	1.9	2.3	1.0
Sr	9.4	11	12
Br	2.5	0.90	0.82
Se	0.79	0.48	N.D.[a/]
As	0.62	1.2	0.82
Ge	2.0	0.90	3.70
Ga	0.02	N.D.[a/]	0.14
Zn	153	143	148
Cu	95	114	130
Ni	28	25	20
Fe	73	110	100
Mn	7.8	8.8	5.8
Cr	31	32	33
Ca	750	750	1150
K	337	700	900
Al	N.D.[a/]	1.0	9.0

[a/] N.D., not detectable.

determine the extent of variation over one year. Elemental concentrations in female hair seem to be rather consistently higher than those for male hair.

Analysis of Human Fingernails. Results from hair analyses led to interest in extending our studies to fingernails as well. These materials have also been shown to store metals that are in excessive concentration in the body. Arsensic poisoning has been established by neutron-activation analysis[14] studies of nail sections. The metal concentration of elements associated with certain diseases has also been studied in nails[15,16], particularly sodium and potassium in cases of children with cystic fibrosis. Little information is found in the literature, however, concerning concentrations in fingernails of elements other than the more common ones.

Sample procurement was again controlled as closely as possible. The sample treatment was similar to that of hair, involving a nonionic detergent wash and drying, followed by a nitric-perchloric wet ash and formation into the previously described sample electrodes.

Table IV shows the results from some typical fingernail analysis by SSMS. A comparison of concentrations over a large number of samples indicates that the elements encountered and their concentrations are rather similar to those in hair, although the generalization cannot be carried too far. Table V shows a comparison of SSMS analysis to atomic absorption analysis on a pooled nail sample split into duplicate portions. Agreement between the two is reasonably good, showing that careful control of experimental parameters and conditions can significantly improve the uncertain precision and accuracy attributed to SSMS.

Elemental concentrations in fingernails have been monitored for certain individuals for 9 to 12 months by both SSMS and

TABLE IV

Typical Results in Mass Spectrometric Analysis of
Two Different Human Fingernail Samples

Element	Sample 1 (µg/g)	Sample 2 (µg/g)
Bi	1.8	N.D.[a]
Pb	3.7	7.2
La	0.17	0.25
Ba	6.8	2.8
Sn	2.3	2.1
Cd	N.D.[a]	0.99
Ag	0.34	N.D.[a]
Mo	7.5	2.7
Zr	0.28	0.44
Se	N.D.[a]	1.7
As	0.24	0.71
Ge	1.2	1.0
Zn	217	127
Cu	17	25
Ni	7.0	8.1
Fe	21	92
Mn	0.21	1.2
Cr	3.0	2.8
Ca	450	690
K	2000	2900
S	2700	4700
P	61	200
Si	83	95
Mg	11	59
Na	760	850

[a] N.D., not detectable.

TABLE V

Comparison of Atomic Absorption to Mass Spectrometric
Analysis of Trace Elements in Fingernails

Element	Sample 1 (μg/g)		Sample 2 (μg/g)	
	AA	SSMS	AA	SSMS
Ca	927	1100	1393	1400
Zn	190	170	147	130
Mg	99	110	119	130
Cu	76	66	62	67
Fe	28	36	26	25

atomic absorption. No clear seasonal variations were observed
in general, although some individuals might appear to have
interesting fluctuations. In a series of auxiliary studies
it was observed that the trace element concentrations in
fingernails were affected by many environmental factors. Wash
conditions were quite critical. Contact of the nails with
doped solutions almost invariably produced concentration
changes. The constant exposure of the nails to water,
detergents, dirt, and so forth, created uncertainty in
evaluation of sample history and its possible pertubing
effect on elemental concentrations.

Male-female differences were less obvious than in the case
of hair. Calcium appeared to be higher in males than females
but a larger number of subjects would be required for evaluation.
In a study of three married couples in which it was considered
that the male and female had lived under somewhat similar
conditions, such as diet, the elemental concentrations within
each pair were too similar to draw any conclusions.

Analysis of Human Blood Serum. Trace element analysis
of blood serum is rather common for a number of elements
that have concentration levels high enough for analysis by
generally available techniques, such as flame emission,
absorption spectrophotometry, or atomic absorption. Many other
elements are present at levels that require laborious
preconcentration steps, if they may be done at all. SSMS has
been applied to blood serum analysis in our laboratories[17] to
demonstrate the range of elements and concentrations that may
be analyzed in a single sample and in a single shooting.

Blood samples were drawn into sterilized polyethylene
syringes and transferred to acid-cleaned glass tubes. After
clotting, the samples were centrifuged and the serum separated;
2 ml of serum were mixed with 100 mg of graphite and the
mixture dried; it was then ashed in a muffle furnace at $475^{\circ}C$.
In addition to removing organic species, ashing also serves
to concentrate the elements in the sample, thereby increasing
the sensitivity of the method and allowing clear detection and
determination of elements present in such low concentration the
serum that they might be undetected or at least not quantitatively
determined otherwise.

After all preliminary method development studies using
mainly pooled serum were complete, individual serum samples
were obtained for analysis. Elements present at relatively
high concentration and showing heavy mass spectral lines even
for the +2 and +3 ionic states include: Na, K, Cl, P, S.
The following trace elements were clearly detected:

Mg	Fe	Zn	I	Mo
Ca	Co	Br	Ba	Al
Mn	Cu	Sr	Pb	As

Spectral isotopic lines were observed for seven other trace
elements that appear to be present, but at the concentrations

encountered these can be identified only with some uncertainty
because of interferences either from matrix components or
molecular species. These elements are Ti, Ni, Rb, Cr, V, Ge,
and Se. Nickel, Cr. V, Rb, and Se have been reported as
present in serum by other investigators.

Table VI shows SSMS data from six normal subjects for
eleven elements for which comparison literature values are
available. Values determined by atomic absorption are probably
the most reliable standard of comparison, and normal values
for serum Mg, Fe, Cu, Zn, and Ca have been rather well
established by this method. The spark-source mass spectrometer
Mg values are somewhat lower than the accepted normals, but the
values for Fe, Cu, Zn, and Ca agree well with the established
levels. Furthermore, the mass spectrometric values for these
four elements in sample 5 agree very closely with specific
normal ranges determined over a 10 month period in our
laboratories by atomic absorption for subject V.

Most of the elements in Table VI other than Fe, Cu, Ca,
Zn, and Mg are difficult, and in some cases impossible, to
determine by atomic absorption. Iodine, being a nonmetal,
cannot be determined, and elements such as Co, Mo, and Ba,
which are present at very low levels, require tedious preconcentration methods to arrive at reasonable working levels.
Aluminum forms refractory compounds in the flame, and is,
therefore, quite difficult to analyze by atomic absorption,
unless high-temperature flames are used. Emission spectroscopy
has been used to determine serum concentrations of Al, Co, Mo,
and Ba, but not without involved sample preparation procedures.
In contrast, spark-source mass spectrometric analysis requires
only dry ashing and preparation of electrodes.

<u>Analysis of Human Aortic Tissue</u>. One of our projects
with the Medical School has involved a study of trace element

TABLE VI

Spark-Source Mass Spectrometric Analysis of Human Blood Serum from Six Different Subjects

(Values in ppm by weight)

Element	Samples						Lit. values	Method
	1	2	3	4	5	6		
Mg	9.5	13	6.7	13	14	7.2	18-27 18.1- 22.8 13	AA [a] AA NAA [b]
Al	0.26		0.44	0.20	0.34	0.60	0.40	ES [c]
Ca	127	92	104	147	133	135	90-110 85-105 39	AA AA NAA
Mn	0.18	0.55	0.30	0.51	0.46	0.90	0.15 0.013 0.0043	AA ES NAA
Fe	1.2	1.9	1.1	3.7	1.7	1.9	0.5-2.0 0.65- 1.75 1.71	AA AA ES
Co	0.08	0.24	0.09	0.24	0.20	0.17	0.061- 0.063	ES

TABLE VI (continued)

Spark-Source Mass Spectrometric Analysis of Human Blood Serum from Six Different Subjects

(Values in ppm by weight)

Element	Samples						Lit. values	Method
	1	2	3	4	5	6		
Cu	1.3	1.6	1.9	1.3	1.9	1.4	0.70–1.65	AA
							0.5–1.5	AA
							1.20	AA
							1.10	ES
							0.85	NAA
Zn	0.36	0.79	0.74	0.67	0.97	0.61	0.6–1.5	AA
							0.8–1.6	AA
							1.30	ES
							0.93	NAA
Mo	0.093	0.13	0.11	(d)	0.19	0.11	0.34	ES
I	0.061	(d)	0.144	(d)	(d)	(d)	0.050–0.120	
Ba	(e)	(e)	(e)	0.017	0.029	0.031	0.071	ES
							0.066	NAA

a/ AA, atomic absorption.

b/ NAA, neutron activation analysis.

c/ ES, emission spectrography.

distribution in aortic tissue using autopsy cases rated at
varying degrees of atherosclerosis. The deposition of elements
in the tissue has been verified by chemical analysis of aortic
tissue and plaque areas, although only limited work has been
reported. Strain and co-workers[18] recently used activation
analysis to determine nine elements in atherosclerotic aortas.
Tipton[19] had earlier used emission spectroscopy for aortic
analysis. The broad capabilities of SSMS offered numerous
advantages as a survey technique to determine the range of
metals and nonmetals present in atherosclerotic tissue.
Further, we were interested in the change in elemental
concentrations as the rated degree of atherosclerosis increased.
Using SSMS, investigators could monitor not only elements of
suspected significance but also all others down to parts per
billion sensitivities.

Tissue samples, which were rated on a 0 to 7 scale as to
degree of visible hemorrhaging and plaque formation, were
rinsed with a small amount of distilled deionized water to
remove any remaining blood. All samples were of the same
physical size with an area taken around the plaque site. Dry
ashing in a muffle furnace was used to remove organic
constituents.

Table VII shows some preliminary experiments in which the
SSMS data was compared to atomic absorption analysis on
duplicate homogeneous samples. Whereas this table shows good
agreement for the compared elements, further studies indicated
that the two techniques could disagree at times by 20 to 50%.
The reproducibility of atomic absorption was considerably better
than SSMS.

Table VIII contains the elemental concentrations obtained
for 10 different cases. The age, tissue grade, and values for
up to 31 elements are shown for each case. We had hoped to see

TABLE VII

Comparison of Analyses of the Same Tissue Sample by Spark-Source
Mass Spectrometry and Atomic Absorption Spectrometry
(Values given in μg/g, dry weight)

Element	Spark-source	Atomic absorption	Percent difference from atomic absorption
Mg	720	764	− 5.7
Ca	11500	11800	− 2.5
Fe	23.8	27.4	−12
Cu	19.6	22.4	−12
Zn	39.2	40.5	− 3.2

a systematic trend in terms of increasing trace element
concentrations with tissue grade, but this is not clear cut.
Whereas tissues of high rating did show generally high elemental
concentrations, this was not consistent within a single rating
group and considerable fluctuation was noted from one rating
to another. A more detailed study by atomic absorption using
approximately 30 cases showed that comparable fluctuations were
still present when using this more accurate technique, indicating
that the nonsystematic nature of the data was not attributable
to SSMS inconsistencies. Our sampling of the atherosclerotic
area in the tissue may require modification to look at specific
regions of the atherosclerotic lesion. It is also possible that
the visual rating of the tissues takes into account factors
that do not linearly involve elemental concentrations.

E. Potential and Limitations of Spark-Source Mass Spectrometry

At this stage of its development, spark-source mass
spectrometry is only beginning to be recognized as a technique

Spark-Source Mass Spectrometric Analysis of Human

(Values in µg/g,

Sample	1	2	3	4
Grade	1.5	2.5	3.5	3.5
Age (year)	36	94	75	56
Be	0.025	0.650	0.003	0.060
B	34.0	0.350	5.24	3.60
F	16.3	0.776	0.110	0.46
Na	45500	684	3450	2403
Mg	844	82.3	671	567
Al	2.39	37.2	7.69	12.2
P	122000	4382	1186	5730
S	769	178	37.1	224
Cl	1082	451	21.1	922
K	2020	1790	827	603
Co	6800	1621	15400	7890
Ti	40.2	1.98	10.1	5.08
V	0.822	19.2	0.060	0.183
Ni	213	15.6	297	1.97
Mn	N.D.[a]	3.43	10.1	1.76
Fe	164	260	54.1	55.5
Cr	N.D.	37.6	24.0	10.8
Cu	10.9	9.77	3.12	1.92
Zn	30.9	11.4	21.4	4.26
Ga	1.83	2.12	0.625	0.149
As	19.1	4.89	2.63	2.76
Se	5.77	2.85	0.794	N.D.
Br	3.40	8.12	0.172	1.29
Sr	17.2	1.69	11.2	10.2
Zr	15.2	1.12	4.00	1.78
Mo	5.34	20.2	0.885	0.331
Ag	4.97	34.0	0.527	0.092
Cd	N.D.	2.71	N.D.	N.D.
Sn	N.D.	3.79	N.D.	1.39
Ba	13.4	4.33	2.06	0.515
Pb	1.79	16.93	6.24	0.518

[a] N.D., not detectable.

VIII

Atherosclerotic Tissue for 10 Subjects

dry tissue)

5	6	7	8	9	10
4.0	4.5	4.5	5.5	6.5	6.5
68	69	79	78	78	78
0.067	0.307	0.433	0.611	0.009	0.169
2.40	3.47	4.34	903	0.042	16.7
1.41	7.13	5.76	43.4	0.088	92.3
13100	16500	1790	12100	2160	26800
522	937	255	549	317	1360
55.1	20.5	4.35	4.13	1.14	11.1
4640	29000	12300	15300	286	104000
287	308	25.5	1030	54.6	438
265	394	466	3930	294	5100
1182	3120	137	5260	1410	16700
2041	102000	269000	15730	46430	442000
7.10	3.59	3.98	N.D.[a]	1.86	142
0.130	0.114	0.391	5.0	0.288	4.94
6.52	10.7	4.24	100	135	158
0.902	7.49	4.22	26.3	N.D.	49.6
47.3	14.3	47.4	1338	157	1121
14.9	31.1	4.45	768	10.1	N.D.
0.877	5.47	2.55	21.7	2.72	33.1
2.37	40.0	36.9	26.1	16.9	197
1.77	0.126	3.85	31.2	0.217	23.7
7.02	13.4	7.78	16.8	3.98	93.4
0.650	0.422	9.45	8.34	N.D.	26.3
0.79	5.73	1.98	3.89	1.00	26.0
9.59	11.5	19.4	2.26	9.57	149
18.3	N.D.	N.D.	25.4	N.D.	37.3
0.455	0.612	0.291	7.14	0.81	18.2
0.153	0.437	0.180	0.634	0.390	5.60
N.D.	N.D.	N.D.	N.D.	N.D.	N.D.
1.65	3.12	2.62	32.3	N.D.	14.9
0.786	N.D.	2.92	2.76	1.25	29.3
2.18	2.10	3.94	12.9	2.00	12.2

that could have great application to the analysis of trace
elements in biological samples. It offers overall capabilities
equaled by no other analytical method and, as more information
is made available in the literature, will be more recognized
and used by trace element researchers.

The limitations of SSMS have been mainly precision and
accuracy problems along with considerable expense of initiating
such a program, with its large capital investment. While
improvement can hardly be expected in the latter regard, a
new electrical detection system[20] promises to dramatically
reduce difficulties encountered with precision and accuracy.
The elimination of the photoplate detector and its concomitant
uncertainties, along with a more careful control of electrode
position, has produced reported consistent precisions in the
range of 2 to 5%. With this increased capability the
importance of SSMS will increase even more, as it will then
be possible to examine chemical problems that require greater
definition than SSMS currently possesses; that is, small
variations in elemental concentrations may then be monitored.

The electrical detection will also facilitate rapid
procurement of data. Processing of the photoplate, densitometric
analysis, and reading the resultant raw data into a computer
program for final calculations require considerable time.
Direct read out of electron-multiplier detector currents with
digital voltmeters will allow much faster and more accurate
analyses. These electrical detection facilities, which are
just now becoming available, promise to be the necessary
advance that will allow full appreciation and utilization of
this most powerful trace analysis technique.

REFERENCES

[1]. Sasaki, N. and Watanabe, E., Thirteenth Ann. Conf. on
Mass Spectry. and Allied Topics, St. Louis, Missouri,
1965.

[2]. Wolstenholme, W. A., Nature, 203, 1284 (1964).

[3]. Evans, C. A. and Morrison, G. H., Anal. Chem., 40, 869
(1968).

[4]. Yurachek, J. P., Clemena, G. G., and Harrison, W. W.,
Anal. Chem., 41, 1666 (1969).

[5]. Owens, E. B. and Giardino, N. A., Anal. Chem., 35, 1172
(1963).

[6]. Clemena, G. G. and Harrison, W. W., unpublished data.

[7]. Harrison, W. W., Netsky, M. G., and Brown, M. D.,
Clin. Chim. Acta, 21, 55 (1968).

[8]. Netsky, M. G., Harrison, W. W., Brown, M. D., and
Benson, C. A., Am. J. Clin. Path., 51, 358 (1969).

[9]. Harrison, W. W., Yurachek, J. P., and Benson, C. A.,
Clin. Chim. Acta, 23, 83 (1969).

[10]. Martin, G. M., Nature, 202, 903 (1964).

[11]. Kopita, L., Byers, R. K., and Schwachman, H., New Engl.
J. Med., 276, 949 (1967).

[12]. Goldblum, R. W., Derby, S., and Lerner, A. B., J. Invest.
Dermatol., 20, 13 (1953).

[13]. Perkins, A. K. and Jervis, R. E., J. Forensic Sci., 11,
50 (1966).

[14]. Shapiro, H. A., J. Forensic Med., 14, 65 (1967).

[15]. Kopita, L. and Schwachman, H., Nature, 202, 501 (1964).

[16]. Antonelli, M., Ballati, G., and Annibaldi, L., Arch.
Dis. Childh., 44, 218 (1969).

[17]. McKernon, M. A., Charlottesville, Virginia: University
of Virginia, 1969, (M. S. Thesis).

[18]. Strain, W. H., Rob, C. G., Pories, W. J., Childers, R. C.,
       Thompson, J. F., Hennessen, J. A., and Graber, J. M.,
       Appl. Spectry., 23, 121 (1969).

[19]. Tipton, I. H., Schroeder, H. A., Perry, H. M., and
       Cook, M. J., Health Phys., 9, 89 (1963).

[20]. Technical Bulletins, Associated Electrical Industries,
       Ltd., Manchester, England.

AUTHOR INDEX

Numbers in brackets are reference numbers and indicate that an author's work is referred to although his name is not cited in the text. Underlined numbers give the page on which the complete reference is listed.

A

Abe, K., 221, [121, 123-125], 246, 247
Adams, J.B., 225 [181], 249
Adams, M.H., 223 [152], 248
Adiga, P.R., 226 [202,-204], 251
Aguillardo, D., 223 [141], 247
Albright, C.H., 216 [13], 239
Allaway, W.H., 57 [2], 60 [25], 61 [2], 79, 81
Allen, S.H., 12 [19], 17
Allison, F., Jr., 223 [147, 148], 248
Aloy, R., 224 [162], 249
Altmann, H., 223 [155, 156], 248
Amaha, M., 217 [69], 243
Anderson, W.A.D., 90, 96 [29], 121
Andersson, N., 196 [17], 213
Andran, R., 269 [15], 309
Angino, E.E., 59 [15], 80
Annibaldi, L., 407 [16], 419
Anthony, W.L., 328 [1,2], 333 [5], 341 [1], 342 [12], 342, 343
Antonelli, M., 407 [16], 419
Antoñev, A.A., 226 [225], 230, 252
Appelgren, L., 196, 213
Aptekar, S.G., 60 [27], 81
Arce, R., 221 [118], 246
Archibald, J.G., 216 [8], 239
Argrett, L.C., 65 [40], 82, 87, 93, 120
Arnold, E.L., 374 [12], 375 [12a], 378, 388, 389,
Arnon, D.I., 217 [49], 242
Assis, L.M., 272 [49], 312
Avtandilov, G.G., 216 [38], 219 [38], 241
Azarnoff, D.L., 197, 201, 212

B

Babicky, A., 86 [2-5], 87 [3,8], 88 [2,20], 90 [20,22,23], 93 [2,4,22,27], 95 [32], 96 [22], 101 [32], 102 [2-5, 32], 103 [5], 104 [5], 119-121
Babskii, E.B., 222, 247
Bagdasarova, L.B., 216 [27], 240
Bakhanova, G.S., 217 [63], 243
Bala, Y.M., 216 [37], 219 [37], 241
Balassa, J.J., 126 [15], 138 [15], 151, 165, 168, 169 [7], 182 [7], 193, 196 [16], 197, 213, 215, 216 [7], 217, 239, 243, 323-325 [10], 326
Ball, E.G., 145 [35], 153
Ballati, G., 407 [16], 419
Barlow, R.M., 18
Barney, G.H., 337, 342
Barreras, R.F., 125 [12], 151
Barron, G.P., 289 [27], 295 [27], 310
Bartter, F.C., 282 [20], 299 [42], 310, 311
Baumann, C.A., 63 [37, 39], 64, 65, 68, 69, 82, 93, 121
Baur, H., 224 [161], 249
Beach, D.J., 226 [210, 217], 251, 252
Beath, O.A., 58 [3], 59 [3], 80, 86 [6], 109 [6], 120
Beck, A.B., 290 [29], 297 [29], 310
Belyaev, V.I., 222 [129, 130, 139], 247
Beneš, I., 86 [2], 88 [2,17, 20], 90 [20,22,23], 93 [2,22,27], 96 [22], 102 [2], 119 [37], 119, 121, 122

421